Review and Reso

Pediatric Nursing

3rd Edition

CONTINUING EDUCATION SOURCE

NURSING CERTIFICATION REVIEW MANUAL

CLINICAL PRACTICE RESOURCE

Mary Jo Gilmer, PhD, MBA, RN-BC, FAAN
Clara J. Richardson, MSN, RN–BC

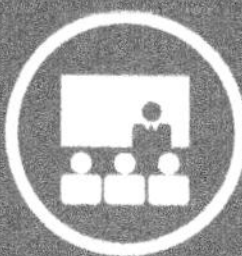

NURSING KNOWLEDGE CENTER

Library of Congress Cataloging-in-Publication Data

Gilmer, Mary Jo.

Pediatric nursing review and resource manual. – 3rd ed. / by Mary Jo Gilmer and Clara Richardson.

p. ; cm.
Rev. ed. of: Pediatric nursing review and resource manual / by Paula Chiplis ... [et al.]. 2nd ed. 2010.
Includes bibliographical references and index.
ISBN 9781935213314 (alk. paper)
I. Richardson, Clara, 1955- II. American Nurses Credentialing Center. III. Pediatric nursing review and resource manual. IV. Title.
[DNLM: 1. Pediatric Nursing–methods–United States–Examination Questions. 2. Pediatric Nursing–methods–United States–Handbooks.
3. Pediatric Nursing–methods–United States–Outlines. WY 18.2]

618.92'00231–dc23

2012047149

The American Nurses Credentialing Center (ANCC), a subsidiary of the American Nurses Association (ANA), provides individuals and organizations throughout the nursing profession with the resources they need to achieve practice excellence. ANCC's internationally renowned credentialing programs certify nurses in specialty practice areas; recognize healthcare organizations for promoting safe, positive work environments through the Magnet Recognition Program® and the Pathway to Excellence ® Program; and accredit providers of continuing nursing education. In addition, ANCC's Institute for Credentialing Innovation provides leading-edge information and education services and products to support its core credentialing programs.

ISBN 13: 9781935213444

8515 Georgia Ave., Suite 400
Silver Spring, MD 20910

PEDIATRIC NURSING REVIEW AND RESOURCE MANUAL, 3RD EDITION

JANUARY 2013

Please direct your comments and/or queries to: revmanuals@ana.org

The healthcare services delivery system is a volatile marketplace demanding superior knowledge, clinical skills, and competencies from all registered nurses. Nursing autonomy of practice and nurse career marketability and mobility in the new century hinge on affirming the profession's formative philosophy, which places a priority on a lifelong commitment to the principles of education and professional development. The knowledge base of nursing theory and practice is expanding, and while care has been taken to ensure the accuracy and timeliness of the information presented in the **Pediatric Nursing Review and Resource Manual,** clinicians are advised to always verify the most current national guidelines and recommendations and to practice in accordance with professional standards of care used with regard to the unique circumstances that apply in each practice situation. In addition, every effort has been made in this text to ensure accuracy and, in particular, to confirm that drug selections and dosages are in accordance with current recommendations and practice, including the ongoing research, changes to government regulations, and the developments in product information provided by pharmaceutical manufacturers. However, it is the responsibility of each nurse practitioner to verify drug product information and to practice in accordance with professional standards of care. In addition, the editors wish to note that provision of information in this text does not imply an endorsement of any particular products, procedures or services.

Therefore, the authors, editors, American Nurses Association (ANA), American Nurses Association's Publishing (ANP), American Nurses Credentialing Center (ANCC), and the Nursing Knowledge Center cannot accept responsibility for errors or omissions, or for any consequences or liability, injury, and/or damages to persons or property from application of the information in this manual and make no warranty, express or implied, with respect to the contents of the **Pediatric Nursing Review and Resource Manual.** Completion of this manual does not guarantee that the reader will pass the certification exam. The practice examination questions are not a requirement to take a certification examination. The practice examination questions cannot be used as an indicator of results on the actual certification.

PUBLISHED BY
Nursing Knowledge Center
8515 Georgia Avenue, Suite 400
Silver Spring, MD 20910-3402
www.nursingknowledgecenter.org

ACKNOWLEDGMENTS

The authors gratefully acknowledge the foundational work provided by Paula Chiplis, PhD, RN, CPNP, and Karen Corlett, MSN, RN-BC, CPNP-AC/PC, PNP-BC, on the previous edition of this manual.

INTRODUCTION TO THE CONTINUING EDUCATION (CE) CONTACT HOUR APPLICATION PROCESS FOR *PEDIATRIC NURSING REVIEW AND RESOURCE MANUAL, 3RD EDITION*

Continuing Education is no longer available for this manual.

Inquiries or Comments

If you have any questions about the CE contact hours, please e-mail the Nursing Knowledge Center at revmanuals@ana.org. You may also mail any comments to Editorial Project Manager, at the address listed below.

Nursing Knowledge Center
American Nurses Association
Attn: Editorial Project Manager
8515 Georgia Avenue, Suite 400
Silver Spring, MD 20910-3492
Fax: (301) 628-5342

CONTENTS

CHAPTER 1

TAKING THE CERTIFICATION EXAMINATION

When you sign up to take a national certification exam, you will be instructed to go online and review the testing and renewal handbook (www.nursecredentialing.org/documents/certification/application/generaltestingandrenewalhandbook.aspx). Review it carefully and be sure to bookmark the site so you can refer to it frequently. It contains information on test content and sample questions. This is critical information; it will give you insight into the nature of the test. The agency will send you information about the test site; keep this in a safe place until needed.

GENERAL SUGGESTIONS FOR PREPARING FOR THE EXAM

Step One: Control Your Anxiety

Everyone experiences anxiety when faced with taking the certification exam.

Step Two: Do Not Listen to Gossip About the Exam

A large volume of information exists about the tests based on reports from people who have taken the exams in the past. Because information from the testing facilities is limited, it is hard to ignore this gossip.

- Remember that gossip about the exam that you hear from others is not verifiable.
- Because this gossip is based on the imperfect memory of people in a stressful situation, it may not be very accurate.

- People tend to remember those items testing content with which they are less comfortable; for instance, those with a limited background in women's health may say that the exam was "all women's health." In fact, the exam blueprint ensures that the exam covers multiple content areas without overemphasizing any one.

Step Three: Set Reasonable Expectations for Yourself

- Do not expect to know everything.
- Do not try to know everything in great detail.
- You do not need a perfect score to pass the exam.
- Learn the general rules, not the exceptions.
- The most likely diagnoses will be on the exam, not questions on rare diseases or atypical cases.
- Think about the most likely presentation and most common therapy.

Step Four: Prepare Mentally and Physically

- While you are getting ready to take the exam, take good physical care of yourself.
- Get plenty of sleep and exercise, and eat well while preparing for the exam.
- These things are especially important while you are studying and immediately before you take the exam.

Step Five: Access Current Knowledge

General Content

You will be given a list of general topics that will be on the exam when you register to take the exam. In addition, examine the table of contents of this book and the test content outline, available at www.nursecredentialing.org/cert/TCOs.html.

- What content do you need to know?
- How well do you know these subjects?

Take a Review Course

- Taking a review course is an excellent way to assess your knowledge of the content that will be included in the exam.
- If you plan to take a review course, take it well before the exam so you will have plenty of time to master any areas of weakness the course uncovers.
- If you are prepared for the exam, you will not hear anything new in the course. You will be familiar with everything that is taught.
- If some topics in the review course are new to you, concentrate on these in your studies.
- People have a tendency to study what they know; it is rewarding to study something and feel a mastery of it! Unfortunately, this will not help you master unfamiliar content. Be sure to use a review course to identify your areas of strength and weakness, then concentrate on the weaknesses.

Depth of Knowledge

- How much do you need to know about a subject?
- You cannot know everything about a topic.
- Study the information sent to you from the testing agency, what you were taught in school, what is covered in this text, and the general guidelines given in this chapter.
- Look at practice tests designed for the exam. Practice tests for other exams will not be helpful.
- Consult your class notes or a clinical diagnosis and management textbook for the major points about a disease. Additional reference books can be found online at www.nursecredentialing.org/cert/refs.html.
- With regard to medications, know the drug categories and the major medications in each. Assume all drugs in a category are generally alike, and then focus on the differences among common drugs. Know the most important indications, contraindications, and side effects. Emphasize safety. The questions usually do not require you to know the exact dosage of a drug.

Step Six: Institute a Systematic Study Plan

Develop Your Study Plan

- Write up a formal plan of study.
  - Include topics for study, timetable, resources, and methods of study that work for you.
  - Decide whether you want to organize a study group or work alone.
  - Schedule regular times to study.
  - Avoid cramming; it is counterproductive. Try to schedule your study periods in 1-hour increments.
- Identify resources to use for studying. To prepare for the examination, you should have the following materials on your shelf:
  - A good pathophysiology text.
  - This review book.
  - A physical assessment text.
  - Your class notes.
  - Other important sources, including: information from the testing facility, a clinical diagnosis textbook, favorite journal articles, notes from a review course, and practice tests.
  - Know the important national standards of care for major illnesses.
  - Consult the bibliography on the test blueprint. When studying less familiar material, it is helpful to study using the same references that the testing center uses.
- Study the body systems from head to toe.
- The exams emphasize health promotion, assessment, differential diagnosis, and plan of care for common problems.
- You will need to know facts and be able to interpret and analyze this information utilizing critical thinking.

Personalize Your Study Plan

- How do you learn best?
  - If you learn best by listening or talking, attend a review course or discuss topics with a colleague.
- Read everything the test facility sends you as soon as you receive it and several times during your preparation period. It will give you valuable information to help guide your study.
- Have a specific place with good lighting set aside for studying. Find a quiet place with no distractions. Assemble your study materials.

Implement Your Study Plan

You must have basic content knowledge. In addition, you must be able to use this information to think critically and make decisions based on facts.

- Refer to your study plan regularly.
- Stick to your schedule.
- Take breaks when you get tired.
- If you start procrastinating, get help from a friend or reorganize your study plan.
- It is not necessary to follow your plan rigidly. Adjust as you learn where you need to spend more time.
- Memorize the basics of the content areas you will be required to know.

Focus on General Material

- Most of what you need to know is basic material that does not require constant updating.
- You do not need to worry about the latest information being published as you are studying for the exam. Remember, it can take 6 to 12 months for new information to be incorporated into test questions.

Pace Your Studying

- Stop studying for the examination when you are starting to feel overwhelmed and look at what is bothering you. Then make changes.
- Break overwhelming tasks into smaller tasks that you know you can do.
- Stop and take breaks while studying.

Work With Others

- Talk with classmates about your preparation for the exam.
- Keep in touch with classmates, and help each other stick to your study plans.
- If your classmates become anxious, do not let their anxiety affect you. Walk away if you need to.
- Do not believe bad stories you hear about other people's experiences with previous exams.
- Remember, you know as much as anyone about what will be on the next exam!

Consider a Study Group

- Study groups can provide practice in analyzing cases, interpreting questions, and critical thinking.
    - You can discuss a topic and take turns presenting cases for the group to analyze.
    - Study groups can also provide moral support and help you continue studying.

Step Seven: Strategies Immediately Before the Exam

Final Preparation Suggestions

- Use practice exams when studying to get accustomed to the exam format and time restrictions.
  - Many books that are labeled as review books are simply a collection of examination questions.
  - If you have test anxiety, such practice tests may help alleviate the anxiety.
  - Practice tests can help you learn to judge the time it should take you to complete the exam.
  - Practice tests are useful for gaining experience in analyzing questions.
  - Books of questions may not uncover the gaps in your knowledge that a more systematic content review text will reveal.
  - If you feel that you don't know enough about a topic, refer to a text to learn more. After you feel that you have learned the topic, practice questions are a wonderful tool to help improve your test-taking skills.
- Know your test-taking style.
  - Do you rush through the exam without reading the questions thoroughly?
  - Do you get stuck and dwell on a question for a long time?
  - You should spend about 45 to 60 seconds per question and finish with time to review the questions you were not sure about.
  - Be sure to read the question completely, including all four answer choices. Choice "a" may be good, but "d" may be best.

The Night Before the Exam

- Be prepared to get to the exam on time.
  - Know the test site location and how long it takes to get there.
  - Take a "dry run" beforehand to make sure you know how to get to the testing site, if necessary.
  - Get a good night's sleep.
  - Eat sensibly.
  - Avoid alcohol the night before.
  - Assemble the required material—two forms of identification and watch. Both IDs must match the name on the application, and one photo ID is preferred.
  - Know the exam room rules.
    - You will be given scratch paper, which will be collected at the end of the exam.
    - Nothing else is allowed in the exam room.
    - You will be required to put papers, backpacks, etc., in a corner of the room or in a locker.

- No water or food will be allowed.
- You will be allowed to walk to a water fountain and go to the bathroom one at a time.

The Day of the Exam

- Get there early. You must arrive to the test center at least 15 minutes before your scheduled appointment time. If you are late, you may not be admitted.
- Think positively. You have studied hard and are well prepared.
- Remember your anxiety reduction strategies.

Specific Tips for Dealing With Anxiety

Test anxiety is a specific type of anxiety. Symptoms include upset stomach, sweaty palms, tachycardia, trouble concentrating, and a feeling of dread. But there are ways to cope with test anxiety.

- There is no substitute for being well prepared.
- Practice relaxation techniques.
- Avoid alcohol, excess coffee, caffeine, and any new medications that might sedate you, dull your senses, or make you feel agitated.
- Take a few deep breaths and concentrate on the task at hand.

Focus on Specific Test-Taking Skills

To do well on the exam, you need good test-taking skills in addition to knowledge of the content and ability to use critical thinking.

All Certification Exams Are Multiple Choice

- Multiple-choice tests have specific rules for test construction.
- A multiple-choice question consists of three parts: the information (or stem), the question, and the four possible answers (one correct and three distracters).
- Careful analysis of each part is necessary. Read the entire question before answering.
- Practice your test-taking skills by analyzing the practice questions in this book and on the ANCC Web site.

Analyze the Information Given

- Do not assume you have more information than is given.
- Do not overanalyze.
- Remember, the writer of the question assumes this is all of the information needed to answer the question.
- If information is not given, it is not relevant and will not affect the answer.
- Do not make the question more complicated than it is.

What Kind of Question Is Asked?

- Are you supposed to recall a fact, apply facts to a situation, or understand and differentiate between options?
  - Read the question, thinking about what the writer is asking.
  - Look for key words or phrases that lead you (see Table 1–1). These help determine what kind of answer the question requires.

TABLE 1-1.
EXAMPLES OF KEY WORDS AND PHRASES

▸ avoid	▸ initial	▸ most
▸ best	▸ first	▸ significant
▸ except	▸ contributing to	▸ likely
▸ not	▸ appropriate	▸ of the following
		▸ most consistent with

Read All of the Answers

- If you are absolutely certain that answer "a" is correct as you read it, mark it, but read the rest of the question so you do not trick yourself into missing a better answer.
- If you are absolutely sure answer "a" is wrong, cross it off or make a note on your scratch paper and continue reading the question.
- After reading the entire question, go back, analyze the question, and select the best answer.
- Do not jump ahead.
- If the question asks you for an assessment, the best answer will be an assessment. Do not be distracted by an intervention that sounds appropriate.
- If the question asks you for an intervention, do not answer with an assessment.
- When two answer choices sound very good, the best one is usually the least expensive, least invasive way to achieve the goal. For example, if your answer choices include a physical exam maneuver or imaging, the physical exam maneuver is probably the better choice, provided it will give the information needed.
- If the answers include two options that are the opposite of each other, one of the two is probably the correct answer.
- When numeric answers cover a wide range, a number in the middle is more likely to be correct.
- Watch out for distracters that are correct but do not answer the question, combine true and false information, or contain a word or phrase that is similar to the correct answer.
- Err on the side of caution.

Only One Answer Can Be Correct

- When more than one suggested answer is correct, you must identify the one that best answers the question asked.
- If you cannot choose between two answers, you have a 50% chance of getting it right if you guess.

Avoid Changing Answers

- Change an answer only if you have a compelling reason, such as you remembered something additional, or you understand the question better after rereading it.
- People change to a wrong answer more often than to a right answer.

Time Yourself to Complete the Whole Exam

- Do not spend a large amount of time on one question.
- If you cannot answer a question quickly, mark it and continue the exam.
- If time is left at the end, return to the difficult questions.
- Make educated guesses by eliminating the obviously wrong answers and choosing a likely answer even if you are not certain.
- Trust your instinct.
- Answer every question. There is no penalty for a wrong answer.
- Occasionally a question will remind you of something that helps you with a question earlier in the test. Look back at that question to see if what you are remembering affects how you would answer that question.

ABOUT THE CERTIFICATION EXAMS

The American Nurses Credentialing Center Computerized Exam

The ANCC examination is given only as a computer exam, and each exam is different.

The order of the questions is scrambled for every test, so even if two people are taking the same exam, the questions will be in a different order. The exam consists of 175 multiple-choice questions.

- 150 of the 175 questions are part of the test, and how you answer will count toward your score; 25 are included to refine questions and will not be scored. You will not know which ones count, so treat all questions the same.
- You will need to know how to use a mouse, scroll by either clicking arrows on the scroll bar or using the up and down arrow keys, and perform other basic computer tasks.
- The exam does not require computer expertise.
- However, if you are not comfortable with using a computer, you should practice using a mouse and computer beforehand so you do not waste time on the mechanics of using the computer.

Know What to Expect During the Test

- Each ANCC test question is independent of the other questions.
  - For each case study, there is only one question. This means that a correct answer on any question does not depend on the correct answer to any other question.
  - Each question has four possible answers. There are no questions asking for combinations of correct answers (such as "a and c") or multiple-multiples.
- You can skip a question and go back to it at the end of the exam.
- You cannot mark key words in the question or right or wrong answers. If you want to do this, use the scratch paper.
- You will get your results immediately, and a grade report will be provided upon leaving the testing site.

Internet Resources

- ANCC Web site: www.nursecredentialing.org
- ANA Bookstore: www.nursesbooks.org (catalog of ANA nursing scope and standards publications and other titles that may be listed on your test content outline)
- National Guideline Clearinghouse: www.ngc.gov

CHAPTER 2

DEVELOPMENTAL AND BEHAVIORAL SCIENCES

Mary Jo Gilmer, PhD, MBA, RN-BC, FAAN, and
Paula Chiplis, PhD, RN, CPNP

Children have unique minds, bodies, and needs. Careful attention to these differences and consideration of psychosocial and physical growth are essential in assessing, analyzing, and planning care for children. In addition, family context and cultural and spiritual dimensions of care affect a child in a multitude of ways; family dynamics, roles, and values should be a part of each plan of care.

PSYCHOSOCIAL, COGNITIVE, AND ETHICAL-MORAL DEVELOPMENT

Psychosocial theorists whose frameworks are useful in pediatric health care are presented below.

Erikson's Life Stages

Erik Erikson, a developmental psychologist and psychoanalyst, presented a now widely accepted theory of personality development in 1963. His theory of psychosocial development emphasizes healthy growth through 8 stages, 5 of which occur in childhood. Through identification of key conflicts or critical periods in personality development, Erikson described a favorable and unfavorable aspect of each psychosocial stage (Table 2–1).

TABLE 2-1.
ERIKSON'S LIFE STAGES

AGE	PSYCHOSOCIAL STAGE
Infant (0-12 months)	Trust vs. mistrust
Toddler (1-3 years)	Autonomy vs. shame, doubt
Preschooler (4-6 years)	Initiative vs. guilt
School age (7-12 years)	Industry vs. inferiority
Adolescent (13-18 years)	Identity vs. role confusion

Piaget's Levels of Cognitive Development

A well-known theory of cognitive development was described by the Swiss developmental psychologist Jean Piaget. According to Piaget, cognitive development consists of age-related changes that occur in an orderly and sequential manner (Table 2–2).

TABLE 2-2.
PIAGET'S LEVELS OF COGNITIVE DEVELOPMENT

AGE	COGNITIVESTAGE	CHARACTERISTICS
0-2 years	Sensorimotor	Learns through senses and motor activity. Object permanence (something exists even when out of sight) develops and is a basis for stranger anxiety.
2-7 years	Preoperational	Egocentrism shifts to social awareness, magical thinking, and animism. Play is essential as a way of understanding the world and working out experiences.
7-11 years	Concrete	Understands cause and effect and conservation of matter.
11-15 years	Formal	Achieves intellectual thought with abstract thinking and ability to consider different outcomes.

Through assimilation, children incorporate new knowledge, skills, ideas, and insights into their familiar cognitive schemas. Through accommodation, children change and organize existing schemas to solve increasingly difficult tasks.

Maslow's Hierarchy of Needs

Abraham Maslow theorized that human needs are hierarchical and range from fundamental physiological needs to higher levels of self-actualization. In prioritizing ways to address child and family needs, ensure the fundamental needs are met before attempting to address higher-level needs. The first four needs are basic or "deficiency needs." Self-actualization is a growth need.

1. Physiological needs include breathing, food, water, sex, sleep, homeostasis, excretion.
2. Safety needs include security of body, employment, resources, morality, family, health, property.

3. Love and belongingness needs include friendship, family, sexual intimacy.
4. Ego and esteem needs include self-esteem, confidence, achievement, respect for others, respect by others.
5. Self-actualization needs include morality, creativity, spontaneity, problem-solving, lack of prejudice, acceptance of facts.

Kohlberg's Moral Development

Lawrence Kohlberg's moral development theory consists of three major levels. The theory allows for prediction of behavior, is principally concerned with justice, and postulates that development continues throughout the individual's lifetime.

- Preconventional (4–7 years): Decisions are based on obedience and avoiding punishment. Morality is external; children conform to rules imposed by authority figures. Present in children and adults.
- Conventional (7–11 years): Children are concerned with conformity and being loyal. Rules are to be followed to "be good." Present in teens and adults as well as children.
- Postconventional (≥ 12 years): Internalized standards and social responsibility are formed. Decisions can be made in conflicting ethical situations. Present in teens and adults.

BEHAVIOR MODIFICATION

The philosophy and techniques of behavior modification are designed to increase adaptive behavior through positive reinforcement and decrease maladaptive behavior by punishing or ignoring the behavior. For example, a toddler refusing food can learn to eat when the behavior is reinforced with minutes of playtime for bites of food. Behavior modification is based on the "operant conditioning" principle of learning, also known as Pavlovian or classical conditioning. Basic assumptions include:

- Problems are defined in terms of measurable behavior.
- Treatment is aimed at altering a person's current environment to help the person function in the desired manner.
- Outcome behaviors are specified.
- Methods of treatment and rationale are precisely described.
- Techniques are applied to behaviors of everyday life: toilet training, eating, and accepting responsibility for self-care.

Expected behaviors must be clearly explained, and rewards must be attractive enough to reinforce desired behavior.

PHYSICAL DEVELOPMENT: NORMAL GROWTH EXPECTATIONS AND DEVELOPMENTAL MILESTONES

Growth is defined as an increase in physical size. Development is an orderly series of events and behaviors that lead to new patterns of behavior. Primary factors influencing growth and development include:

- Genetics
- Nutrition
- Prenatal and environmental factors
- Family and community
- Culture

Preterm (gestational age < 37 weeks)

- Minimal subcutaneous fat
- Relaxed posture with limbs extended
- Proportionately large head, reflecting cephalocaudal development
- Smooth and shiny skin with visible blood vessels
- Abundant fine lanugo on body
- Soft, pliable ear cartilage (pinnae)
- Palms and soles have minimal creases
- Skull and ribs feel soft
- Head is subject to "preemie head," positional molding that can be minimized by frequent repositioning and use of a gel mattress
- Scarf sign—preterm elbow is easily brought across chest

Newborn (neonate, birth to 28 days)

- **Respiratory system:** Chemical and thermal stimuli initiate respirations. Surface tension of fluid is reduced by surfactant, which facilitates breathing. Respirations are shallow and irregular, with typical rate of 40–60/min.
- **Circulatory system:** Inspired oxygen dilates pulmonary vessels, which decreases pulmonary vascular resistance and increases pulmonary blood flow. Ductus arteriosus closes as a result of increased oxygen and decreased prostaglandins. Foramen ovale closes with compression of two portions of atrial septum.
- **Thermoregulation:** Heat regulation is important because of the neonate's large body surface area, thin layer of subcutaneous fat, and lack of shivering.
- **Fluid and electrolytes:** Rapid metabolism can lead to acidosis. Immature kidneys cannot concentrate urine well.
- **Gastrointestinal (GI) system:** Deficiency of lipase limits ability to absorb fats. Immature liver decreases storage of glycogen and makes the newborn prone to hypoglycemia. Regurgitation and frequent stooling are common.

- **Renal:** Decreased ability to concentrate urine, voids ~200–300 cc/day
- **Integumentary:** Plugging of sebaceous glands causes milia. Low melanin causes light skin.
- **Musculoskeletal:** Mostly cartilage rather than bone

Infant (1 to 12 months)

- Period of most rapid growth of a person. Typically, an infant:
  - Doubles birth weight by 6 months
  - Triples weight by 12 months
  - Grows approximately 9–11 inches in first year
  - Erupts first tooth at ~6 months
  - Needs breastmilk or formula for first year of life
  - Begins solid foods at 4–6 months, starting with rice cereal
- Posterior fontanelle closes at 6–8 weeks.
- Milestones of development typically occur in order:
  - 1 month: Head lag, grasp reflex strong, hands closed, quiets when hears a voice, fixes on an object at 8–10 inches away, cries and watches faces intently
  - 2 months: Posterior fontanel fuses, lifts head when prone, visually searches for sounds, cries are differentiated, social smile
  - 3 months: Focuses on an object with both eyes (binocular vision), regards own hand, hands loosely open, squeals to show pleasure, coos, babbles, shows interest in surroundings, is aware of strange surroundings
  - 4 months: Holds head erect in vertical position, rolls from back to side, grasps objects with both hands, makes consonant sounds (n, k, g, p, b), recognizes familiar faces and objects
  - 4–6 months: Sits with support, grasps objects with palm, rolls from stomach to back, plays with toes, grasps and manipulates small objects, prefers complex visual stimuli
  - 6 months: Rolls from back to stomach, may chew and bite, begins to imitate sounds, begins to fear strangers, searches for dropped object (concept of object permanence begins), laughs when head is hidden
  - 7–8 months: Sits erect momentarily, beginning pincer grasp, reaches for toys out of reach, responds to "no," bears weight on feet with support
  - 8–9 months: Crawls on hands and knees, pulls self to standing, hand dominance evident, responds to simple commands, beginning of fears of going to bed and being left alone
  - 10 months: Says "dada"
  - 12 months: Walks, drinks from cup
- Infant's play is solitary and favorite toys are mobiles, teething toys, plastic blocks, rattles, unbreakable mirror

Toddler (1 to 3 years)

Physical development slows as the toddler's appetite decreases, but he or she needs a diet high in protein for brain development. Typically:

- Drinks whole milk until the age of 2 years, when 2% milk is recommended
- Toddlers gain ~3–5 inches and 5 pounds per year.
- The anterior fontanelle fuses between 12 and 18 months.
- Birth weight quadruples by 24 months.
- Height at 2 years is approximately half adult height.

Psychosocial development includes curiosity, gaining sense of autonomy. A toddler typically:

- Generalizes concepts
- Learns to differentiate self from others
- Learns to tolerate separation from primary caregiver
- Engages in parallel play; favorite toys are manipulation toys, blocks, shapes, telephones, kitchens (imitative play)

Preschooler (3 to 6 years)

Growth continues at about 5 pounds and 3 inches per year.

- Appetite decreases
- Needs ~1,800 calories per day
- Has strong food preferences
- Respiratory movement is principally abdominal or diaphragmatic (as opposed to thoracic) in children younger than 6–7 years old.

Development is more refined with increased strength and agility.

- Likes to explore
- 3 years: Rides tricycle, copies circle
- 4 years: Throws ball overhand and catches ball; copies a square
- 5 years: Jumps rope, balances on one foot, ties shoes, uses scissors
- Uses associative and cooperative play; favorite toys are creative, educational

School Age (6 to 12 years)

During the school-age years, growth in height and weight are slower and steadier than in earlier years.

- Gains ~2 inches and 4–5 pounds per year
- Loses deciduous teeth beginning at 6 years, with 26 of the 32 permanent teeth erupting by age 12
- Moves gracefully and is steadier than earlier
- Has more mature GI system, so fewer stomach upsets and better maintenance of blood sugar levels
- Prepubescence occurs at ~9 years in girls and ~10 years in boys

This time is often called the *latency period*; the school-age child is typically in a period of relative tranquility.

- Engages in cooperative play
- Has a sense of industry
- Maintains relationships with same-sex peers

Adolescent (12 to 18 years)

The teen years are a period of profound biologic, intellectual, psychosocial, and economic change.

- Goes through puberty (growth spurt, sexual maturation with secondary sex characteristics)
- Refines motor skills
- Blood volume and systolic blood pressure increase
- Lung size increases
- Respiratory rate decreases to adult rate
- Neural system is fine-tuned as support cells brace and nourish the neurons.

Adolescent development brings advances in cognition with abstract thinking and increasing emotional independence from parents.

- Engages in increasingly competitive play
- Goes through a period of identity formation
- Uses formal operational thought with abstract reasoning
- Is preoccupied with body image
- Generally conforms to group norms
- Has wide mood swings
- Uses principled moral reasoning

FAMILY CONCEPTS AND ISSUES

Families have been defined in many different ways for many different purposes. A family is the mainstay of society and is described as what an individual considers the family to be. This may, but does not necessarily, include relationships between dependent children and one or more protective adults. Healthcare personnel and services support the family's strength and competence with family-centered philosophy in caring for the child, recognizing that the family is the constant in the child's life.

Five major family structures exist, according to the U.S. Census Bureau:

- Traditional nuclear family, which includes a married couple and biological children
- Nuclear family, which includes two parents who may or may not be married, with their children who may be biological, adopted, step, or foster
- Blended family or household, which includes at least one stepparent, stepsibling, or half-sibling
- Extended family or household, which includes at least one parent, one child, and one or more related or unrelated members. Parent–child and sibling relationships may be biologic, step, adoptive, or foster.
- Single-parent family, which is increasingly common and usually headed by a single mother, although fathers may also head single-parent families
- Same gender parents, who may be male or female, are also becoming increasingly common.

Family theories are used to describe how families respond to events both within and outside the family. Combinations of theories have relevance for nursing practice because each theory has strengths and limitations.

- **Family systems theory:** A change in one part of the family system affects all other parts of the family; families have periods of rapid changes and growth as well as periods of relative stability.
- **Family stress theory:** Families encounter normative, expected, and unexpected stressors and cope with a range of responses and effectiveness. Coping is using learned cognitive or behavioral strategies, or both, to relieve stress, and families cope and respond to stressors with great variability.
- **Family developmental theory:** Families change over time in similar and consistent ways. There are eight developmental stages of the family throughout the life span:
    1. Beginning family that is a newly married or formed couple
    2. Child-bearing family with infant
    3. Family with preschoolers
    4. Family with school-age children
    5. Family with teenagers
    6. Family launching young adults

7. Middle-aged family—empty nest
8. Family in retirement and old age

The age of the oldest child indicates the stage. Each stage helps identify transitions and potential stressors. Blended (step), low-income, single-parent, dual-career, and divorcing families also have typical developmental stages.

- **Structural-functional theory:** The family's major goal is socialization of the child. Family serves to
  - Meet psychological needs of members
  - Socialize and help children become productive members of society
  - Perpetuate the species through reproduction
  - Work as an economic unit
  - Provide for physical necessities

Families play a vital role in society as they produce and consume goods and services; replace dying members of society; and transmit knowledge, customs, values, and beliefs to the young. In working with children, nurses must include family members in the plan of care; the family is the patient.

FAMILY-CENTERED CARE

For effective family-centered care, it is essential to

- Assess individual and family health needs and strengths
- Identify problems influencing health of the family as a whole
- Identify problems influencing individual family members
- Use family resources, teaching, counseling, and evaluating of progress toward goals

CULTURAL AND SPIRITUAL DIVERSITY

Culture is the totality of socially transmitted values, behavior patterns, institutions, arts, and other products of human work characteristic of a society that organize the society's childrearing system and are transmitted to the next generation by family. Culture provides the context in which families experience health and illness. To provide holistic care, nurses must be culturally sensitive and develop some understanding and appreciation for the ways culture influences childrearing practices and attitudes toward health.

- **Demographic changes:** More than 1 in 5 U.S. children are foreign born or the child of foreign-born parents because of immigration (Mather, 2007). The migration of people requires nurses to be transcultural in their approach to caring for diverse populations. By 5 years old, children can identify persons belonging to their cultural background. Cultures vary in the extent to which they tolerate divergence from the norm.
- **Ethnicity:** A population differentiated from others by customs, characteristics, language, or similar factors. Differences may also include family structure, language, food preferences, moral codes, and expression of emotion.
- **Gender**, or the characteristics describing masculinity or femininity, may influence the family's perception of the implication of illness or disability. Male children are valued more than female children in some cultures.
- Nurses need to adapt practices to the health needs of families rather than attempt to change longstanding beliefs.
- Nurses need to listen with the goal of understanding rather than agreement.
- Beliefs about health and illness in many cultures vary from the values of Western healthcare professionals and healthcare institutions.

Religion and *spirituality* are often used interchangeably, but spirituality is broader than religion. An individual's orientation dictates a code of morality and influences the family's attitude towards education and male/female role identity. Religion may influence choice of life companion(s), profession, diet, acceptability of healthcare options, and rites at birth, transition to adulthood, illness, and death.

- Religion is an integrated system of beliefs that is associated with a code of morality and often influences the family's attitude toward education, gender role identity, professional aspirations, and food choices.
- Spirituality is often defined as an individual's sense of peace, purpose, and connection to others, and beliefs about the meaning of life. While spirituality may be found and expressed through organized religion, many people find meaning in nature or in relationships.

SUMMARY

Psychosocial, cognitive, moral, and physical development occur within a social context typically consisting of one or two parents and their children. Genetic traits and the family environment play a large role in shaping the physical make-up and identity of children as they grow into adolescence and become adults. Family interactions and modeling can shape a child's self-esteem, socialization, and cultural identity.

REFERENCES

Ball, J. W., Bindler, R. C., & Cowen, K. J. (2010). *Child health nursing: Partnering with children and families* (2nd ed.). East Rutherford, NJ: Prentice Hall.

Bowden, V. R., & Greenberg, C. S. (2010). *Children and their families: The continuum of care* (2nd ed.). Philadelphia: Lippincott Williams & Wilkins.

Hagan, J. F., Shaw, J. S., & Duncan, P. M. (Eds.). (2007). *Bright futures: Guidelines for health supervision of infants, children, and adolescents* (3rd ed.). Elk Grove Village, IL: American Academy of Pediatrics.

Hockenberry, M. J., & Wilson, D. (2011). *Wong's nursing care of infants and children* (9th ed.). St. Louis, MO: Elsevier/Mosby.

Mather, M. (2007). *U.S. racial/ethnic and regional poverty rates converge but kids are still left behind.* Retrieved from www.prb.org/Articles/2007/USRacialEthnicAndRegionalPoverty.aspx

National Association of Pediatric Nurse Practitioners, Society of Pediatric Nurses, American Nurses Association. (2008). *Pediatric nursing: Scope and standards of practice.* Silver Spring, MD: Nursesbooks.org.

Pillitteri, A. (2010). *Maternal & child health nursing: Care of the childbearing and childrearing family* (6th ed.). Philadelphia: Lippincott Williams & Wilkins.

CHAPTER 3

COMMUNICATION

Mary Jo Gilmer, PhD, MBA, RN-BC, FAAN, and
Karen Corlett, MSN, RN-BC, CPNP-AC/PC, PNP-BC

Communication is an essential part of health care. Accurate communication between and among nurses, physicians, other members of the healthcare team, patients, families, and caregivers improves the process and delivery of health care.

We communicate with patients and families at every encounter. Some of our encounters are mundane and some involve sharing of quite personal patient or family information. We communicate when taking a patient history, when conveying what we are doing, and when providing instruction. Communication is important to assessing health and disease, and to educating others about necessary care. Regardless of what we are communicating, the process and structure of communication is much the same. To receive and convey content effectively, we should consider the elements of ideal communication.

CULTURALLY SENSITIVE COMMUNICATION

- Assessment of and respect for
  - Usual healthcare providers and systems
    - Complementary and alternative medicine practices and providers
  - Definition of family
    - Make-up of family
    - Family functioning
  - Decision-making processes within the family
  - Attitude toward physical contact
  - Cultural implications of eye contact
  - Native language or dialect
  - Gender of caregiver in relation to gender of patient or parent
  - Religious preferences
  - Tenets or beliefs that affect healthcare choices
- Nurses can improve their cultural awareness through personal education regarding cultural beliefs, lifestyle differences, and religious practices
  - Do not assume that skin color implies culture.

COMPONENTS OF THERAPEUTIC COMMUNICATION

- Establish rapport
  - Honesty, commitment, and caring
- Build trust
  - Commitment of time and availability
- Show respect
  - Address formally unless given permission to use informal levels of address
  - Assess, acknowledge, and respect culture
- Empathy
  - Understanding of and respect for situation
  - Convey concern and caring
- Active listening
  - Verbal content and nonverbal context
  - Clarification of understanding
  - Listener's nonverbal actions are important cues for speaker

- Feedback
  - Verbal and nonverbal encouragement
  - Clarification of content and meaning of verbal and nonverbal communication
- Managing conflict
  - Goal is for both parties to come away feeling satisfied
  - Clarify and acknowledge thoughts and feelings of participants
  - Create alternative solutions
  - Negotiate toward acceptable solution with input from all stakeholders
    - Avoid a win-lose situation
    - Goal is win-win
    - Ideal is situation in which each party feels comfortable with compromises made
- Maintain professional boundaries
  - Challenging because of stress or emotions felt during relationship
  - Limit contact with patient and family outside of workplace
  - Avoid sharing personal information with patients and families
- Therapeutic modes of communication with children
  - Talking and listening
  - Role-play, acting
  - Storytelling
  - Artwork, drawing, painting, sculpting
  - Music
  - Humor

COMMUNICATION BARRIERS

- Physical barriers
  - Space between participants
  - Qualities of the room
    - Acoustics
    - Audiovisual equipment
    - Temperature
    - Lighting
    - Arrangement of furniture

- Noise distractions
- Sensory impairments
    - Hearing, vision, or speech deficits
    - Drug or disease effects
- Medical terminology

- Psychosocial barriers
    - Developmental age or stage
        - Consider regression with stress or illness
    - Personal state
        - Emotional state
        - Preconceived ideas
            - About caregiving role
            - Related to disease or diagnosis
        - Previous experiences
            - With healthcare system
            - With persons with similar diagnosis or needs
        - Personal or societal beliefs
            - Values, morals, judgments
        - Body language, facial expressions

MODES OF COMMUNICATION

- Conveying information
    - Talking, lecturing
        - Inflection, tone, and emphasis influence the message
        - One-on-one, small group, large group
    - Written
    - Audio or video recordings, or both
    - Interactive programs
- Nonverbal communication
    - Nonverbal message is just as, or more, important than verbal message
    - Body language
        - Open, relaxed posture (avoid crossed arms and knees)
        - At same level as listener

        - Sitting, standing, or kneeling as appropriate
        - Eye contact within constraints of cultural norms
    - Personal space between speakers and listeners
        - Defined differently among cultures
        - Be aware of physical barriers that may be between speaker and recipients such as crib railings or the hospital bed
    - Appearance
        - Clothing, hairstyle, body art, jewelry, and so on
    - Hand gestures
    - Touch
- Receiving information
    - Listening
        - Active process
        - Give feedback regarding degree of understanding
            - Restate
            - Summarize
            - Ask for clarification
- Formal communication
    - Preplanned
    - Organized
    - Objectives predetermined
- Informal communication
    - Just as powerful as formal communication
    - Spontaneous
        - Taking advantage of teachable moments
    - Often occurs during other events or tasks
    - Can be a less intimidating process
        - Fewer barriers
        - Often yields more feelings
- Group dynamics (Tuckman, 1965)
    - Forming
        - Politeness prevails
        - Getting to know—not much revealed as yet
        - Group members get along well or pretend to

- Storming
    - Maneuvering for position within the group
    - Informal role assignments (leader, negotiator, defender, etc.)
    - Attempts at doing the work of the group
- Norming
    - Trust develops
    - Issues revealed
    - The group starts to work well together
- Performing
    - Active work predominates
    - Cooperation and efficiency
    - The group works smoothly
- Adjourning and mourning
    - A formal dissolution of the group
    - Important for participants to sense that the purpose or work of group is completed
- Groups work through these stages at different speeds
    - May spend more time in one stage than another
    - May cycle through all these stages in one efficient meeting
    - Groups that cannot get through "norming" rarely perform well

PATIENT CONFIDENTIALITY

- Health Insurance Portability and Accountability Act (HIPAA)
    - National mandate to protect the privacy of patient information
    - Structures in place to protect the privacy of the medical record
    - All written and verbal communication about patient status is protected.
        - Computers and portable access devices must have protection in place.
    - Appropriate sharing of information
        - Between healthcare providers and family members with patient's permission
        - Among healthcare providers to facilitate safe care
        - Among healthcare entities, billing departments, and insurers
        - Only necessary information should be shared.
    - Mandatory reporting

      - Reportable diseases to health departments or government agencies
      - Police reports, such as for gunshot injuries
      - Suspected or documented nonaccidental injury, neglect, abuse

WRITTEN COMMUNICATION IN NURSING PRACTICE

- A part of the medical record
- Legal document
- Documentation of nursing care delivered
- Documentation of patient status
- Principles of documentation
  - Accurate
  - Clear: Use only approved abbreviations, correct any errors appropriately
  - Timely: Dated, timed, and entered into record in a timely fashion
  - Legible: Content and signature
  - Patient-specific: Related to child and family needs
- Documentation systems
  - Medical activity report (MAR): A computerized schedule for administering medications to a patient for a defined period of time, including providers' orders and time to administer the drugs
  - Clinical pathways (CP): Also known as care pathways, critical pathways, integrated care pathways, or care maps, clinical pathways are useful in managing the quality and standardization of care processes and promote organized and efficient patient care based on evidence. They are useful as guides for evidence-based documentation.
  - Electronic medical record (EMR): A computerized system for the storage, retrieval, and modification of medical records
  - Dispensing system: Automated medication-dispensing systems offer medications safely to patients on-site.

PROFESSIONAL COMMUNICATION

- With other care team providers
  - Healthcare jargon is appropriate.
    - Precise meanings conveyed
- Much of communication is verbal.
  - Document important elements of verbal exchanges in the medical record

- Transfer of care
  - When transferring care of patient temporarily or permanently
  - Concise yet complete
  - SBAR is a mnemonic useful for change of shift communication:
    - **S**ituation
    - **B**ackground
    - **A**ssessment
    - **R**ecommendations
    - Include issues, tests, and results that are in process or pending
  - Can be verbal or written process
    - Must have opportunity to clarify information and ask questions as part of transfer of care process
- Dealing with difficult people
  - Address behavior privately
    - Away from patient's family members and other patients or families
    - Away from patient care areas if conflict between providers
    - May be helpful to have neutral third party present
  - Describe issue, conflict, behavior
    - Remain calm; use "I" statements
    - Describe effects of words or actions
  - If issues unresolved, seek resolution via appropriate chain of command
    - Nursing chain of command
    - Family services chain of command
    - Medical staff office chain of command
    - State nurses association
    - Union negotiations

ADVOCACY

- Professional advocacy
  - For the growth of the profession of nursing
    - Expand your personal knowledge base
    - Know what it is to be a nurse and how to explain the profession to families and other providers
      - Address myths or incorrect beliefs

        - Differentiate between provider orders and nursing care plans
            - Highlight the practice of nursing
        - Join a professional organization
            - Participate in committees
            - Seek office
        - Contact government representatives in support of the nursing profession
            - Become aware of proposed regulations affecting nurses
    - For patients and families
        - Advocate for family-centered care in your facility
        - Ensure patient rights are respected
        - Provide developmentally appropriate care for the child
        - Support community endeavors beneficial to children's health
        - Lobby for change to support children's health care
            - At the community, state, and national levels
            - Get involved with child advocacy organizations
            - Become aware of and involved with legislative changes

SUMMARY

Trust and respect are important building blocks for successful communication in helping nurses understand a situation, care for one another, and resolve differences. Effective communication extends far beyond the exchange of words and includes creation of a safe environment, attentive listening, nonverbal interactions, and mutual understanding.

REFERENCES

Ball, J. W., Bindler, R. C., & Cowen, K. J. (2010). *Child health nursing: Partnering with children and families* (2nd ed.). East Rutherford, NJ: Prentice Hall.

Bowden, V. R., & Greenberg, C. S. (2010). *Children and their families: The continuum of care* (2nd ed.). Philadelphia: Lippincott Williams & Wilkins.

Fischbach, F., & Dunning, M. B. (2009). *A manual of laboratory and diagnostic tests* (8th ed.). Philadelphia: Lippincott Williams & Wilkins.

Hagan, J. F., Shaw, J. S., & Duncan, P. M. (Eds.). (2008). *Bright Futures: Guidelines for health supervision of infants.* (3rd ed.). Elk Grove Village, IL: American Academy of Pediatrics.

Hockenberry, M. J., & Wilson, D. (2011). *Wong's nursing care of infants and children* (9th ed.). St. Louis, MO: Elsevier Mosby.

Institute for Healthcare Improvement (n.d.). *SBAR technique for communication: A situational briefing model.* Retrieved from http://www.ihi.org/IHI/Topics/PatientSafety/SafetyGeneral/Tools/SBARTechniqueforCommunicationASituationalBriefingModel.htm

Pillitteri, A. (2010). *Maternal & child health nursing: Care of the childbearing and childrearing family* (6th ed.). Philadelphia: Lippincott Williams & Wilkins.

United States Department of Health and Human Services. (2003). *Summary of the HIPAA privacy rule.* Retrieved from http://www.hhs.gov/ocr/privacy/hipaa/understanding/summary/privacysummary.pdf

Tuckman, B. (1965). Developmental sequence in small groups. *Psychological Bulletin (6),* 384–399.

CHAPTER 4

THE NURSING PROCESS

Clara J. Richardson, MSN, RN-BC

The nursing process is a standardized method of identifying patient needs and problems and then utilizing a problem-solving approach to meet those needs. The six steps of the nursing process are assessment, diagnosis, outcome identification, planning, implementation, and evaluation.

NURSING ASSESSMENT

Assessment of the Child and Family

The pediatric health history may be altered based on setting, age of the child, and focus of care. In the ambulatory setting, the history is extensive and expanded with each visit as the practitioner strives to provide comprehensive well-child care. At the hospital, the focus is on the areas of history most relevant to the present condition. Prenatal and birth history tends to become briefer with older children. The nurse should involve the child in obtaining data as much as developmental level allows. This is especially important with adolescents. As they mature, adolescents should have time alone with their healthcare provider to share pertinent history and have privacy during the physical examination. Ideally, in an integrated healthcare system, the individual's lifetime health history would be available to all providers in all settings.

Identifying Data

- Child's nickname
- Informant's relationship to the child

Reason for Seeking Care

- Progression of symptoms
- Exposure to communicable disease

Past Medical History

- Immunization record
- Communicable diseases
- Past illnesses, surgeries, hospitalizations, emergency room visits
- Allergies to medications, foods, animals, insects, dust, etc.
- Current medications, vitamins, nutritional supplements

Birth History

- Prenatal history
    - Maternal health
        - Age and extent of prenatal care
        - Past pregnancies
        - Illnesses, exposure to diseases or environmental toxins
        - Attitudes toward the pregnancy
    - Maternal medications
        - Prescribed medications
        - Vitamins and over-the-counter medications
        - Illicit drugs, alcohol, smoking
    - Length of gestation, problems encountered
    - Parents' blood types

Natal History

- Labor and delivery
    - Length of labor
    - Spontaneous or induced
    - Vaginal or cesarean
    - Forceps
    - Medications, epidural anesthesia
- Infant's condition at birth
    - Apgar scores
    - Gestational age assessment
    - Birth weight, length, head circumference

Neonatal History

- Problems
    - Respiratory problems, jaundice, seizures

    - Thermoregulation or glucose problems
    - Neonatal intensive care unit
    - Any other problems
- Length of hospital stay
- First weeks at home
    - Feeding
    - Sleeping
    - Elimination
- Family bonding
    - Parent–child
    - Siblings
    - Extended family, friends

Dietary History

- Infant feeding
    - Duration of breastfeeding
    - Formula brand, preparation, storage
    - Introduction of solids, finger foods
    - Vitamin, iron, or fluoride supplements
- Older child
    - Age of weaning from breast or bottle
    - Self-feeding skills
    - 24-hour recall, usual diet
    - Vitamins, nutritional supplements
    - Food preferences, foods avoided
    - Food allergies

Developmental History

- Developmental milestones
    - Age of holding head up steadily
    - Age of sitting independently
    - Age of walking independently
    - Age of saying meaningful words
    - Any concerns about development
    - Differences from siblings or other children

- Toilet training
  - Age
  - Methods
  - Problems
- Dentition
  - Number of teeth
  - Age at first tooth eruption
  - Age at first tooth loss
  - Dental hygiene
  - Visits to dentist
- Sleep patterns
  - Amount and timing
  - Place, bedtime rituals
  - Nightmares, terrors, waking
- Habits
  - Thumbsucking, nail biting, hair twisting
  - Repetitive motions such as rocking or head banging
  - Temper tantrums
  - Alcohol, drug use
  - Inhalant abuse (sniffing, huffing)
  - Smoking, smokeless tobacco

Sexual History

- Peers, dating
- Sexual experiences
- Pregnancy prevention
- Prevention of sexually transmitted infections
- Risk of partner abuse

Social History

- Residence
  - Home type, condition, size, safety precautions
  - City or well water
  - Urban or rural
  - Neighborhood, play area safety

    - Residents and relationships
    - Pets
- Financial situation
    - Parents' occupations
    - Source of healthcare payment
        - Private insurance
        - Medicaid
    - Social service agency assistance
    - Unmet needs
- Family relationships
    - Family roles and organization
    - Languages spoken and read
    - Childrearing practices, discipline
    - Extended family
    - Support systems
- Community involvement
    - Childcare, school
    - Social clubs, sports, activities
    - Religious involvement

Family Health History

- Ages and health problems
- Genetic or familial health problems
- Genetic screening for hereditary diseases

Health Practices

- Usual healthcare providers, medical home
- Regularity of well-child visits
- Lay providers, folk healers
- Religious or cultural practices related to health
- Illness prevention and treatment
    - Special foods, beverages, herbs, spices, supplements
    - Ointments, creams, steam, heat, cold, massage
    - Other forms of complementary and alternative medicine
    - Over-the-counter medications

Physical Assessment

Age Variations and Tips

- Infants and toddlers
    - Keep on parent's lap as much as possible
    - Complete auscultation, pulse, respirations while child quiet
    - Save intrusive activities (temperature, throat, ears) until the end
    - Keep security objects near
    - Use distraction
- Preschoolers
    - Short, simple verbal explanations
    - Demonstrate on dolls, stuffed animals
    - Let child handle equipment
    - Save genital assessment until the end
- School-age children
    - Explain purpose of assessment and body functioning
    - Use pictures, body diagrams
    - Save genital assessment until the end
- Adolescents
    - Provide privacy and assure confidentiality
    - Keep conversation nonjudgmental, nonconfrontational
    - Save genital assessment until the end

Growth Measurements

- Gender-specific growth charts may be downloaded from the National Center for Health Statistics
    - Infants, birth to 24 months
        - Length for age and weight for age
        - Head circumference for age
        - Weight for length
    - Children and adolescents, 2–20 years
        - Stature for age and weight for age
    - Body mass index (BMI) for age
- Height
    - Length is measured in lying position

- Stature is measured in standing position
- Result is within normal limits if between 3rd and 97th percentiles
- Child should follow a steady curve on a standardized growth chart
- Use gestation-adjusted age for preterm infants up to 24 months of age when using a standardized growth chart

- ▶ Weight
  - Children younger than 3 years are weighed nude for most precise measurement, or with minimal clothing
  - Older children wear underwear or a light gown
  - Result is within normal limits if between 3rd and 97th percentiles
  - Child should follow a steady curve on a standardized growth chart
  - Use gestation-adjusted age for preterm infants up to 24 months of age when using a standardized growth chart
  - Ask about recent weight gain or loss
- ▶ Head circumference
  - Measured in children up to 36 months

Vital Signs

- ▶ Temperature
  - Axillary recommended for infants younger than 1 month
  - Rectal measurement is most accurate for children between 1 and 3 months
  - Rectal site should not be used in infants younger than 1 month of age, with recent rectal surgery, with diarrhea or anorectal lesions, or receiving chemotherapy
  - Temporal artery not accurate for infants younger than 3 months with acute illness or fever
  - Tympanic has much variability and is not a precise measurement
  - Oral for cooperative children
- ▶ Pulse
  - Apical for children younger than 2 years
  - Count for full minute
  - Usual rates
    - Newborn 100–180
    - < 2 years 80–130
    - 2–6 years 70–120
    - 6–10 years 70–110
    - 10–16 years 60–100

- Respirations
  - Count for full minute
  - Usual rates
    - Newborn 30–60
    - 1 year 20–40
    - 2–5 years 20–30
    - 6–9 years 18–30
    - 10 years 16–20
    - 11–17 years 12–16
- Blood pressure
  - Cuff bladder width 40% of upper arm circumference
  - Cuff bladder length 80%–100% of upper arm circumference
  - Percentile charts available from Centers for Disease Control and Prevention (www.cdc.gov)
  - Estimate of usual value
    - Diastolic
      - Ages 1–5 years = 56
      - Ages 6–18 years = age in years + 52
    - Systolic
      - Ages 1–7 years = age in years + 90
      - Ages 8–18 years = (2 × age in years) + 83

Pediatric Variations of Adult Physical Assessment Findings

- Lymph nodes
  - Small, nontender, movable nodes are usually normal in children
- Head
  - Flatness on one side often denotes lying in one position
  - Infant should hold head erect and midline by age 4 months
  - Anterior fontanel closes at 12–18 months of age
- Neck
  - Neck short until age 3–4 years
  - Any mass can easily obstruct airway
- Eyes
  - Permanent eye color by age 6–12 months
  - Presence of red reflex rules out many serious defects

  - Infant should be able to fixate on one visual field by age 3–4 months
  - Visual acuity testing should begin by age 3 years
    - Snellen letter charts
    - Tumbling E chart
    - HOTV chart
    - Allen picture test
- Ears
  - For otoscopic exam
    - Pull pinna down and back for children younger than 3 years.
    - Pull pinna up and back for children older than 3 years.
  - Variety of auditory tests for newborns and older children
- Chest
  - Children younger than 6 years use abdominal, rather than diaphragmatic, breathing.
  - Breast changes of puberty commonly start in girls at 10–14 years.
  - Gynecomastia in boys may be the result of hormonal conditions or obesity.
  - See Chapter 9 for additional respiratory assessment.
  - See Chapter 10 for additional cardiac assessment.
- Abdomen
  - To check for inguinal hernia in a child too young to cough, have the child blow hard through a straw or laugh
  - Palpate tender areas last
- Extremities
  - Absence of femoral pulse may indicate coarctation of the aorta
  - Bowleg appearance is normal in children younger than 3 years
  - Knock-knee appearance is normal until 7 years of age

Pain Assessment Tools Based on Age of Child

- Premature Infant Pain Profile Scale (PIPPS): Neonates with gestational ages from 28 to 36 weeks' gestation
  - Gestational age
  - Behavioral state
  - Heart rate
  - Oxygen saturation
  - Brow bulge
  - Eye squeeze

- Nasolabial furrow
- CRIES Scale: 0–6 months
  - Crying
  - Requires O_2 for $SaO_2 < 95\%$
  - Increased vital signs (blood pressure and heart rate)
  - Expression
  - Sleepless
- Neonatal Infant Pain Scale (NIPS): < 1 year
  - Facial expression
  - Cry
  - Breathing patterns
  - Arms
  - Legs
  - State of arousal
- FLACC Scale: 2 months–7 years
  - Face
  - Legs
  - Activity
  - Cry
  - Consolability
- Children's Hospital Eastern Ontario Pain Scale (CHEOPS): 1–7 years
  - Cry
  - Facial
  - Child verbal
  - Torso
  - Touch
  - Legs
- Oucher Scale: 3–12 years
  - Six photograph faces, ranging from not hurt to biggest hurt you could ever have
  - White, Black, Hispanic forms
- Wong-Baker Faces Pain Rating Scale (FACES): > 3 years
  - Six cartoon faces, ranging from no hurt to hurts worst
  - English and Spanish forms
- Noncommunicating Children's Pain Checklist: 3–18 years with cognitive impairment

  - Vocal
  - Social
  - Facial
  - Activity
  - Body and limbs
  - Physiological
  - Eating and sleeping
- Numeric Pain Scale: > 9 years
  - None
  - Mild: 0–3
  - Moderate: 4–6
  - Severe: 7–10
- COMFORT Scale: Infants, children, adults
  - Alertness
  - Calmness
  - Respiratory distress
  - Crying
  - Physical movement
  - Muscle tone
  - Facial tension
  - Blood pressure
  - Heart rate

Fall Risk Assessment Tools

- CHAMPS Fall Risk Assessment Scale
  - Presence of risk factors related to
    - C: change in or altered mental status
    - H: history of falls
    - A: age less than 3 years
    - M: altered mobility
    - P: parental involvement
    - S: safety interventions
- Humpty Dumpty Falls Scale (HDFS)
  - Presence of risk factors related to

- Age
- Gender
- Diagnosis
- Cognitive impairments
- Environmental factors
- Response to surgery, sedation, or anesthesia
- Medication usage

Family Assessment Tools

- Calgary Family Assessment Model: An in-depth evaluation
  - Structural category: family members, caregivers, supports outside of immediate family
  - Developmental category: life stage events (divorce, childbirth, etc.)
  - Functional category: interaction of family members
- Family Adaptability and Cohesion Evaluation Scales IV (FACES IV): In-depth evaluation of balanced (healthy) and unbalanced (problematic) family functioning
  - Balanced
  - Rigidly cohesive
  - Midrange
  - Flexibly unbalanced
  - Chaotically disengaged
  - Unbalanced
- Family Apgar: Very brief five-item scale to measure family members' satisfaction
  - Family problem-solving
  - Shared responsibility and decision-making
  - Physical and emotional maturation, self-fulfillment
  - Commitment to share time, space, and material resources
- Friedman Family Assessment Model: Variable depth of assessment through short and long forms
  - Identifying data
  - Developmental stage and history
  - Environmental data
  - Family structure
  - Family functions
  - Family stress, coping, adaptation

- Home Observation for Measurement of the Environment (HOME): Short and long forms depending on depth of assessment desired
  - Measure quality and quantity of stimulation and support available to child in the home
    - Infant/Toddler (IT) HOME
    - Early Childhood (EC) HOME
    - Middle Childhood (MC) HOME
    - Early Adolescent (EA) HOME
    - Child Care (CC) HOME
    - Disability (DA) HOME

NURSING DIAGNOSIS AND TREATMENT

Diagnosis

Nursing diagnosis is a standardized language to communicate patient needs and problems, which may be actual or potential problems based on the patient's risk factors. The North American Nursing Diagnosis Association (NANDA) produced the first taxonomy in 1986. Renamed NANDA International (http://www.nanda.org), the organization remains committed to the continued development of nursing diagnostic terminology.

The Nursing Interventions Classification (NIC) provides a standardized list of more than 500 research-based physiological and psychosocial interventions. The Nursing Outcome Classification (NOC) contains more than 300 outcomes that can be used to evaluate the effects of nursing interventions. These classifications are available from the University of Iowa's Center for Nursing Classification & Clinical Effectiveness at http://www.nursing.uiowa.edu/excellence/nursing_knowledge/clinical_effectiveness/index.htm.

Outcome Identification

After identifying the appropriate nursing diagnoses, the nurse specifies the expected changes in physical condition or behavior that the patient will exhibit after interventions are implemented. Patient outcomes should consist of specific behaviors that can be seen, measured, or evaluated. They should also include a time frame for attainment. Nurses usually develop their own outcomes, but NOC could certainly be used and may provide a usable format for computerized charting.

Planning

Once the nurse defines expected outcomes, he or she describes specific nursing interventions that will assist the patient in attaining those outcomes. Evidence-based interventions come from data the nurse gathers from the child's and family's statements, from the nurse's own observations, and from current research information. The nurse uses critical thinking to plan care based on the evidence and his or her own clinical expertise. Searching for evidence requires that the nurse be able to access information using appropriate computer search engines. Again, nurses usually develop their own interventions, but using NIC language may have some advantages if standardization is desired.

Implementation

Implementation is the nurse fulfilling the role of care provider, putting plans into action. It must be noted that all nursing care in pediatrics is family-centered care. The entire family, not just the child, is the patient. The nurse implements interventions for all family members to enable them to show their present competencies and develop new competencies with the ultimate goal of empowering families to control their own lives.

Evaluation

In the evaluation step of the process, the nurse decides if the patient outcomes were met, if the nursing interventions were effective, and if the plan needs modification. If alterations are required and the nurse–patient interaction continues, the last step of the nursing process may not actually be the end.

REFERENCES

Breau, L., McGrath, P., Finley, A., & Camfield, C. (2004). *Non-communicating children's pain checklist-revised (NCCPC-R).* Retrieved from http://pediatric-pain.ca/files/02/78/NCCPCR_200901.pdf

Caldwell, B., & Bradley, R. (1984). *Home observation for measurement of the environment (HOME) inventory.* Retrieved from http://www.ualr.edu/case/index.php/home/home-inventory/

Faulds, S., & Moore, J. (2007). *Pediatric pain assessment tools.* Retrieved from http://www.anes.ucla.edu/pdf/assessment_tool-cheops.pdf

Faulds, S., & Moore, J. (2007). *Pediatric pain assessment tools.* Retrieved from http://www.anes.ucla.edu/pdf/assessment_tool-nips.pdf

Graf, E. (2011). Magnet children's hospitals: Leading knowledge development and quality standards for inpatient pediatric fall prevention programs. *Journal of Pediatric Nursing, 26*(2), 122–127.

Hill-Rodriguez, D., Messmer, P. R., Williams, P. D., Zeller, R. A., Williams, A. R., Wood, M., & Henry, M. (2009). The Humpty Dumpty Falls Scale: A case-control study. *Journal for Specialists in Pediatric Nursing, 14*(1), 22–32.

Hockenberry, M. J., & Wilson, D. (2011). *Wong's nursing care of infants and children* (9th ed.). St. Louis, MO: Mosby.

Manworren, R. C. B., & Hynan, L. S. (2003). Clinical validation of FLACC: Preverbal patient pain scale. *Pediatric Nursing, 29,* 140–146.

National Center for Health Statistics. *Clinical growth charts.* Retrieved from http://www.cdc.gov/nchs/about/major/nhanes/growthcharts/clinical_charts.htm

National Institutes of Health. *Pain intensity instruments.* Retrieved from http://painconsortium.nih.gov/pain_scales/

Oucher Organization. (n.d.). *Oucher!™.* Retrieved from http://www.oucher.org/the_scales.html

Pasero, C. (2002). Pain assessment in infants and young children: Premature infant pain profile. *American Journal of Nursing, 102,* 105–106.

Razmus, I., & Davis, D. (2012). The epidemiology of falls in hospitalized children. *Pediatric Nursing, 38*(1), 31–35.

Willis, M. H. W., Merkel, S. I., Voepel-Lewis, T., & Malviya, S. (2003). FLACC behavioral pain assessment scale: A comparison with the child's self-report. *Pediatric Nursing, 29,* 195–198.

CHAPTER 5

BASIC AND APPLIED SCIENCES

Mary Jo Gilmer, PhD, MBA, RN-BC, FAAN, and
Paula Chiplis, PhD, RN, CPNP

TRAUMA AND DISEASE PROCESSES

An understanding of age-specific anatomy and physiology, common genetic disorders, transmission of infectious diseases, and the use of traction to treat fractures is essential to the pediatric nurse.

Age-Specific Anatomy and Physiology

Defined and predictable patterns in growth and development are universal to all children, but they follow the patterns in a manner and time that is unique to each child.

- Directional trends
    - Cephalocaudal (head→down)
    - Proximal to distal (inside→outside)
    - Differentiation (simple→complex)
- Biologic growth
    - Skeletal maturation occurs over ~20 years, beginning with centers of ossification in an embryo and concluding when the last epiphysis is fused to the shaft of a bone. Bone fractures may be difficult to discover and may affect subsequent growth and development.
    - Intentional movements replace neurologic primitive reflexes as the brain develops. Growth of the brain is reflected in increasing head circumference, possible until fontanelles close.
    - Lymphoid tissues are relatively small in infants, but are well developed and grow quickly.
    - Kidneys and liver are immature at birth and in early childhood, leading to decreased metabolism of medications and fairly dilute urine.

- Physiological changes
    - *Metabolism* describes all chemical and energy transformations in the body. Basal metabolic rate (BMR) is slightly higher in boys than in girls and further increases over girls in pubescence.
    - Thermoregulation is an important adaptation to extra-uterine life, and even young children are susceptible to temperature fluctuations. Infections can result in either a rapid temperature elevation or a decrease in temperature in young children. Young children can also become overheated during active play.

COMMON GENETIC DISORDERS

Prenatal diagnosis is available for many disorders, leading to ethical dilemmas such as whether to use the option of abortion.

- Cystic fibrosis is an autosomal recessive condition with abnormal exocrine gland function and excessive salt in sweat. It is the most common lethal disease in Whites, with a median life span of 25 years.
    - Chronic pulmonary involvement: Excessive mucus, reduced cilia function, recurrent infections
    - Pancreatic compromise: Lack of trypsin, malabsorption; also rectal prolapse, meconium ileus, liver cirrhosis, gallbladder tones, salivary gland obstruction
    - Prenatal diagnosis available at chromosome 7q31.2; sweat chloride test used for postnatal diagnosis
- Sickle cell disease (SCD) is an autosomal recessive, chronic hemolytic anemia from production of abnormal hemoglobin (HbS) with reduced oxygen-carrying capacity.
    - Causes infarction of lungs, kidneys, spleen, bones, painful leg ulcers, dactylitis, priapism, renal failure, and increased risk for pneumococcal infections and salmonella osteomyelitis
    - Incidence is 1:400–600 Blacks and 1:1,000 Hispanics; also seen in individuals from India, Middle East, and Mediterranean
    - Prenatal diagnosis available with chorionic villi sampling or amniocentesis
    - Postnatal screening test is Sickledex; electrophoresis provides definitive diagnosis.
    - Life expectancy is mid-40s, but with more comprehensive care and better therapeutic options, life expectancy is increasing
- Trisomy 21 (Down syndrome) is compatible with live birth, but physical and mental abnormalities vary greatly.
    - Characterized by mental retardation, craniofacial abnormalities, low-set ears, ventricular and atrial septal defects, patent ductus arteriosus, hypotonia, respiratory infections, acute leukemia, malformed kidneys, hydronephrosis, cryptorchidism, seizures, apneic events
        - IQ 25–75

        - 50% die by 60 years
        - Males are sterile
    - Frequency 1:1,500 for mothers 20 years old and 1:30 for mothers 45 years old
    - Prenatal and postnatal diagnoses available at chromosome 21.
- Achondroplasia is an autosomal dominant common form of dwarfism
    - Adult stature 48–52 inches
    - Characterized by shortened limbs, normal-length torso, lordosis, sleep apnea, possible hydrocephalus, prominent forehead, flattened nasal bridge, short stubby fingers, normal IQ and life span
    - Women may have backaches from enlarged breasts, premature menarche and menopause
    - Prenatal diagnosis available on chromosome 4p16.3
- Huntington's disease is an autosomal dominant, progressive neurological deterioration caused by neuron atrophy, with death approximately 15 years from onset
    - Onset at 15–50 years
    - Characterized by psychiatric symptoms, choreoathetoid movements, progressive dementia, intellectual decline, seizures, rigidity, and dystonia
    - Prenatal diagnosis available on chromosome 4p16.3
- Familial hypercholesterolemia is an autosomal dominant, common single-gene disorder with early onset atherosclerotic disease of coronary, cerebral, and peripheral arteries and xanthomas (cholesterol deposits in skin and tendons)
    - Incidence 1:200–500
    - Diagnosis available on chromosome 19p13.2
- Osteogenesis imperfecta is an autosomal dominant osteoporosis with recurrent fractures of long bones
    - Life span normal in spite of repeated fractures
    - Characterized by blue sclera, conductive deafness, discolored teeth, and multiple fractures
    - Diagnosis available on chromosome 17q21.31
- Polycystic kidney disease is an autosomal dominant condition with development of cysts in kidneys, liver, pancreas, and spleen; renal failure; and hypertension
    - Cysts remain asymptomatic until 3rd or 4th decade
    - Incidence 1:1,000
    - Accounts for 10% of adult cases of renal failure
    - Diagnosis available on chromosome 4121

COMMON CHILDHOOD DISEASES

Newborn

- Conjunctivitis of the newborn (ophthalmia neonatorum) < 30 days
  - Characteristics: red conjunctiva, swollen with yellow or white discharge
  - Complications: periorbital cellulitis, brain abscess, and decreased vision
  - Treatment: usually optic antibiotics because the condition is caused by *Chlamydia, Neisseria gonorrhea,* or both
  - Nursing management: instilling antibiotics, teaching parents careful handwashing, and limiting exposure to other children until on antibiotics for 24 hours
- Atopic dermatitis (eczema)
  - Characteristics: chronic red, pruritic crust or vesicles on face, scalp, and/or extensor aspects of arms and legs
  - Complications: secondary skin infections
  - Treatment: avoid allergy-causing foods and environmental factors; lubricate with moisturizing ointments and creams (Eucerin, Elidel, Aquaphor, Cetaphil, Protopic, Vaseline) 3–4X/day; apply topical steroids (ointment preferred) such as hydrocortisone .5%–2.0%
  - Nursing management
    - Reduce frequency of bathing to a few times per week in tepid, not hot, water
    - Lubricate skin after bathing or swimming
    - Apply hydrocortisone 0.5%–2%
    - Use Benadryl or Atarax for pruritus

Infancy

- Cow's milk allergy (CMA)
  - Characteristics: crying, pallor, irritability, diarrhea, vomiting, colic, wheezing, bloody stools, rhinitis, asthma, sneezing, coughing, eczema, or a combination within first 4 months of life
  - Complications: slow growth, possible anaphylaxis
  - Treatment: eliminate cow's milk–based formula and switch to a casein hydrolysate milk formula such as Pregestimil, Nutramigen, or Alimentum, in which milk proteins are broken down into amino acids
  - Nursing management
    - Reassure and educate parents
    - Maintain infants on a milk-free diet for 1–2 years, after which small quantities of milk are reintroduced; many children outgrow sensitivity by 3–4 years old

- Diaper dermatitis
    - Incidence is 50% of young children, peak age 9–12 months, and caused by wetness, pH, and fecal irritants. Risk factors for *Candida albicans* infection are compromised skin, altered immune status, and antibiotic therapy.
    - Characteristics: bright red rash with raised borders, often with satellite lesions in skin folds
    - Complications: scarring, systemic infections
    - Treatment: topical glucocorticoids or antifungals if nursing management not successful
    - Nursing management
        - Superabsorbent disposable diapers
        - Change diapers frequently
        - Expose to air (minor diaper dermatitis) or use thick zinc oxide or petroleum to protect skin (moderate–severe)

Early Childhood

- Chickenpox (varicella-zoster virus [VZV])
    - Transmission: spread by respiratory secretions and direct contact with skin lesions, although scabs are not infectious; incubation 2–3 weeks
    - Characteristics: rash on trunk with less on limbs
    - Complications: secondary bacterial infections (e.g., abscesses, cellulitis, necrotizing fascitis, pneumonia, sepsis), encephalitis, hemorrhagic varicella, chronic or transient thrombocytopenia
    - Treatment: antiviral acyclovir and VZIG in high-risk children, diphenhydramine to relieve itching
    - Vaccine available; see the Centers for Disease Control and Prevention's Web site, www.cdc.gov/vaccines
    - Nursing management
        - Isolation until vesicles are dry to prevent spread
        - Daily tepid baths and skin care
        - Calamine lotion for itching; keep fingernails short and clean; keep child cool to decrease itching
- Diphtheria (Corynebacterium diphtheriae)
    - Transmission: direct contact with discharge from nose, skin, or lesions
    - Characteristics: fever; malaise; highly pruritic rash that starts as macule and progresses to vesicle that breaks and crusts; lymphadenopathy; pseudomembrane in nasal, pharyngeal, or laryngeal areas
    - Complications: myocarditis, neuritis

- Treatment: penicillin or erythromycin, complete bed rest to prevent myocarditis, tracheostomy for airway obstruction
- Vaccine available; see the Centers for Disease Control and Prevention's Web site, www.cdc.gov/vaccines
- Nursing management
    - Maintain isolation
    - Have epinephrine available
    - Observe respirations for obstruction; suction as necessary
    - Administer humidified oxygen

- Fifth disease or erythema infectiosum (human parvovirus B19)
    - Transmission: unknown route, possibly respiratory secretions of infected persons
    - Characteristics: facial rash with "slapped face" appearance, maculopapular red spots on upper and lower extremities
    - Complications: self-limited arthritis and arthralgia
    - Treatment: symptomatic antipyretics and analgesics
    - Vaccine: none available
    - Nursing management: isolation is important if exposed to pregnant women because virus can be teratogenic. Isolation is not necessary except in child with immunosuppression and aplastic crises.
- Roseola (exanthema subitum)
    - Transmission: unknown but limited to children 6 months to 3 years
    - Characteristics: high fever in child who looks well; rose-pink macules on trunk that spread to neck, face, and extremities; nonpruritic, cervical, and postauricular lymphadenopathy; inflamed pharynx; cough; coryza
    - Complications: recurrent febrile seizures and, rarely, encephalitis
    - Treatment: nonspecific; antipyretics for fever
    - Vaccine: none available
    - Nursing management: discuss precautions if child is prone to febrile seizures
- Measles (rubeola)
    - Transmission: respiratory droplet spread; direct contact with respiratory tract secretions, blood, or urine
    - Characteristics: fever, malaise, cough, conjunctivitis, photophobia, Koplik spots in mouth, red rash on face that spreads downward, anorexia, lymphadenopathy, and desquamation
    - Complications: otitis, pneumonia, bronchiolitis, obstructive laryngitis, encephalitis
    - Treatment: supportive care
    - Vaccine available; see the Centers for Disease Control and Prevention's Web site, www.cdc.gov/vaccines

- Nursing management
  - Respiratory isolation until 5th day of rash
  - Antipyretics
  - Dim lights for photophobia
  - Examine cornea for signs of ulceration
  - Vaporizer
  - Tepid baths

- Mumps
  - Transmission: direct contact or airborne via droplet
  - Characteristics: fever, headache, anorexia followed by earache, swollen parotid gland(s) accompanied by pain and tenderness
  - Complications: sensorineural deafness, postinfectious encephalitis, myocarditis, arthritis, hepatitis, sterility (in men; rare), meningitis, epididymo-orchitis (inflammation of testes)
  - Treatment: analgesics, antipyretics, fluids
  - Vaccine available; see the Centers for Disease Control and Prevention's Web site, www.cdc.gov/vaccines
  - Nursing management
    - Isolation, analgesics, antipyretics, fluids, and hot or cold packs to neck
    - For orchitis, support with tight-fitting underwear

- Pertussis or whooping cough (Bordetella pertussis)
  - Transmission: direct contact or droplet spread from infected person
  - Characteristics: upper respiratory infection (URI) symptoms for 1–2 weeks, followed by severe hacking cough (paroxysmal stage), sneezing, low-grade fever; coughing is more frequent at night, associated with high-pitched crowing or whoop that lasts 4–6 weeks
  - Complications: atelectasis, otitis media, pneumonia, seizures, weight loss, hernia, prolapsed rectum
  - Vaccine available; see the Centers for Disease Control and Prevention's Web site, www.cdc.gov/vaccines
  - Treatment: azithromycin, pertussis immunoglobulin
  - Nursing management
    - Isolation, bed rest, and hospitalization may be required for infants and dehydrated children
    - Assess respiratory function for possible intubation; have oxygen available
    - Encourage fluids; use high humidity

- Poliomyelitis (enteroviruses)
  - Transmission: direct contact with infected person via fecal-oral and pharyngeal-oropharyngeal routes
  - Characteristics are in three forms:
    1. Fever, sore throat, headache, anorexia, vomiting, abdominal pain lasting hours to days
    2. All previous symptoms with pain and stiff neck, back, and legs
    3. Same as 2) with recovery, then signs of central nervous system (CNS) paralysis
  - Complications: permanent paralysis, respiratory arrest, hypertension, kidney stones from demineralization of bones during immobility
  - Treatment: respiratory assistance for respiratory paralysis, physical therapy after acute phase
  - Vaccine available; see the Centers for Disease Control and Prevention's Web site, www.cdc.gov/vaccines
  - Nursing management
    - Maintain complete bed rest during acute phase
    - Administer mild sedatives
    - Use moist hot packs, range of motion (ROM) exercise
    - Observe for respiratory paralysis
- Rubella (German measles)
  - Transmission: nasopharyngeal secretions, blood, stool, and urine
  - Characteristics: low-grade fever, headache, malaise, lymphadenopathy, sore throat, and then rash. Rash on face spreads downward in red-pink maculopapular exanthema that disappears by day 3.
  - Complications: teratogenic effects on fetus; condition may lead to arthritis, encephalitis, or purpura (rare)
  - Treatment: antipyretics for fever
  - Vaccine available; see the Centers for Disease Control and Prevention's Web site, www.cdc.gov/vaccines
  - Nursing management includes isolating client from pregnant women
- Scarlet fever (Group A β-hemolytic streptococci)
  - Transmission: direct contact, droplet spread, or contact with articles contaminated with Group A β-hemolytic streptococci
  - Characteristics: abrupt high fever, vomiting, headache, chills, malaise, abdominal pain, enlarged tonsils
  - Complications: peritonsillar and retropharyngeal abscess, sinusitis, glomerulonephritis, carditis, polyarthritis

- Treatment: penicillin or erythromycin
- Vaccine not available; see the Centers for Disease Control and Prevention's Web site, www.cdc.gov/vaccines
- Nursing management: respiratory precautions until 24 hours after start of antibiotics

Middle Childhood

- Impetigo (Staphylococcus)
    - Transmission: auto-inocular and contagious by contact
    - Characteristics: reddish macule that becomes vesicular, ruptures easily leaving moist erosion, sharply marginated irregular outlines; exudates form honey-colored crusts; pruritus
    - Complications: secondary infections
    - Treatment: topical bactericidal ointment; oral or parenteral antibiotics (penicillin) when severe
    - Nursing management: careful removal of crusts, comfort care
- Scabies (infestation with scabies mite, *Sarcoptes scabiei*)
    - Transmission: prolonged contact with the mite—it requires about 45 minutes for the mite to burrow under the skin
    - Characteristics: intense itching, which may lead to excoriations secondary to scratching; maculopapular lesions occur interdigitally and in axillary, popliteal, and inguinal areas
    - Complications: secondary infections
    - Treatment: application of a scabicide such as Elimite; persons in close proximity to an infested person should be treated
    - Nursing management: educate families about accurately following directions for use of scabicide. Elimite should be applied to all skin surfaces, with care to avoid eye contact. Touching and holding child should be minimized, and nurses should wear gloves.
- Head lice (Pediculosis capitis)
    - Transmission: person to person or sharing of personal items
    - Characteristics: scalp itching and irritation
    - Complications: scratch marks and inflammatory papules caused by secondary infections
    - Treatment: application of pediculicides (Nix or RID) and manual removal of nits. Daily removal of nits should continue until no longer found.
    - Nursing management: educate families that anyone can get lice
        - Lice do not jump or fly and are not transmitted by pets.

  - Lice survive for 48 hours away from the host, but nits are shed into the environment and can hatch in 7–10 days.
  - Recurrent lice are a problem that necessitates proactive family and school education

- Lyme disease (spirochete *Borrelia burgdorferi*)
  - Transmission: Tick bite, especially the deer tick
  - Characteristics in Stage 1: Erythema chronicum migrans at bite with raised doughnut-like border, pain described as burning, warm to touch, occasionally pruritic; fever, headache, malaise, anorexia, stiff neck, generalized lymphadenopathy, splenomegaly, sore throat, conjunctivitis, cough
  - Complications in Stage 2: Neurologic, cardiac, and musculoskeletal involvement 2–11 weeks after cutaneous symptoms
  - Complications in Stage 3: Musculoskeletal pains occur months or years later; chronic arthritis; late neurological problems may include deafness, encephalopathy, and keratitis
  - Treatment: Amoxicillin or penicillin < 8 years of age; doxycycline or amoxicillin ≥ 8 years of age; cefuroxime and erythromycin if allergic
  - Vaccine: None available
  - Nursing management:
    - Education to protect from tick exposure through avoidance
    - Use of repellent such as DEET (diethyltoluamide) or permethrin for children > 1 year old
- Cat scratch disease
  - A common regional lymphadenitis in children and teens; benign and self-limited, resolves spontaneously in 2–4 months
  - Transmission: 90% of the time follows scratch or bite of an animal leading to infection with *Bartonella henselae,* gram-negative bacteria
  - Characteristics: erythematous papule at inoculation—painless and nonpruritic
  - Complications: encephalitis, hepatitis
  - Treatment: supportive care
  - Vaccine: none available
  - Nursing management
    - Limit activity to prevent trauma to enlarged lymph nodes; bed rest for those with fever
    - Analgesics for discomfort, but there is no need to get rid of pet

Adolescence

- Acne vulgaris
  - Increased sebum production causing inflamed papules, pustules, nodules, and cysts; begins in early adolescence and gradually increases until late teens
  - Characteristics: formation of blackheads (open comedones) or whiteheads (closed comedones); proliferation of *P. acnes*, a benign organism always present on the skin
  - Complications: secondary infection, scarring
  - Treatment: supportive care and specific treatments determined by type of lesions. Resolves slowly over 6+ weeks. Topical benzoyl peroxide inhibits bacterial growth. Accutane may be used in severe cases, but pregnancy must be prevented when using this medication.
  - Nursing management
    - Explanation of disease process
    - Education about gentle cleansing

TRACTION

The purpose of traction is immobilization to maintain proper alignment of fractures.

- Types
  - Skin traction: pull is applied to skin and indirectly to skeletal structures
  - Skeletal traction: pull is applied directly to bone by pins, wires, or tongs through the diameter of the bone
  - External fixators: portable devices attached by percutaneous pins or wires to the leg bone for correction of deformities, limb lengthening, or pseudoarthroses
  - Bryant traction: running traction in which the pull is in one direction only. The legs are flexed at 90° angle at the hips and the buttocks are raised slightly off the bed, resulting in countertraction.
  - Buck extension: used for short-term immobilization (e.g., for dislocation, Legg-Calvé-Perthes disease); the legs are extended
  - Russell traction: skin traction applied to lower leg with padded sling under the knee, creating two lines of pull (longitudinal and perpendicular) and allowing some position changes without malalignment
  - Cervical traction: helps prevent dislocation or fracture of the vertebrae, which may result in spinal cord injury (Halo; Crutchfield, Barton, or Gardner-Wells tongs)
  - Care of child with traction
    - Ensure equipment is properly positioned with correct amount of weight, weights freely hanging, pulleys correctly aligned, body in alignment

- ▷ Assess skin under straps and pin insertion sites for redness, edema, skin breakdown, and drainage
- ▷ Assess extremity for neurovascular status
- ▷ Monitor for pain and skin condition of prominences lying on bed
- ▷ Sterile pin care
- ▷ Provide skin care every 4 hours, using sheepskin under affected extremity

PHARMACOLOGY

Growth and maturation of children contribute to the bodies' capacity to metabolize and excrete medications. Immaturity of organs, or problems with absorption, distribution, metabolism, or excretion, can significantly alter effects of medications. Newborn and premature babies with immature enzyme systems in the liver are particularly vulnerable to harmful effects of drugs.

Drug Interactions

Nurses and parents need to be aware of possible drug interactions, particularly with antihistamines. One example is the use of astemizole (Hismanal), which, if given with erythromycin, can lead to life-threatening cardiac dysrhythmias. Stevens-Johnson syndrome (erythema multiforme), sometimes associated with ingestion of drugs used for upper respiratory infection, manifests as a rash and lesions and has a mortality rate of about 10%.

- ▶ *Over-the-counter:* Concern over the use of antihistamines, decongestants, antitussives, and expectorants has been growing among pediatricians. Pharmaceutical companies continue to market the drugs for children, but the efficacy is not well documented and therefore, these should not be given to any child under the age of 2 years.
- ▶ *Herbal:* In recent years, investigators have reported widespread use of alternative medicines. Some herbal therapies have potentially harmful side effects as well as adverse interactions with medications. It is therefore important for healthcare providers to have knowledge about herbal medications, to inquire about their use, and to educate families about the risks and benefits, as well as potential interactions these products may have with over-the-counter and prescription medications.
- ▶ *Complementary and alternative medicine (CAM)* includes a variety of products and practices not currently a part of conventional medicine. They are primarily used for chronic medical conditions, and evidence to determine safety and effectiveness is often lacking. There are five classes of therapy:

  1. Biologically based: foods, diets, vitamins, herbal or plant preparations
  2. Manipulative treatment: chiropractic, osteopathy, massage
  3. Energy-based: Reiki, magnetic treatment, pulsed fields current
  4. Mind–body techniques: mental healing, relaxation, hypnosis, expressive

5. Alternative medical systems: homeopathy, naturopathy, ayurvedic, traditional Chinese medicine (including acupuncture and moxicombustion)

Prescription

After a drug is prescribed to a child, careful diligence is needed to determine the correct dose, watching for side effects or complications. Antiarrhythmics, anticoagulants, chemotherapeutic agents, electrolytes, and insulin should be double-checked by another nurse prior to being administered to a child; they may be hazardous or even lethal at incorrect doses.

- *Therapeutic drug levels* need to be monitored because children respond to drugs so differently. Evaluation of side effects and toxic effects is also useful to determine correct dosages.
- *Medication reconciliation* is a formal process for creating the most complete and accurate list possible of a patient's current medications and comparing the list to those in the patient record or medication orders. The process includes
  - Identify the kind of patient medication information that will be collected outside of 24-hour settings.
  - Collect the patient's medication information.
  - Compare the patient's medication information with newly prescribed medications to ensure no contraindications.
  - Explain to the patient and/or family the importance of maintaining updated medication information.
  - Provide the patient and/or family with a complete list of all medications the patient should be taking for future reference.
- *Weight-specific dosing* has been used to determine safe doses for children. Most often the method used is mg/kg. The most reliable method is to calculate the body surface area (BSA), using a nomogram derived from the height and weight of a child.
- *Administering medications*
  - Oral: preferred route whenever possible
    - Risk for aspiration with either pill or liquid; use liquid if patient is unable to swallow
    - Use spoon, plastic cup, plastic dropper, or plastic syringe (without needle)
  - Intramuscular (IM): ensure syringe can measure precise amounts
    - Use smallest gauge needle possible to deliver fluid safely, and proper length to deposit the medication into the body of the muscle
    - Sites
      - Infants: vastus lateralis until child has been walking for a year
      - Young children > 2 years and adolescents: Deltoid for small amounts of medication
  - Subcutaneous: useful for insulin, hormone replacement, allergy desensitization

- Intradermal: tuberculin testing, local anesthesia, and allergy testing given into the volar surface of the forearm
- Rectal: less reliable, but may be used when oral route is difficult or contraindicated
- Optic, otic, and nasal: similar to adult administration, but gain child's cooperation through use of helpful techniques
    - Eye: apply finger pressure to lacrimal punctum to prevent drainage of medication to the nasopharynx, with subsequent unpleasant taste
    - Ear: allow medication stored in refrigerator to warm to room temperature before administration
    - Nose: position child with head hyperextended to prevent medication from trickling into the child's throat

- *Monitoring response to medication*
    - Calculate safe dosage
    - Know expected action, possible side effects, and signs of toxicity
    - Toxic effects may be difficult to evaluate (e.g., tinnitus in preverbal child)
    - Immaturity or capacity to metabolize and excrete drugs may alter effects
        - Newborn and premature infants have immature liver and kidney function
        - Medical conditions may affect body's ability to detoxify and excrete

NUTRITION

Early eating habits are especially important in developing healthy children. Nutrition is often regarded as the most important determinant of growth. The nurse can be instrumental in guiding parents in food selection for their children. During early childhood, a child is growing rapidly with an associated demand for calories, particularly protein. There are many plateaus and growth spurts, and a child's nutritive needs may change, but habits are developed early and care should be taken to ensure that those are healthy habits.

Nutrition Guidelines

Nutritional assessment can be completed through careful clinical exams, evaluating hair, skin, and mouth particularly. In addition, diet intake records can be used, but may be inaccurate. Finally, biochemical analysis helps inform adequate nutrition.

Routes

While oral feedings are the most satisfying to young children, they also may be fed by nasogastric tube or intravenously.

Formulas

Breastfeeding or formula is recommended during the first year of life because of infants' inability to tolerate cow's milk. For the first 6 months, human milk is the most desirable and complete diet. Even though breastmilk is relatively low in iron, it is absorbed better than iron-fortified formula. Additional iron (400 IU daily) may be added if a mother's iron intake is inadequate. Addition of solid foods may begin at 4–6 months and should be added one food at a time when infant shows signs of solid-food readiness. Rice cereal is generally the first food introduced to an infant. Tooth eruption begins at about 6 months of age. Finger foods such as crackers, raw fruit, or vegetables can be added.

Vitamins and Supplements

Necessary for specific metabolic activity, vitamins are an essential food element and important in growth and development. A deficiency of a vitamin can affect metabolic activity, and excessive amounts of vitamins may have a toxic effect on a child because of organ immaturity. As long as a child maintains a balanced diet in adequate amounts, vitamin deficiencies are rare in the United States. Fat-soluble vitamins (A, D, E, and K) are found in many foods and stored in the liver. Vitamin K is also synthesized by intestinal bacteria, and vitamin D becomes available to the body through exposure to sunlight.

Therapeutic and Alternative Diets

Vegetarian and other alternative diets are becoming more common, and care must be taken to ensure children maintain adequate nutrition while excluding meat and other foods from their diets. Various types of diets include:

- Lacto-ovo-vegetarians exclude animal flesh but eat dairy products and eggs.
- Lacto-vegetarians exclude animal flesh and eggs but eat dairy products.
- Vegans exclude animal flesh, dairy products, and eggs.
- Zen macrobiotics exclude meat, poultry, milk, and eggs, and eat large amounts of leafy, root, and sea vegetables, brown rice, fruit, and fish.
- Semivegetarians avoid red meat but eat fish, poultry, eggs, and dairy products.

Weight Gain or Loss

Changes in children's assessment parameters on the growth chart should be carefully evaluated because excessive weight gain may be associated with:

- Congestive heart failure
- Nephrotic syndrome (severe edema)

Weight loss may be associated with:

- Adrenocortical insufficiency
- Bacterial endocarditis (or any other severe infection)
- Diabetes insipidus
- Graves' disease
- Cystic fibrosis

Growth Charts

An important aspect of a child's physical exam is growth in relation to previous growth patterns and in relation to other children's growth. The National Center for Health Statistics has revised growth charts to include body mass index, heights, weights, and head circumferences for ages birth to 20 years. Three important indicators for further evaluation are:

- Widely disparate height and weight percentiles
- Failure to show expected growth rates
- Sudden increase or decrease in previously steady growth (except in puberty)

Body Mass Index

Body mass index (BMI), is equal to [weight in pounds/height in inches × height in inches] × 703. This measurement represents the relationship between height and weight. It can be either calculated or found on a nomogram. A child is described as overweight if she or he falls above the 85th percentile. The BMI is helpful in detecting early signs of risk for overweight and obesity. The prevalence of overweight and obesity among children has greatly increased over the past decade. The most prevalent physical complication of childhood obesity is diabetes. However, self-esteem and psychosocial problems may also occur. Obesity may persist into adulthood, with the additional risks of heart disease and joint problems.

Total Parenteral Nutrition (TPN)

TPN is also known as IV alimentation or hyperalimentation and provides for the nutritional needs of infants or children. Total nutrient admixture (TNA) may refer to 1) minerals, water, trace elements, and other additives in a single container; or 2) dextrose, amino acids, and lipids in a single solution. TPN often refers to dextrose and amino acids with additives to which lipids are piggybacked into the system.

- Indications for use: include chronic intestinal obstruction or conditions preventing bowel function, malabsorption, severe diarrhea, extensive body burn
- Requirements: for infusion, include use of a large vessel such as superior vena cava, innominate vein, or internal jugular vein to minimize phlebitis and irritation

- Caveats
    - Use strict aseptic technique to prevent bacterial growth with high-glucose, high-protein solutions
    - Avoid adding other solutions or medicines in the line
- Complications
    - Liver disease, especially in preterm infants
    - Imbalance in elements, such as hypoglycemia
    - Catheter-related events, such as infection, sepsis, venous thrombosis, embolization, endocarditis, or both
- Nursing management
    - Monitor for blood sugar changes
    - Allow infants to suck nonnutritively to fulfill oral needs
    - Monitor for liver changes
    - Reassess requirements for growth
    - Monitor social and motor development because IV infusion may reduce mobility and socialization

CHEMISTRY

Body Fluid Balance and Imbalance

Infants and young children are more susceptible to fluid and electrolyte imbalance because it develops rapidly in children and they adjust less quickly. Children tend to run higher fevers than adults because of:

- Increased surface area (skin) relative to size: preemie has 5×, infant has 2–3× body surface area/kg compared to an adult
- Higher metabolic rate
- Immature kidney of infant doesn't concentrate or dilute urine, conserve or excrete sodium, or acidify urine

Children may experience dehydration, water intoxication, or edema.

- Dehydration is classified as isotonic, hypotonic, or hypertonic. The most common causes of dehydration are loss of fluid from vomiting, diarrhea, diabetic ketoacidosis, and extensive burns.

Electrolyte Balance and Imbalance

- Hyponatremia occurs with loss of sodium (Na) through sweating, replaced with water, resulting in weakness, dizziness, nausea, apathy, weak pulse, decreased blood pressure, lethargy, Na < 130 mEq/L.

- Hypernatremia results in intense thirst; dry, sticky mucous membranes; flushed skin; oliguria; nausea; hoarseness; increased temperature; Na > 150 mEq/L.
- Hypokalemia (low serum potassium [K]) manifests as muscle weakness, cramping, hypotension, cardiac arrhythmias, ileus, tachy- or bradycardia, irritability, apathy or drowsiness, fatigue, K < 3.5 mEq/L.
- Hyperkalemia can result in hyperreflexia, twitching, muscle weakness, flaccid paralysis, bradycardia, ventricular fibrillation and arrest, oliguria, apnea, and respiratory arrest, K ≥ 5.5 mEq/L.
- Hypocalcemia manifests as tingling of nose, ears, toes, fingers; tetany, convulsions, laryngospasm, neuromuscular irritability; hypotension, cardiac arrest; Ca < 8.5 mg/dL.
- Hypercalcemia results in constipation, weakness, fatigue, nausea, anorexia, thirst, bradycardia or cardiac arrest, increased calcium in urine causing kidney stones, muscle hypotonicity.

CLINICAL SIGNS ASSOCIATED WITH ISOTONIC DEHYDRATION IN INFANTS

- Children with isotonic dehydration typically display symptoms of hypovolemia, reduced size of vascular compartment
- Falling blood pressure
- Low central venous pressure
- Poor capillary filling

Clinical observations important with fluid balance

- Intake and output
- Heart rate—tachycardia
- Temperature—elevated
- Respirations—rapid
- Blood pressure—children compensate, so decreased BP is critical
- Skin color, turgor, temperature, elasticity
- Edema
- Mucous membranes
- Fontanel
- Salivation and tearing
- Eyeballs
- Muscle cramps
- Behavior

- Weight
- Urine output—should be at least 1cc/kg/hr

Basic metabolic panel (BMP): A group of blood tests completed as part of a routine physical or to assist with diagnosing a medical concern.

- Glucose
- Calcium
- Sodium, potassium, carbon dioxide, and chloride
- Blood urea nitrogen (BUN) and creatinine

Acid–base balance: Disturbances in acid–base balance include respiratory acidosis, respiratory alkalosis, metabolic acidosis, and metabolic alkalosis.

- Normal laboratory values
  - pH: 7.35–7.45
  - pO_2: 80–100
  - pCO_2: 35–45
  - HCO_3: 22–26
  - Electrolytes
    - K: 3.5–5.0 mEq/L
    - Na: 136–149 mEq/L
    - Cl: 98–106 mEq/L

SUMMARY

Vulnerability to trauma, infection, and malnutrition may be mitigated with proactive family education and maximing access to care. It is incumbent upon the pediatric nurse to partner with families to enhance the growth and development of children.

REFERENCES

Ball, J. W., Bindler, R. C., & Cowen, K. J. (2010). *Child health nursing: Partnering with children and families* (2nd ed.). East Rutherford, NJ: Prentice Hall.

Bowden, V. R., & Greenberg, C. S. (2010). *Children and their families: The continuum of care* (2nd ed.). Philadelphia: Lippincott Williams & Wilkins.

Hagan, J. F., Shaw, J. S., & Duncan, P. M. (Eds.). (2007). *Bright futures: Guidelines for health supervision of infants, children, and adolescents* (3rd ed.). Elk Grove Village, IL: American Academy of Pediatrics.

Hockenberry, M. J., & Wilson, D. (2011). *Wong's nursing care of infants and children* (9th ed.). St. Louis, MO: Elsevier/Mosby.

Pillitteri, A. (2010). *Maternal & child health nursing: Care of the childbearing and childrearing family* (6th ed.). Philadelphia: Lippincott Williams & Wilkins.

Wilson, B. A., Shannon, M. T., Shields, K., & Geoff, W. (2011). *Pearson nurse's drug guide 2012*. New York: Pearson.

CHAPTER 6

EDUCATIONAL PRINCIPLES AND STRATEGIES

Mary Jo Gilmer, PhD, MBA, RN-BC, FAAN, and
Karen Corlett, MSN, RN-BC, CPNP-AC/PC, PNP-BC

This chapter provides a framework to describe the process and components of child and family teaching, which is undertaken by nurses on a daily basis from the time of admission through discharge. The actual content of patient and family education will be discussed in the sections devoted to the major health problems.

PATIENT EDUCATION

- Begins at first contact
  - Emergency department
  - Preoperative visit
  - Admission
  - Well-child visit
  - Clinic visit
- Necessary for health promotion and disease prevention
  - Basic understanding of the workings of their body
  - Knowledge of how to access components of the healthcare system such as wellness centers, clinics, hospitals
- Important in management of acute and chronic disease

- Increasing importance as more care is undertaken in the home

- Preprocedure teaching
  - Assessment of learning needs
    - Age, developmental stage
      - Affects timing of preparation, depth of information, and word choices
    - Background
      - Past history and experience with healthcare system
      - Culture, religion
      - Family attitudes and family dynamics
      - Previous information supplied
    - Current knowledge and expectations
  - Planning and delivery of patient education
    - Encourage participation of child
    - Encourage parental involvement
      - May have different interdisciplinary personnel or physical spaces to meet developmental and educational needs of both child and caregivers
    - Developmentally appropriate play as learning tool
      - Coloring, painting
      - Dolls, toys
    - Medical play with safe medical equipment
      - Familiarize child with the environment
  - Reinforcement of learning
    - Through daily activities, nursing care, and play activities
    - Support parents and family in their ability to reinforce education
  - Evaluation of learning
    - Ask child (preschooler and older) to explain plan of care or upcoming tests and procedures
    - Correct and reinforce as indicated
    - Teach back method
- Patient and family teaching as one component of the education process
  - Assessment of learning needs
    - Prioritized objectives
      - Need to know vs. nice to know
      - Consider time available and attention span

- Assessment of barriers to learning
  - For patient
  - For family or other caregivers
- Planning and delivery of patient education
  - Multisensory teaching methods based on preference and abilities of learner
    - Verbal information
    - Printed materials: flyers, posters, books, articles
    - Audio or video presentations, or both
    - Interactive computer programs
    - Demonstration
      - Simulations
      - Return demonstration of learned skills
    - Individual vs. group learning environment
- Reinforcement of education
  - Targeted to priority knowledge and skills
  - Positive feedback for gained skill or knowledge
  - Constructive correction where indicated
- Evaluation of learning
  - Pre- and posttest comparisons
  - Recitation of knowledge
  - Return demonstration of skills
    - Simulations
    - Actual performance
- Revision of teaching methods, plan, target knowledge
  - Based on evaluation of learning
    - Input from teacher and learner(s)
  - Implementation of revised plan

- Barriers to effective learning
  - Lack of readiness for change or learning
    - Acceptance of illness or deficit is necessary before being motivated to take care of new needs
  - Differences in health beliefs or practice
  - Visual, cognitive, auditory, language, or learning disabilities or deficits
  - Use of healthcare jargon

- Anxiety, drug or disease effects, environmental distractions
- Culturally insensitive teaching
- Developmental stage or educational abilities of the learner not taken into account
    - Consider regression of developmental maturity and limited learning abilities in times of stress or illness
- Organizational barriers to effective patient and family education
    - Space, noise, privacy, time, and resource constraints

- Support in place to continue necessary learning; although education is important in positively influencing compliance, it does not ensure compliant behavior. In order to enhance understanding and provide support to retain material, complying with the following guidelines is essential.
    - Provide written materials to which families can refer for reinforcement of information.
    - Use "teachable moments"—times when family is most likely to accept information.
    - Use wristwatch alarms for medication reminders.
    - Coordinate medications with mealtimes.
    - Use sticker charts or tokens with younger children.
    - Community resources and support
    - Specific resources and support for disease management or lifestyle change
        - Leukemia and Lymphoma Society
        - Juvenile Diabetes Association
        - National Organization of Rare Diseases
        - Cystic Fibrosis Foundation
        - Curesearch
        - Caring Bridge
        - Sickle Cell Disease Association of America

SUMMARY

Education is a key component of comprehensive care of a child and family and prerequisite to health promotion and disease prevention strategies. With shortened clinic visits and hospitalizations, teaching becomes increasingly important.

REFERENCES

Badarudeen, S., & Sabharwal, S. (2008). Readability of patient education materials from the American Academy of Orthopaedic Surgeons and Pediatric Orthopaedic Society of North America web sites. *Journal of Bone and Joint Surgery, 90*(1), 199–204. doi: 10.2106/JBJS.G.00347

Ball, J. W., Bindler, R. C., & Cowen, K. J. (2010). *Child health nursing: Partnering with children and families* (2nd ed.). East Rutherford, NJ: Prentice Hall.

Bowden, V. R., & Greenberg, C. S. (2010). *Children and their families: The continuum of care* (2nd ed.). Philadelphia: Lippincott Williams & Wilkins.

Coffman, J. M., Cabana, M. D., Halpin, H. A., & Yelin, E. H. (2008). Effects of asthma education on children's use of acute care services: A meta-analysis. *Pediatrics, 121*(3), 575–586.

Hagan, J. F., Shaw, J. S., & Duncan, P. M. (Eds.). (2007). *Bright futures: Guidelines for health supervision of infants, children, and adolescents* (3rd ed.). Elk Grove Village, IL: American Academy of Pediatrics.

Hockenberry, M. J., & Wilson, D. (2011). *Wong's nursing care of infants and children* (9th ed.). St. Louis, MO: Elsevier/Mosby.

Joint Commission, The. (2010). *Meeting the Joint Commission's 2011 national patient safety Goals*. Oakbrook Terrace, IL: Joint Commission Resources.

Marquis, B. L., & Huston, C. J. (2011). *Leadership roles and management functions in nursing* (7th ed.). Philadelphia: Lippincott Williams & Wilkins.

National Association of Pediatric Nurse Practitioners, Society of Pediatric Nurses, American Nurses Association. (2008). *Pediatric nursing: Scope and standards of practice*. Silver Spring, MD: Nursesbooks.org.

Pillitteri, A. (2010). *Maternal & child health nursing: Care of the childbearing and childrearing family* (6th ed.). Philadelphia: Lippincott Williams & Wilkins.

Polit, D. F., & Beck, C. T. (2009). *Essentials of nursing research: Appraising evidence for nursing practice* (7th ed.). Philadelphia: Lippincott Williams & Wilkins.

Russell, S. S. (2006). An overview of adult-learning processes. *Urologic Nursing, 26*(5), 349–352, 370.

CHAPTER 7

LIFE SITUATIONS AND ADAPTIVE AND MALADAPTIVE RESPONSES

Mary Jo Gilmer, PhD, MBA, RN-BC, FAAN, and
Karen Corlett, MSN, RN-BC, CPNP-AC/PC, PNP-BC

PALLIATIVE CARE

- Care for those with life-threatening or life-limiting conditions for which there is no cure
  - Risk of death need not be imminent
  - Often an interdisciplinary approach
    - Physicians, nurses, social workers, psychiatrists, pain management specialists, pharmacists, dietitians, child life specialists, and others may be represented on the team.
- Can begin at any time from diagnosis to near end of life
  - Ideally begun early in course of disease or condition
- Assist with care and planning for best possible life, despite potential limitations from disease
  - Does not imply limitation of care or avoidance of resuscitation
  - Care choices emphasize management of physical and emotional pain and symptoms, including comfort and function.
  - Patients and families may cycle in and out of aggressive vs. comfort care during the course of the disease.
  - Palliative care can coexist with hospice care toward end of life.

END-OF-LIFE CARE

- Physical care and emotional support of the dying child and grieving family
- Understanding death
    - Children's concepts of death
        - Infant, toddler (sensorimotor); 1–3 years: Reacts to separation and changes in routine, but no concept of death
        - Preschooler (preoperational); 4–6 years: Sees death as reversible and temporary
        - Early school-age (concrete); 7–9 years: Depending on life experiences, begins to see death as real and inevitable but usually unable to understand own mortality
        - Later school-age (concrete to early formal operations); 10–12 years: Sees death as final, irreversible; fascinated with details about death
        - Adolescence (formal operations); 13–18 years: Sees death as inevitable, universal, and irreversible; frequently denies own mortality through risk-taking
    - Age-appropriate education
        - Developmentally targeted books, stories, role play
            - Child life, social work, chaplain, and psychiatry departments can be helpful.
            - Can also help parents and caregivers with developmentally appropriate explanations for children
        - Sensitivity to parents' desires regarding cultural or religious philosophies
    - Family education
        - Process of death
            - Assistance with physical care needs
            - Developmentally appropriate explanations of physical symptoms and activity changes associated with the dying process
        - Impact of death on family unit, siblings
        - Grief support
            - In anticipation of death
            - Once death occurs
                - Community resources
                - After care for the bereaved
    - Stages of grief (Kübler-Ross)
        - Denial
            - Denial of risk of death or actual death
        - Anger

- Why me, why my child?
- Bargaining
  - Desire to trade places with the dying child
  - Bargaining to live until a certain time, holiday, or special event
- Depression
  - Not wanting to go on
  - Not caring about life, grieving parent not caring about remaining family
- Acceptance
  - Of death or probability of death

RESPONSE TO CRISIS

- Diagnosis or hospitalization
  - Response of patient
    - Dependent on age and developmental stage
    - Understanding of disease process and outcomes
    - Change from usual routines
      - Physiologic
        - Nutrition, sleep, pain
      - Psychologic and environmental
        - Few familiar or comforting objects or people
        - Pain
        - Change in daily routine
        - Inability to be held or comforted in usual manner
        - Separation from family and peers
          - Promote family-centered care
  - Response of family
    - Change in family unit
      - Patient's role in family prior to illness
      - Change in family members' roles because of illness
        - Breadwinner to caregiver
        - Stay-at-home parent to hospital caregiver, with financial implications
        - Sibling becomes caregiver or household manager in absence of stay-at-home parent

    - Grandparent becomes primary caregiver of well siblings
    - Neighbor becomes chauffeur for well siblings or patient
  - Temporary vs. permanent adjustment to new roles
    - May be difficult for some to flex in and out of roles as needs wax and wane
    - May be difficult transition to new or old role once crisis is resolved

- The vulnerable child syndrome
  - Parental perception that the child is at higher risk of illness, injury, or death
    - After full recovery from a perceived or actual life-threatening illness
    - Difficult conception, pregnancy, or birth
    - When the child reminds the parent of someone who experienced premature death
  - Parental behaviors toward the "vulnerable child"
    - Treating the child as younger than chronologic or developmental age
    - Difficulty with discipline and limit-setting
    - Overindulgent or controlling parenting
    - Excessive concern about child's health and wellness and frequent visits to healthcare providers
    - Difficulty separating from child
  - Nursing management
    - Gather data regarding child and family risks for vulnerable child syndrome
      - Ask about previous serious illness (real or perceived)
      - Ask about parental fears for the child
      - Observe parenting behaviors
    - Assess for presence of risk factors for vulnerable child syndrome
    - Parental awareness of issues may bring change in behavior
    - Family counseling for those with continued parenting difficulties
- Coping mechanisms
  - Behaviors intended to decrease stress
  - Action-oriented behaviors
    - Planning
    - Learning
    - Limiting competing activities
      - Preserving energy for the stressor
    - Restraint or self-control

        - Confrontation
        - The problem causing the stress is addressed, improved, or eliminated.
    - Emotion-based behaviors; can be adaptive or maladaptive depending upon situation and frequency
        - Denial
        - Avoidance
        - Sleep or relaxation
        - Hope, positive thinking
        - Repression
        - Distraction
        - Humor
- Maladaptive responses
    - Suicide or suicidal ideation
        - Teens have highest incidence
        - Risks and warning signs
            - Major life stressor
            - Depression
            - Talk of suicide
            - Suicide event in community
            - Giving away possessions or making a will
            - Failure in school
            - Mood swings
            - Loss of interest in food, personal appearance, relationships
        - Assessment of lethality and risk
            - Does the child have a plan?
                - Time, method, access to method
                - Rescue opportunity in place
                    - Remote location for event vs. knowing parent will arrive home shortly after attempt
            - Referral for inpatient psychiatric hospitalization if danger to self or others
    - Substance abuse
        - Alcohol, tobacco, prescription, over-the-counter, or illicit drugs
        - Warning signs
            - Change in habits

        - Change in hygiene, appearance, food preferences, appetite
      - Change in mood
      - Failure in school
      - Change in peer group
      - Smell of drugs or alcohol
        - Finding drugs, alcohol, or paraphernalia of use
      - Illegal acts
- Depression
  - May be situationally appropriate depression of mood
    - Limited duration
    - Return to full functionality
  - Clinical depression
    - Refer for professional care and counseling
    - Entire family may need to be part of counseling
  - Signs and symptoms of depression
    - Depressed mood
    - Inability to enjoy usual activities
    - Weight gain or loss
    - Difficulty concentrating
    - Insomnia or hypersomnia
    - Lack of self-worth
    - Thoughts of, or attempts at, suicide
    - Change in family or peer relationships
    - Change in school performance
    - Change in appearance, clothing, hygiene
  - Assessment
    - Reliable tools for measurements of childhood depression
    - Children's Depression Inventory
    - Children's Depression Rating Scale
- Posttraumatic stress disorder
  - Anxiety disorder following a life-threatening or traumatic event
    - Natural disasters
    - Accidents
    - Conflict incidents

        - War, murder, abuse, rape
    - Symptoms
        - Reexperiencing the trauma or event
            - Dreams, intrusive thoughts
            - May be expressed in child's play
        - Avoidance of situation that triggers memories of event
            - Avoidance of feelings related to event
            - Numbing of feelings
            - Lack of enjoyment
        - Hypervigilance
            - Startles easily
            - Difficulty sleeping
    - Nursing care
        - Referral for specialty care
        - Build trusting relationship
        - Explore trauma and meaning
            - Validate child's experience of and reaction to traumatic event
            - Lift responsibility for event from child
        - Increase coping repertoire
- Eating disorders
    - Complex set of behaviors related to food
        - Multifactorial causation
        - Most common in teens but age at onset decreasing
        - More common in girls than boys
    - Anorexia nervosa
        - Severe food restriction
        - Altered body image
        - Weight loss
            - Irrational fear of weight gain or becoming fat
        - Underweight
        - Physical manifestations of weight loss
            - Hypothermia and cold intolerance
            - Hair loss and brittle nails
                - May grow fine hair on body (lanugo)

            - Skipping or stopping of menstrual cycles
            - Cardiac dysrhythmia
        - Significant morbidity and mortality
            - Fluid and electrolyte abnormalities can be life-threatening
    - Bulimia
        - Cycle of bingeing (excessive calorie intake) and subsequent purging
            - Laxative use
            - Induced vomiting
            - Excessive exercise
            - Fasting
        - Feeling of lack of control over food
        - Underweight not required for diagnosis; child may actually be overweight
    - Psychological diagnoses
        - DSM criteria for diagnosis
        - Require ongoing treatment of patient and family
- Child maltreatment
    - Intentional injury of a child
        - 1,750 reported child deaths from abuse and neglect in 51 states and territories in 2009
        - An underreported statistic
    - Child neglect
        - Lack of provision for physical, emotional, or educational needs
            - Nutrition, health care, safe environment, school attendance
            - Due to intentional abuse, neglect, or lack of knowledge
        - Chronic neglect
            - Lack of clean environment, inadequate nutrition
        - Acute neglect resulting in injury (e.g., lack of supervision around a pool, bathtub, lake, or river resulting in a drowning)
    - Physical abuse
        - Results in bodily injury
            - Bruises, bites, burns, broken bones, brain injury
    - Emotional abuse
        - Lack of affection or emotional support
        - Continued belittling of the child

  - Can affect physical growth and development in addition to emotional growth and maturation
  - All forms of abuse have emotional effects on the child
- Sexual abuse
  - Inappropriate touching or sexual behavior between an adult and a child
- Most perpetrators of abuse are caregivers
  - Relatives next most common
  - Nonrelatives in position of authority
    - Coach, minister, teacher, group leader, and so on
  - Strangers are rarest of perpetrators
- Children at risk
  - The very young
    - Children < 3 years old have highest rates of abuse
    - Dependent neglect highest in this age group
  - General risks
    - Stress events
    - Living below the poverty level
    - Caretaker has experienced abuse or violence
    - Caretaker with limited coping strategies for stress
    - Caregiver depression
- Injuries that should raise concern about abuse
  - Any injury not consistent with the reported story
    - Discrepancies in story
    - Repeated injuries
  - Fractures
    - Ribs, scapula, sternum, or metacarpals
  - Burns
    - Multiple healed or healing burns
    - Immersion burns
      - Flexor areas spared as child tries to protect self from hot liquid
    - Contact burns
      - May have shape of identifiable object
        - Cigarette, curling iron, brand, and so on
  - Shaken baby syndrome

- Subdural hematoma
- Retinal injury
- Rib or other occult bone fractures
- Caused by vigorous shaking of the child
    - Child's large head for body size causes coup-countercoup injury and shear injury to blood vessels and brain tissue
- 1/3 of affected children die, 1/3 have serious residual injury from the shaking

- Munchausen syndrome by proxy
    - Psychological disorder of the parent
        - Parent creates illness in child
        - Parent has secondary gain from interaction with healthcare professionals
            - Parent often has some type of healthcare background
        - Parent may take elaborate measures to continue the symptoms and appearance of chronic illness in the child
            - Child may become technology-dependent due to parental claims of symptoms
        - Difficult to diagnose; symptoms often subjective
            - Apnea, feeding intolerance, seizures are common complaints
        - As with most cases of abuse, child will protect the parent

- Nurses are mandatory reporters
    - MUST report documented or suspected child maltreatment to authorities
    - Can be reported by another discipline in the institution, such as social work
        - Reports can be anonymous
        - Reports must be investigated by state agency
- Prevention
    - Education
        - Nationally, locally, and individually
        - Prenatal and postnatal education
        - Stress management
        - Community services and resources
    - In-home support
        - By nurses, social workers, or other agency representatives

    - Education, evaluation, and connection to community resources
- Regular visits to healthcare provider
    - Physical exam
    - Psychosocial assessment
        - Review of effective coping strategies
        - Depression or other psychological disorders
        - Respite opportunities
- Out-of-home childcare
    - As respite for continuous childcare responsibilities
    - Model for child of healthy interactions
- Life skills training
    - For new parents
    - For older children who have experienced abuse
- Family support services
    - Community agencies
    - Facilitating personal support networks
- Public education
    - Awareness of problem
    - Risk factors to be aware of
    - Ways to support those at risk
    - Solicitation of financial support for agencies

SUMMARY

Life situations can lead to adaptive and maladaptive responses, but assessment of risk factors, family education, and availability of support may help families cope with stress without resorting to violence and other harmful outcomes.

REFERENCES

American Academy of Pediatrics, & Pickering, L. K. (Eds.). (2009). *Red book: 2009 report of the Committee on Infectious Diseases* (28th ed.). Elk Grove Village, IL: American Academy of Pediatrics.

Ball, J. W., Bindler, R. C., & Cowen, K. J. (2010). *Child health nursing: Partnering with children and families* (2nd ed.). East Rutherford, NJ: Prentice Hall.

Bowden, V. R., & Greenberg, C. S. (2010). *Children and their families: The continuum of care* (2nd ed.). Philadelphia: Lippincott Williams & Wilkins.

Fischbach, F., & Dunning, M. B. (2009). *A manual of laboratory and diagnostic tests* (8th ed.). Philadelphia: Lippincott Williams & Wilkins.

Gilmer, M. J. (2002). Pediatric palliative care: A family-centered model for critical care. *Critical Care Nursing Clinics of North America, 14*(2), 207–214.

Hagan, J. F., Shaw, J. S., & Duncan, P. M. (Eds.). (2007). *Bright futures: Guidelines for health supervision of infants, children, and adolescents* (3rd ed.). Elk Grove Village, IL: American Academy of Pediatrics.

Hockenberry, M. J., & Wilson, D. (2011). *Wong's nursing care of infants and children* (9th ed.). St. Louis, MO: Elsevier/Mosby.

Huff, S., Friebert, S., Gilmer, M. J., Remke, S., Riggs, M., Steinhorn, D., & Toce, S. (2009). *Standards of practice for pediatric palliative care and hospice.* Alexandria, VA: National Hospice and Palliative Care Organization.

Joint Commission, The. (2010). *Meeting the Joint Commission's 2011 national patient safety goals.* Oakbrook Terrace, IL: Joint Commission Resources.

Jones, B., Gilmer, M. J., Raley, J., Dokken, D., Fryer, D., & Sydnor-Greenberg, N. (2011). Parent and sibling relationships and the family experience. In J. Wolfe, B. Sourkes, & P. Hinds (Eds.), *Textbook of interdisciplinary pediatric palliative care*. Philadelphia: Elsevier Saunders.

Kübler-Ross, E., & Kessler, D. (2005). *On grief and grieving: Finding the meaning of grief through the five stages of loss.* New York: Simon & Schuster.

Marquis B. L., & Huston C. J. (2011). *Leadership roles and management functions in nursing* (7th ed.). Philadelphia: Lippincott Williams & Wilkins.

National Association of Pediatric Nurse Practitioners, Society of Pediatric Nurses, American Nurses Association. (2008). *Pediatric nursing: Scope and standards of practice*. Silver Spring, MD: Nursesbooks.org.

Pillitteri, A. (2010). *Maternal & child health nursing: Care of the childbearing and childrearing family* (6th ed.). Philadelphia: Lippincott Williams & Wilkins.

Polit, D. F., & Beck, C. T. (2009). *Essentials of nursing research: Appraising evidence for nursing practice* (7th ed.). Philadelphia: Lippincott Williams & Wilkins.

Stuart, G. W. (2009). *Principles and practice of psychiatric nursing* (9th ed.). Philadelphia: Mosby.

Tschudy, M. M., Arcara, K. M., Johns Hopkins Hospital, & Children's Medical and Surgical Center. (2012). *The Harriet Lane handbook: A manual for pediatric house officers* (19th ed.). Philadelphia: Elsevier Mosby.

U.S. Department of Health and Human Services, Children's Bureau. (2010). *Child maltreatment 2009.* Retrieved from http://www.acf.hhs.gov/programs/cb/pubs/cm09/cm09.pdf#page=66

Wilson, B. A., Shannon, M. T., & Shields, K. (2012). *Pearson's nurse's drug guide 2012.* New York: Pearson Education.

CHAPTER 8

SENSORY DISORDERS

Clara J. Richardson, MSN, RN-BC

DEVELOPMENTAL CHARACTERISTICS OF THE PEDIATRIC SENSORY SYSTEM

- Visual acuity at birth ranges from 20/100 to 20/400.
- Visual acuity at 1 year of age is 20/40 to 20/60; it becomes 20/20 between the ages of 3 and 5 years.
- Binocularity, the ability to focus on one visual field with both eyes simultaneously, developes by 4 months of age.

HEARING DISORDERS

Description

Hearing disorders in children involve hearing impairment that ranges from slight (16–25 dB loss) to profound (91 dB loss). The loss may be unilateral or bilateral. A conductive hearing loss is due to dysfunction of the external or middle ear. Sensorineural loss is caused by impairment of the inner ear or auditory nerve. A mixed loss has both sensory and conductive components.

Etiology

Causes of conductive loss are malformation of the outer or middle ear and, more often, infections of the middle ear. Sensorineural loss is caused by hereditary factors in about half of the cases. In many instances, the cause is unknown. The more common causes include complications from viral infection, bacterial meningitis, head trauma, perinatal disorders, and genetic disorders.

Incidence and Demographics

Unilateral hearing loss occurs in 30–56 of 1,000 children and bilateral loss in 10–15 of 1,000 children. Approximately 1.5% of school-age children have low-frequency loss, and 3% have high-frequency loss.

Risk Factors

- Family history
- Viral infections
- Bacterial meningitis
- Chronic otitis media with effusion
- Exposure to loud environmental noise
- Head injury
- Intracranial hemorrhage
- Cleft palate
- Neonatal hyperbilirubinemia
- Low birth weight
- Cerebral palsy
- Down syndrome
- Maternal substance abuse
- Maternal infections during pregnancy
  - Rubella
  - Cytomegalovirus (CMV)
  - Toxoplasmosis
  - Herpes virus
  - Syphilis
- Ototoxic antibiotics
  - Kanamycin (Kantrex)
  - Gentamicin (Garamycin)
  - Vancomycin (Vancocin)
  - Tobramycin (Nebcin)
- Chemotherapeutic drugs
  - Cisplatin
  - Carboplatin
  - Vincristine

Prevention and Screening

- Avoidance of loud environmental noise
- Ear protection during exposure to loud noise
- Monitor school classroom acoustics
- Newborn screening identifies moderate to profound loss
- Screen at-risk children and children who exhibit signs of loss

Assessment

History

- History of risk factors
- Inability to localize sound by 6 months
- Delayed consonant-vowel babbling by 7 months
- Absence of well-formed syllables (da, na, yaya) by 11 months
- Failure to respond to verbal instructions not accompanied by gestures by 16 months
- Delayed comprehensible speech by 24 months

Physical Exam

- Infants
  - No reaction to loud noise
  - Delayed developmental communication milestones
- Older children
  - Use of gestures rather than words
  - Asking for repetition
  - Decreased response to verbal expression
  - Avoidance of social interaction
  - Confused or inattentive facial expression

Diagnostic Studies

- Pure-tone air conduction hearing test
- Speech testing such as speech reception threshold
- Middle ear tests such as tympanometry
- Automated auditory brainstem response (AABR)
- Otoacoustic emissions (EOAE)

Management

Invasive Treatment

- Cochlear implant to stimulate the auditory nerve
- Bone-anchored hearing apparatus implanted in temporal bone

Nonpharmacologic Treatment

- Amplification with hearing aids or assistive listening devices
- Speech–language therapy
- American Sign Language (ASL)
- Assistive technology such as teletypewriters or telecommunication devices
- Strategies to enhance communication
  - Get child's attention before speaking
  - Position: close, eye level, and in front of child
  - Speak clearly, at even rate, and in short sentences
  - Use facial expressions

Pharmacologic Treatment

- No pharmacologic management indicated

Patient and Family Education

- Nature of defect and extent of hearing loss
- Amplification options
- Communication options
- Child and family support groups
- Advocacy for school-based services
- Hearing aid battery safety to prevent ingestion

Outcomes and Follow-up

- The child will have early identification of hearing impairment.
- The child will participate in an early intervention program.
- The child will utilize amplification devices.
- The child will show increased hearing with cochlear implant.
- The child will experience optimal communication.
- The family will demonstrate strategies to enhance communication with the child.

- The family will verbalize understanding of disability and treatment options.
- The family will access available resources to support the child's development and school experience.

VISION DISORDERS

Description

Vision disorders in children refer to any defect in structure or function that causes impairment of vision. The degree of impairment ranges from low vision (partial sight) with visual acuity better than 20/200 but worse than 20/70 to legal blindness with acuity of 20/200 or worse.

Etiology

- *Cerebral visual impairment (CVI)* due to damage of the visual cortex in the occipital lobe or damage in some other area of the brain that affects vision
    - Hypoxia
    - Infection of the central nervous system
    - Traumatic brain injury
- *Retinopathy of prematurity (ROP)*
    - Immature retinal vasculature
    - Blood vessels grow abnormally, die, and form scar tissue
    - Scar tissue can cause retinal detachment and loss of vision
- *Optic nerve hypoplasia*
    - Nerve is small and thin and transmits impaired information to brain
    - Results in sensory nystagmus, jiggling movement of the eyes
    - Occurs with neurological impairment
- *Strabismus*
    - Misalignment of eyes or deviation of one eye
    - Results in amblyopia, "lazy eye," with reduced visual acuity in one or both eyes that cannot be resolved with glasses

Incidence and Demographics

One half to two thirds of children with developmental disabilities have a significant vision disorder. Approximately 25% of newborns weighing less than 2,500 grams will have some degree of retinopathy of prematurity; 2%–3% of children have amblyopia.

Risk Factors

- Family history
- Prematurity
- Cerebral palsy
- Cognitive disability
- Autism spectrum disorders
- Eye trauma
- Traumatic brain injury
- Maternal smoking, antiepileptic medications, alcohol use
- Maternal infections such as sexually transmitted infections, rubella, syphilis, or toxoplasmosis

Prevention and Screening

- Prevention
  - Early prenatal care
  - Prenatal screening for risk factors
  - Avoid exposing premature infants to high concentrations of oxygen
  - Rubella immunization for all children
  - Safety education to prevent eye trauma
  - Compliance with treatment of vision impairment
- Regular vision screening with age-appropriate screening tool
  - Assessment of normal vision parameters in infants and young children
  - Acuity charts

Assessment

History

- See Risk Factors above.

Physical Exam

- Infant does not fixate on face or follow objects
- Wandering eye or nystagmus
- Eyes that gaze in one direction
- No reaction to bright light or movement of object toward eye
- Visual field losses
- Accommodation disorders
- Reduced acuity, color, and contrast sensitivity

Diagnostic Studies

- See Screening above.

Management

Invasive Treatment

- Strabismus: surgical strengthening or weakening of eye muscles
- Retinopathy of prematurity: retinal ablation by cryotherapy or laser photocoagulation

Nonpharmacologic Treatment

- Corrective lenses
- Textured, sound-producing toys
- Verbal cues before touching, moving from space to space
- Orientation to environment
- Self-care education
- Optical aids to enhance vision
- Braille education
- Books on tape
- Computer training, voice recognition software
- Strabismus: occlusion therapy with patching of stronger eye to promote use of weaker eye

Pharmacologic Treatment

- Strabismus: atropine to blur vision in stronger eye

Patient and Family Education

- Nature of defect and extent of vision impairment
- Treatment options and plans
- Strategies to promote normal development
- Information about nonpharmacologic management, above
- Child and family support groups
- Advocacy for school-based services

Outcomes and Follow-up

- The child will experience maximum vision, depending on condition.
- The child will participate in an early intervention program.
- The child will develop independence in self-care activities and mobility.
- The child will develop skills in other senses to compensate for lack of vision.

- The child will demonstrate socialization at home and school.
- The family will maintain a safe environment for the child.
- The family will orient the child to its surroundings.
- The family will demonstrate strategies to promote optimal development.

CONJUNCTIVITIS

Description

Conjunctivitis is inflammation of the conjunctiva, the membrane lining the eyelid and covering the exposed surface of the sclera.

Etiology

The condition may be bacterial, viral, or allergic. Newborns may become infected during the birth process with *Chlamydia trachomatis, Neisseria gonorrhoeae*, or herpes simplex virus. Common causes of bacterial conjunctivitis in children are *Streptococcus pneumoniae, Staphylococcus aureus, Haemophilus influenzae*, and *Moraxella catarrhalis*. The usual viral cause is adenovirus. Conjunctivitis is spread by direct contact or contact with contaminated objects and surfaces.

Incidence and Demographics

About 15% of the population will have an episode of conjunctivitis at some time.

Risk Factors

Exposure to causative organism

Prevention and Screening

- Hand hygiene
- Avoidance of contact with affected eye drainage
- Environmental cleaning of surfaces and shared toys

Assessment

History

- Maternal infection

Physical Exam

- Eye drainage

    - Bacterial: thick, mucopurulent
    - Viral: serous, watery
    - Allergic: thick, stringy
- Redness of the conjunctiva
- Swollen eyelid
- Crusting of eyelid
- Burning sensation
- Tearing

Diagnostic Studies

- Diagnosis based on symptoms
- Culture if no improvement

Management

Invasive Treatment

- No invasive management indicated

Nonpharmacologic Treatment

- Warm, moist compresses to loosen crusty drainage
- Cold compresses to decrease swelling
- Avoid eye makeup during infection

Pharmacologic Treatment

- Bacterial: antibacterial eye ointment or drops
- Viral: topical antihistamines and decongestants
- Allergic: artificial tears for dry eyes, topical or systemic corticosteroids

Patient and Family Education

- Prevention of spread of infection
- Medication administration
- Nonpharmacologic comfort measures

Outcomes and Follow-up

- The child will show decrease in redness, swelling, and drainage.
- The child and family will verbalize an understanding of strategies to prevent spread of infection.
- The family will demonstrate medication administration.
- The family will utilize comfort measures.

OTITIS MEDIA AND OTITIS EXTERNA

Description

Acute otitis media (AOM) is a viral or bacterial infection of the middle ear. *Otitis media with effusion* (OME) is fluid in the middle ear without acute infection. *Otitis externa* (OE), commonly called swimmer's ear, is bacterial infection of the outer ear.

Etiology

Obstruction of the Eustachian tube allows fluid to accumulate in the middle ear. The fluid may be contaminated from the nasopharynx, resulting in acute otitis media. If the fluid does not drain, otitis media with effusion results. The effusion may last for weeks or months after the infection has resolved. Bacterial otitis media is often caused by *Streptococcus pneumoniae, Hemophilus influenzae*, and *Moraxella catarrhalis.*

The outer ear canal is ordinarily protected from infection by cerumen, but when the canal is altered by water, humidity, or insufficient cerumen, invasion by bacteria may occur. Common causative organisms of otitis externa are *Pseudomonas aeruginosa, Staphylococcus epidermidis,* and *Staphylococcus aureus.*

Incidence and Demographics

Acute otitis media is most prevalent during infancy. By age 1 year, 60%–80% of infants experience at least one episode. Children are more prone to develop otitis media than adults for several reasons. The child's Eustachian tube is shorter, wider, lies more parallel, and consists of underdeveloped cartilage. They have larger adenoids that prevent drainage, have immature humoral defense mechanisms leading to increased infection risk, and spend more time lying down, which allows fluid to pool at the back of the throat with easy access to the Eustachian tube. AOM occurs infrequently in school-age children and adolescents. Occurrence is higher in Native American children, Alaskan and Canadian Eskimos, and indigenous Australian children.

Otitis externa occurs in all age groups, and about 10% of people will experience OE at some point. It is more likely to occur during the summer months.

Risk Factors

- Acute otitis media
    - Lack of or limited breastfeeding
    - Daycare attendance
    - Exposure to tobacco smoke and air pollution
    - Pacifier use
    - Previous episode of AOM

- Family history
- Allergic rhinitis
- Cleft palate
- Down syndrome
- Otitis externa
  - High humidity and warm temperatures
  - Swimming
  - Trauma to the ear canal
  - Devices that occlude ear canal such as hearing aids or earphones
  - Allergic contact dermatitis from earrings, hair products, cosmetics

Prevention and Screening

No screening is indicated, but some prevention is possible.

- Acute otitis media prevention
  - Breastfeeding
  - Decrease use of pacifier in infants older than 6 months
  - Avoid propping bottle
  - Avoid exposure to tobacco smoke and pollution
  - Avoid forceful nose blowing
- Otitis externa prevention
  - Avoid objects in ear such as cotton swabs
  - Ear plugs for swimming
  - Use hair dryer on lowest setting to dry canal after swimming or bathing
  - Prophylaxis with acidifying or alcohol ear drops before swimming

Assessment

History

- Acute otitis media with or without effusion
  - Upper respiratory infection
- Otitis externa
  - Water in ear

Physical Exam

- Acute otitis media

- Pain evidenced by ear pulling, head rolling, irritability in infants
- Immediate relief of pain if tympanic membrane ruptures
- Fever, rhinitis
- Decreased appetite, vomiting, diarrhea
- Postauricular and cervical lymph gland enlargement
- Tympanic membrane appears red, bulging, with no visible landmarks or light reflex; decreased mobility with pneumatic otoscopy

- Otitis media with effusion
  - Intermittent ear discomfort
  - Feeling of fullness, popping, fluid motion
  - Conductive hearing loss
  - Tympanic membrane appears dull gray, slightly injected, with obscured landmarks and visible fluid level; decreased mobility with pneumatic otoscopy
- Otitis externa
  - Pruritis
  - Pain
  - Erythema
  - Grayish, greenish, cheesy discharge
  - Swelling with conductive hearing loss

Diagnostic Studies

- Tympanometry
- Tympanocentesis with aspiration and culture of middle ear fluid with multiple antibiotic failures

Management

Invasive Treatment

- Myringotomy with pressure-equalizing tube insertion

Nonpharmacologic Treatment

- Acute otitis media
  - Application of heat or cold
- Otitis externa
  - Clean canal of debris with curette
  - Clean drainage from outer canal and skin around ear
  - Apply petroleum jelly to skin around ear to prevent excoriation from drainage

    - Gauze wick if canal is very edematous, to get medication inside canal

Pharmacologic Treatment

- Otitis media
    - Amoxicillin (Amoxil)
    - Amoxicillin-clavulanate (Augmentin)
    - Cephalosporin (cefdinir, cefpodoxime, cefuroxime, ceftriaxone)
    - Levoflaxacin
    - Analgesics for pain
- Otitis externa
    - Polymycin B/neomycin/hydrocortisone (Cortisporin otic drops)
    - Ofloxacin (Floxin otic drops)
    - Ciprofloxacin-dexamethasone (Ciprodex)
    - Analgesics for pain

Patient and Family Education

- Diagnosis and treatment plan
- Medication administration
- Strategies for nonpharmacologic management
- Strategies for prevention
- Strategies for dealing with temporary conductive hearing loss
- Keeping water out of ears of children who have pressure-equalizing tubes

Outcomes and Follow-up

- The child will experience effective pain management.
- The child will recover without complications such as:
    - Persistent hearing loss
    - Perforation of tympanic membrane
    - Acute mastoiditis
    - Delayed language development
- The family will verbalize understanding of diagnosis and treatment plan.
- The family will demonstrate medication administration, nonpharmacologic management, and strategies for dealing with hearing loss.
- The family will verbalize strategies for prevention.

RETINOBLASTOMA

Description

Retinoblastoma is a primary intraocular cancer arising from the retina.

Etiology

The disease begins with gene mutation of one or more retinal cells. If untreated, retinoblastoma grows causing retinal detachment and necrosis. Invasion continues into the orbit, into the optic nerve, and then into the central nervous system. Sites of metastasis are lungs, bone, and brain.

Incidence and Demographics

The incidence of retinoblastoma is 1 in 14,000–18,000 live births. It is usually diagnosed in children between 1 and 2 years of age, and onset after 5 years old is rare. 20%–30% of children have bilateral tumors. The survival rate, with at least one eye having normal vision, is 99%.

TABLE 8-1.
INCIDENCE OF RETINOBLASTOMA IN CHILDREN PER 100,000

	< 1 YEAR	1-4 YEARS
Retinoblastoma	0.26	0.88

Risk Factors

- Family history

Prevention and Screening

- No prevention
- Screening for red reflex should be done at every well-child visit

Assessment

History

Family History

- Family often first to notice whitish glow

Physical Exam

- Leukokoria, white reflex called "cat's-eye reflex"
- Red reflex may be absent, asymmetrical, blunted on one side, or have dark spots
- Strabismus

- Discoloration of iris
- Glaucoma
- Pain

Diagnostic Studies

- Indirect ophthalmoscopic exam to determine size and location of tumor
- Ultrasound
- CT scan
- MRI with contrast
- Lumbar puncture and bone scan in advanced disease

Management

Invasive Treatment

- Laser photoablation to destroy tumor with ultraviolet radiation
- Cryotherapy to destroy tumor with extremely cold temperature
- Enucleation for advanced disease

Nonpharmacologic Treatment

- Radioactive plaques: high-dose radiation therapy
- External beam radiation therapy

Pharmacologic Treatment

- Chemotherapy
  - Vincristine (Oncovin)
  - Cyclophosphamide (Cytoxan)
  - Doxorubicin (Adriamycin)
  - Cisplatin (Platinol)
  - Carboplatin (CBDCA)
  - Etoposide (VP-16, VePesid)

Patient and Family Education

- Diagnosis and treatment plan
- Care of surgical site
- Care of prosthetic eye
- Strategies for dealing with side effects of chemotherapy

Outcomes and Follow-up

- The child will recover without metastasis.
- The child will maintain vision in at least one eye.
- The family will verbalize understanding of diagnosis and treatment plan.
- The family will demonstrate care of surgical site.
- The family will demonstrate care of prosthetic eye.

TRAUMA TO THE EYE

Description

Eye trauma involves injury to the orbit, eyeball, eyelids, conjunctiva, or lacrimal glands.

Etiology

Orbital fractures are often caused by all-terrain (ATV) crashes, paintball injuries, and fireworks. Children most commonly sustain trapdoor, hinged orbital floor fractures. Penetrating injuries may be the result of contact with sharp objects such as scissors or knives, propulsive objects such as firecrackers or guns, or blunt objects such as small paintballs. Nonpenetrating trauma may be caused by foreign objects, chemical or thermal burns, or large balls. Trauma to the eye can lead to hyphema, an accumulation of blood in the anterior chamber, accompanied by increased intraocular pressure. After a few days, a secondary hemorrhage may occur with further increase in pressure and poorer chance of vision recovery. This secondary injury can cause glaucoma, vitreous hemorrhage, retinal detachment, choroidal rupture, scleral rupture, or otic atrophy. Another common result of trauma is corneal abrasion from mechanical trauma, contact lenses, foreign bodies, or chemicals. Corneal abrasion may lead to ulceration and erosion of the cornea with resulting visual impairment.

Incidence and Demographics

Traumatic eye injuries in children are more common in adolescents and in boys. The majority of injuries are sports-related.

Risk Factors

- Lack of protective eyewear
- Participating in activity inappropriate for developmental age
- Contact lenses

Prevention and Screening

- Protective eyewear

- Adult supervision of dangerous activity
- Appropriate care of contact lenses

Assessment

History

- History of trauma

Physical Exam

- Orbital fracture
  - Intraorbital pain on eye movement
  - Diplopia, double vision, or blurred vision
  - Periocular bruising
  - Swelling
  - Nausea and vomiting
- Hyphema
  - Pain
  - Blurred vision
  - Loss of vision
  - Photophobia
  - Tearing
  - Nausea and vomiting
- Corneal abrasion
  - Pain or foreign body sensation
  - Tearing
  - Photophobia
  - Hazy gray cornea

Diagnostic Studies

- Visual acuity
- Radiography
- CT scan
- Ultrasound
- Ophthalmic examination with fluorescein stain
- Slit lamp ophthalmic examination
- Tonometry to measure intraocular pressure

Management

Invasive Treatment

- Suturing for lacerations
- Surgical repair of fractures
- Surgical evacuation of hyphema
- Intraocular lens implantation for cataracts, a complication of trauma

Nonpharmacologic Treatment

- Orbital fracture
  - Cold compresses
  - Elevate head of bed 30°
  - Avoid nose blowing and sniffing
- Hyphema
  - Eye patch and shield on affected eye
  - Elevate head of bed 30° to promote settling of hyphema
  - Activity limited to bed rest with bathroom privileges, no reading
  - Dim, quiet room
- Corneal abrasion
  - Cold compresses for 24–48 hours, then warm compresses
  - Rest eyes

Pharmacologic Treatment

- Orbital fracture
  - Prophylactic antibiotics such as amoxicillin-clavulanate (Augmentin) or azithromycin
- Hyphema
  - Topical cyclopentolate (Cyclogyl) eye drops for pain
  - Acetaminophen with or without codeine for pain
  - Avoid aspirin and nonsteroidal antiinflammatory drugs (NSAIDs)
  - Topical glucocorticosteroids such as prednisolone or dexamethasone
  - Topical beta-adrenergic blockers for elevated intraocular pressure
  - Ondansetron (Zofran) to prevent vomiting
- Corneal abrasion
  - Topical antibiotic to prevent infection
    - Erythromycin (Ilotycin)

        - Ofloxacin (Ocuflox)
        - Polymyxin B/trimethoprim (Polytrim)
        - Ciprofloxacin (Cipro, Ciloxan)
    - Topical cyclopentolate (Cyclogyl) eye drops for pain
    - Analgesics such as acetaminophen or ibuprofen
    - Ondansetron (Zofran) to prevent vomiting

Patient and Family Education

- Diagnosis and treatment plan
- Medication administration
- Nonpharmacologic management
- Signs of complications
- Prevention of future injury

Outcomes and Follow-up

- The child will recover without permanent visual changes.
- The child and family will verbalize understanding of diagnosis and treatment plan.
- The child and family will verbalize understanding of nonpharmacologic management.
- The child and family will identify strategies to prevent future injury.
- The family will demonstrate medication administration.

REFERENCES

American Speech-Language-Hearing Association. (n.d.). *Hearing and balance.* Retrieved http://www.asha.org/public/hearing/Hearing-Loss/

Andreoli, C. M., & Gardiner, M. F. (2010). Traumatic hyphema. *UpToDate.* Retrieved from http://www.uptodate.com/contents/traumatic-hyphema-clinical-features-and-management?source=search_result&search=hyphema+children&selectedTitle=1%7E30#H19

Epelman, S. (2012). Preserving vision in retinoblastoma through early detection and intervention. *Current Oncology Reports, 14,* 213–219.

Fink, C., & Borchert, M. (2011). Optic nerve hypoplasia and autism: Common features of spectrum diseases. *Journal of Visual Impairment and Blindness, 105*(6), 334–338.

Goguen, L. A. (2011). External otitis. *UpToDate.* Retrieved from http://www.uptodate.com/contents/external-otitis-treatment?source=see_link

Golnik, K. C. (2011). Congenital anomalies and acquired abnormalities of the optic nerve. *UpToDate.* Retrieved from http://www.uptodate.com/contents/congenital-anomalies-and-acquired-abnormalities-of-the-optic-nerve?source=search_result&search=optic+nerve+hypoplasia&selectedTitle=1%7E12

Hockenberry, M. J., & Wilson, D. (2011). *Wong's nursing care of infants and children* (9th ed.). St. Louis, MO: Elsevier Mosby.

Jacobs, D. S. (2011). Conjunctivitis. *UpToDate.* Retrieved from http://www.uptodate.com/contents/conjunctivitis?source=search_result&search=conjunctivitis+in+children&selectedTitle=1%7E150

Jacobs, D. S. (2011). Corneal abrasions and corneal foreign bodies. *UpToDate.* Retrieved from http://www.uptodate.com/contents/corneal-abrasions-and-corneal-foreign- bodies?source=search_result&search=corneal+abrasion+in+children&selectedTitle=%7E43

Kaufman, P. L., & Teed, R. G. W. (2012). Overview of retinoblastoma. *UpToDate.* Retrieved from http://www.uptodate.com/contents/overview-of-retinoblastoma?source=search_result&search=retinoblastoma+children&selectedTitle=1%7E68

Klein, J. O., & Pelton, S. (2012). Acute otitis media in children. *UpToDate.* Retrieved from http://www.uptodate.com/contents/acute-otitis-media-in-children-epidemiology-microbiology-clinical-manifestations-and-complications?source=search_result&search=otitis+media+children&selectedTitle=3%7E150

Lueck, A. H. (2010). Cortical or cerebral visual impairment in children: A brief overview. *Journal of Visual Impairment and Blindness, 104*(10), 585–592.

McKay, S., Gravel, J. S., & Tharpe, A. M. (2008). Amplification considerations for children with minimal or mild bilateral hearing loss and unilateral hearing loss. *Trends in amplification, 12*(1), 43–54.

Neuman, M. I., & Bachur, R. G. (2011). Orbital fractures. *UpToDate.* Retrieved from http://www.uptodate.com/contents/orbital-fractures?source=search_result&search=orbital+fracture&selectedTitle=1%7E16

Rao, R. C., & Poole Perry, L. J. (2011). Decreased vision following eye trauma. *JAMA, 306*(23), 2606–2607.

Rodriguez-Galindo, C. (2011). The basics of retinoblastoma: Back to school. *Pediatric Blood Cancer, 57,* 1093–1094.

Ross, D. S., Holstrum, W. J., Gaffney, M., Green, D., Oyler, R. F., & Gravel, J. S. (2008). Hearing screening and diagnostic evaluation of children with unilateral and mild bilateral hearing loss. *Trends in Amplification, 12*(1), 27–34.

Smith, G. (2010). Differential diagnosis of red eye. *Pediatric Nursing, 36*(4), 213–215.

Tharpe, A. M., & Sladen, D. P. (2008). Causation of permanent unilateral and mild bilateral hearing loss in children. *Trends in Amplification, 12*(1), 17–25.

Tianjing, L., & Shotton, K. (2010). Conventional occlusion versus pharmacologic penalization for amblyopia. *Evidence-Based Child Health, 5,* 1873–1909.

CHAPTER 9

RESPIRATORY DISORDERS

Clara J. Richardson, MSN, RN-BC

LESSONS FROM NURSING THEORISTS, FIELD OF COMMUNICATION, AND PSYCHOLOGY

- Obligates nose breathing: easily obstructed
- Smaller airways: small reduction of lumen size by secretions or inflammation significantly increases airway resistance and work of breathing
- Pliable chest wall: attempts to breathe more deeply result in retractions and counter-productive chest movement
- Fewer and smaller alveoli: less surface area for gas exchange

BRONCHIOLITIS

Description

Bronchiolitis is an acute viral infection of the lower airways resulting in inflammation, necrosis of epithelial cells lining small airways, and bronchospasm.

Etiology

Most cases are caused by respiratory syncytial virus (RSV). The virus is transmitted by direct contact with respiratory secretions. RSV can survive for 30 minutes on skin and for several hours on surfaces. Other common causative organisms include adenoviruses, rhinoviruses, influenza and parainfluenza viruses, and human metapneumonvirus.

Incidence and Demographics

Occurrence of bronchiolitis typically begins in autumn, peaks in winter, and declines in spring. It most commonly occurs in children less than 2 years of age and the peak age of occurrence is 6 months. It is more common in boys and occurs less frequently in breastfed infants.

Risk Factors

- Young age
- Prematurity
- Immunodeficiency
- Cardiopulmonary disease
- Exposure to virus-carrying contacts
- Crowded living conditions
- Exposure to tobacco smoke

Prevention and Screening

- Hand hygiene
- Avoidance of ill contacts
- Environmental cleaning of surfaces and shared toys
- Palivizumab (Synagis) prophylaxis for infants at high risk of developing disease complications
    - Premature birth or chronic cardiopulmonary compromise
    - Monthly administration during season

Assessment

History

- Presence of upper respiratory infection for several days
- Progressive worsening of symptoms
- Onset of cough
- Difficulty feeding

Physical Exam

- Harsh gagging cough
- Copious respiratory secretions
- Tachypnea
- Increased work of breathing: retractions, nasal flaring, prolonged respiratory phase
- Adventitious breath sounds: coarseness, wheezes, crackles
- Decreased oxygen saturations
- Intermittent cyanosis
- Low-grade fever
- Signs of dehydration

Diagnostic Studies

- Viral studies identify causative organism, but are no longer routinely recommended because identification does not change management plan
- Viral studies may be done in infants younger than 3 months to limit use of additional studies and unnecessary antibiotics
- Chest radiography only for severe disease or if another disease is suspected

Management

Invasive Treatment

- No invasive management is indicated.

Nonpharmacologic Treatment

- Nasal suction with bulb syringe or aspirator before feedings, respiratory treatments, or as needed
- Supplemental oxygen as indicated
- Intravenous hydration as indicated
- Contact and droplet precautions
- Hold oral feeding for respirations greater than 60 breaths/minute to decrease aspiration risk

Pharmacologic Treatment

- Racemic epinephrine as needed based on documented clinical improvement
- Albuterol as needed based on documented clinical improvement
- Antipyretic for fever

Patient and Family Education

- Disease process and treatment plan
- Use of bulb syringe
- Strategies to prevent transmission
- Signs of increasing respiratory difficulty
- Signs of dehydration
- Disease progression: cough may last for several weeks, reinfection is possible

Outcomes and Follow-up

- The child will demonstrate adequate oxygenation.
- The child will exhibit signs of adequate hydration.
- The family will demonstrate use of bulb syringe.
- The family will demonstrate strategies to prevent transmission.
- The family will verbalize understanding of disease process.
- The family will verbalize reasons to call healthcare provider.

COMMUNITY-ACQUIRED PNEUMONIA (CAP)

Description

Pneumonia is an acute inflammation of lung tissue resulting in damage to pulmonary mucous membranes, accumulation of debris and exudates in the airways, and ventilation–perfusion ratio abnormalities. Community-acquired pneumonia refers to disease occurring outside of the hospital in a previously healthy child with no contributing disorder or disease.

Etiology

- Newborns
  - Group B streptococcus, gram-negative enteric bacteria, *Ureaplasma urealyticum, Listeria monocytogenes, Chlamydia trachomatis*
  - Cytomegalovirus
- Older children
  - *Streptococcus pneumoniae, Haemophilus influenzae, Mycoplasma pneumoniae, Mycobacterial tuberculosis*
  - RSV, parainfluenza, influenza, adenovirus, metapneumovirus

Incidence and Demographics

Pneumonia is common in children, especially in younger children and in boys. Annual incidence of pneumonia in children younger than 5 years is estimated to be 33 per 10,000 children. Viral pneumonia has a higher incidence than bacterial pneumonia, but bacterial pneumonia is a more serious infection and a more common reason for hospitalization. Approximately 50% of children younger than 5 years of age with CAP require hospitalization. Pneumonia occurs throughout the year, but is more prevalent during colder months.

Risk Factors

- Perinatal transmission from mother
- Congenital heart disease
- Chronic pulmonary disorders such as bronchopulmonary dysplasia, asthma, cystic fibrosis
- Gastrointestinal disorders such as gastroesophageal reflux, tracheoesophageal fistula
- Neuromuscular disorders
- Sickle cell disease
- Congenital and acquired immunodeficiency disorders
- Crowded living conditions
- Exposure to tobacco smoke

Prevention and Screening

- No screening indicated
- Prevention includes
    - *Haemophilus influenzae* type b (Hib) vaccine
    - Pneumococcal conjugate vaccine
    - Annual influenza vaccine for those over 6 months of age
    - Annual influenza vaccine for parents
    - Hand hygiene

Assessment

History

- Anorexia, vomiting, diarrhea, abdominal pain
- Headache, chills, fever
- Decreased activity level

Physical Exam

- High fever
- Infants: cyanosis or apnea
- Cough: hacking and nonproductive to productive
- Increased work of breathing: tachypnea, nasal flaring, retractions
- Adventitious breath sounds: rhonchi or crackles
- Diminished breath sounds
- Shallow respirations
- Chest or abdominal pain
- Dullness to percussion
- Shortness of breath

Diagnostic Studies

- Chest radiograph for more severe illness
- Gram stain and culture of sputum or nasopharyngeal specimen
- Blood cultures for more severe illness or incomplete immunization
- Elevated white blood cell count
- Elevated antistreptolysin O titer if due to streptococcus

Management

Invasive Treatment

- No invasive management indicated

Nonpharmacologic Treatment

- Supplemental oxygen as indicated
- Intravenous hydration as indicated
- Nasal suction
- Elevate head of bed
- Deep breathing exercises
- Ambulation
- Transmission precautions (droplet, contact, airborne) depending on cause

Pharmacologic Treatment

- Infants: amoxicillin, cefdinir, clindamycin
- Amoxicillin
- Azithromycin

- Analgesics for pain
- Antipyretics for fever
- In hospital: ampicillin, cefotaxime, ceftriaxone, nafcillin, vancomycin

Patient and Family Education

- Disease process and treatment plan
- Medication administration
- Importance of rest and hydration
- Signs of increasing respiratory difficulty

Outcomes and Follow-up

- The child will maintain effective airway clearance and gas exchange.
- The child will exhibit signs of adequate hydration.
- The child will recover without complications such as pleural effusion or empyema.
- The family will verbalize understanding of disease process and treatment plan.
- The family will verbalize reasons to call healthcare provider.

LARYNGOTRACHEOBRONCHITIS (LTB)

Description

LTB is one of the croup syndromes affecting the larynx, trachea, and bronchi. It is characterized by inflammation, secretions, and muscle spasms, resulting in airway obstruction, collapse of the glottis on inspiration, and respiratory distress.

Etiology

- Parainfluenza most common cause
- Respiratory syncytial virus (RSV), adenoviruses, measles

Incidence and Demographics

Croup commonly occurs in children between 6 and 36 months of age and is rare in children over 6 years. It is more common in boys and most cases occur in the autumn or early winter.

Risk Factors

- Family history
- Past history of croup

Prevention and Screening

- No specific prevention or screening
- Maintaining complete immunization status and annual influenza vaccine may decrease susceptibility

Assessment

History

- Family or past history
- Signs of upper respiratory infection
- Gradual progression over 1–2 days

Physical Exam

- Hoarseness
- Stridor
- Barking cough
- Tachypnea with prolonged inspiratory phase
- Retractions
- Nasal flaring
- Agitation
- Decreased oxygen saturation

Diagnostic Studies

- Chest radiography only if diagnosis is uncertain
- Laboratory studies only in severe illness

Management

Invasive Treatment

- No invasive management indicated

Nonpharmacologic Treatment

- Supplemental oxygen as needed
- Elevate head of bed
- Intravenous fluid as needed
- Contact precautions
- Rarely, intubation

Pharmacologic Treatment

- Dexamethasone
- Racemic epinephrine
- Antipyretics for fever

Patient and Family Education

- Disease process and treatment plan
- Medication administration
- Signs of increasing respiratory difficulty
- Home management: humidity, hydration, fever management

Outcomes and Follow-up

- The child will maintain effective airway clearance.
- The child will exhibit signs of adequate hydration.
- The family will verbalize an understanding of disease process and treatment plan.
- The family will verbalize an understanding of home care.
- The family will verbalize reasons to call healthcare provider.

EPIGLOTTITIS

Description

Epiglottitis is a life-threatening bacterial infection of the epiglottis with rapid progression of respiratory obstruction leading to hypoxia, hypercapnia, and acidosis. It is considered a medical emergency.

Etiology

- Most commonly caused by *Haemophilus influenzae* type b, so the incidence has decreased dramatically with routine administration of the Hib vaccine
- Other causative organisms include streptococci and *Staphylococcus aureus.*

Incidence and Demographics

Prior to Hib vaccine, the annual incidence was 5 per 100,000 children 5 years and younger. The more recent rate is 0.6 to 0.8 per 100,000 immunized children.

Risk Factors

- Incomplete immunization status for Hib
- Immune deficiency

Prevention and Screening

- Prevention is completing the recommended Hib immunization series
- No screening is indicated

Assessment

History

- Mild upper respiratory illness
- Sore throat that rapidly progresses to respiratory distress

Physical Exam

- Difficulty swallowing
- Drooling
- Muffled voice
- Severe sore throat
- High fever
- Agitation
- Tripod or sniffing position
- Suprasternal and substernal retractions
- Conduct throat examination only in emergency department, intensive care unit, or operating room with emergency personnel present

Diagnostic Studies

- Soft tissue lateral neck radiograph shows enlarged epiglottis
- Visualization via laryngoscopy and bronchoscopy in operating room
- Complete blood cell count, blood culture, epiglottal culture after airway is secured

Management

Invasive Treatment

- Endotracheal intubation

Nonpharmacologic Treatment

- Humidified supplemental oxygen
- Intravenous fluids
- Elevate head of bed

Pharmacologic Treatment

- Ceftriaxone or cefotaxime and clindamycin or vancomycin

- Corticosteroids for difficulty extubating
- Antipyretics for fever

Patient and Family Education

- Disease process and treatment plan
- Specific explanation of emergency care and procedures
- Implications of incomplete immunization status

Outcomes and Follow-up

- The child will maintain patent airway.
- The child will receive necessary vaccines.
- The family will experience psychosocial support during emergency situation.
- The family will verbalize an understanding of disease process, treatment, and importance of immunization status.

FOREIGN BODY ASPIRATION

Description

A condition that involving aspiration of a foreign body into the respiratory tract, causing partial or complete obstruction. Complete obstruction constitutes a medical emergency. Partial obstruction may lead to atelectasis and air trapping.

Etiology

Accidental inhalation of food, toys, coins, or other small objects

Incidence and Demographics

More common among infants and children under the age of 3 years.

Risk Factors

- Young children explore with their mouths
- Mobility while eating
- Presence of small toys or objects

Prevention and Screening

- No screening indicated

- Strategies for prevention
  - No small round foods such as hot dogs, hard candies, nuts, grapes, popcorn
  - No small toys such as marbles or beads
  - No small objects such as coins, pebbles, small batteries
  - Supervision of young children

Assessment

History

- Witnessed aspiration
- Sudden onset of cough and wheezing
- Persistent cough

Physical Exam

- Cough
- Stridor
- Difficulty breathing
- Tachypnea
- Wheezing
- Retractions
- Cyanosis
- Unilateral diminished breath sounds

Diagnostic Studies

- Radiographs
- Bronchoscopy

Management

Invasive Treatment

- Removal via thoracotomy

Nonpharmacologic Treatment

- Endoscopic removal

Patient and Family Education

- Strategies for prevention
- Care of choking child
- Basic life support

Outcomes and Follow-up

- The child will maintain patent airway.
- The child will experience successful removal of the foreign body.
- The family will verbalize an understanding of strategies for prevention.
- The family will verbalize an understanding of care of choking child.
- The family will participate in Basic Life Support class.

TONSILLITIS

Description

Tonsillitis is inflammation and infection of the palatine tonsils in the oropharynx and is often associated with pharyngitis. May involve inflammation of the adenoids, the pharyngeal tonsils.

Etiology

The majority of cases are caused by viruses. The most common bacterial etiology is group A beta-hemolytic streptococcus (GABHS).

Incidence and Demographics

Tonsillitis is common in children, but rare in children younger than 2 years.

Risk Factors

- Exposure to ill contacts
- Frequent upper respiratory infections
- Children have a large amount of pharyngeal lymphoid tissue.

Prevention and Screening

- No specific prevention or screening indicated

Assessment

History

- Upper respiratory infection
- Sore throat
- Difficulty swallowing

Physical Exam

- Tonsils red, swollen, with exudates
- Headache, nausea, vomiting, diarrhea, abdominal pain
- Cervical adenopathy
- Foul-smelling breath
- Fever

Diagnostic Studies

- Rapid streptococcal antigen test
- Throat culture
- Clotting and bleeding times for surgical candidates

Management

Invasive Treatment

- Tonsillectomy for documented recurrent streptococcal infection or history of peritonsillar abscess
- Adenoidectomy for airway obstruction, recurrent infection, sleep disorder

Nonpharmacologic Treatment

- Warm salt water gargles
- Throat lozenges for older children
- Cool mist vaporizer
- Fluids to prevent dehydration
- Postoperative care
    - Side-lying position while asleep
    - Ice collar for comfort
    - Monitor throat for bleeding; frequent swallowing is a sign
    - Cool, noncarbonated liquids and soft diet
    - Avoid red or brown liquids that may look like blood
    - Avoid straws that may injure operative site

Pharmacologic Treatment

- Antibiotics for group A streptococcus
    - Amoxicillin
    - Cephalosporins (cefuroxime, cefdinir)
    - Macrolides (azithromycin, erythromycin)
    - Clindamycin
- Analgesics for pain
- Antipyretics for fever

Patient and Family Education

- Nonpharmacologic comfort measures
- Medication administration
- Postoperative care at home: rest, hydration, diet
- Reasons to call healthcare provider

Outcomes and Follow-up

- The child will report pain relief.
- The child will maintain adequate hydration.
- The child will recover from surgery without complications such as bleeding.
- The family will verbalize an understanding of comfort measures and medication administration.
- The child and family will verbalize an understanding of surgical procedure.
- The family will verbalize an understanding of postoperative education.

RESPIRATORY DISTRESS AND FAILURE

Description

Respiratory distress is characterized by abnormal respiratory rate and effort ranging from mild to severe. Respiratory distress can progress to respiratory failure: inadequate oxygenation or ventilation, or both.

Etiology

Respiratory status may be compromised by any disorder that causes inadequate airway clearance, inability to maintain ventilation or oxygenation, or failure to breathe.

Incidence and Demographics

- No specific defining statistics

Risk Factors

- Young age
- Preexisting respiratory or cardiac disease

Prevention and Screening

- Progression from respiratory distress to respiratory failure may be prevented by early intervention

Assessment

History

- Diagnosis of respiratory disorder
- Progression of symptoms

Physical Exam

- Early tachypnea progressing to bradypnea or apnea
- Early tachycardia progressing to bradycardia
- Early adventitious sounds progressing to absence of sounds
- Poor to absent distal air movement
- Early mood changes with progressive loss of consciousness
- Increased, decreased, or no respiratory effort
- Hypertension
- Hypoxia
- Cyanosis

Diagnostic Studies

- Blood gas analysis is not diagnostic, but useful for monitoring
- Respiratory acidosis
  - pH less than 7.35
  - $PaCO_2$ greater than 45
  - May be due to hypoventilation, respiratory arrest, or central nervous system depression
- Respiratory alkalosis
  - pH greater than 7.45

    - $PaCO_2$ less than 35
    - May be due to hyperventilation

Management

Invasive Treatment

- Possible tracheostomy

Nonpharmacologic Treatment

- Positioning to open airway
- Supplemental high concentration oxygen with nonrebreather mask
- Suctioning as needed
    - Noninvasive positive-pressure ventilation such as continuous positive airway pressure (CPAP), intermittent positive pressure breathing (IPPB), or bilevel positive pressure breathing (BiPAP)
- Early endotracheal intubation
- Mechanical ventilation
- Cardiopulmonary resuscitation

Pharmacologic Treatment

- Dependent on underlying cause
- Intravenous therapy to correct fluid and electrolyte imbalances
- Mild sedatives

Patient and Family Education

- Disease process and treatment plan
- Specific explanation of emergency care and procedures
- Reasons for intubation and expected results

Outcomes and Follow-up

- The child will experience airway maintenance and adequate oxygenation and ventilation.
- The child will recover without complications.
- The family will verbalize an understanding of disease process, treatment plan, and emergency care.
- The family will experience psychosocial support during emergency situation.

BRONCHOPULMONARY DYSPLASIA (BPD)

Description

BPD is a chronic lung disease associated most often with premature birth. It is characterized by chronic inflammation, resulting in recurrent lung injury with abnormal healing. Pulmonary changes involve interstitial edema, thickening and fibrosis of alveolar walls, and squamous metaplasia of bronchiolar epithelium.

Etiology

- Surfactant deficiency
- Meconium aspiration
- Prenatal infection
- Positive-pressure ventilation

Incidence and Demographics

Incidence of BPD increases as survival of immature preterm infants increases and as birth weight decreases

Risk Factors

- Low birth weight
- Gestation less than 28 weeks
- Assisted ventilation
- Need for supplemental oxygen
- Fluid imbalance
- Patent ductus arteriosus
- Pre- or postnatal infections

Prevention and Screening

- No screening
- Strategies for prevention
  - Early and regular prenatal care
  - Glucocorticosteroids to increase surfactant production and promote lung development
  - Surfactant administration for infants with respiratory distress syndrome
  - Lowest peak inspiratory pressure possible with positive-pressure ventilation
  - Lowest level of supplemental oxygen possible

- High-frequency oscillary ventilation
- Avoid fluid overload
- Vitamin A administration

Assessment

History

- Lack of prenatal care
- History of risk factors

Physical Exam

- Tachypnea
- Nasal flaring
- Shallow respirations
- Adventitious lung sounds such as wheezing, crackles, rhonchi
- Grunting respirations
- Inability to wean from supplemental oxygen

Diagnostic Studies

- Chest radiograph
- Echocardiography to rule out heart defect or pulmonary hypertension

Management

Invasive Treatment

- Possible tracheostomy for long-term ventilator support

Nonpharmacologic Treatment

- Supplemental oxygen
- Nasal continuous positive airway pressure
- Intubation
- Mechanical ventilation
- Small, frequent feedings
- Nutritional supplements to add protein and calories

Pharmacologic Treatment

- Corticosteroids
- Bronchodilators

- Diuretics to control interstitial fluid
- Electrolyte supplements
- Vitamin D, calcium, and phosphorus supplements to prevent osteopenia
- RSV prophylaxis with palivizumab

Patient and Family Education

- Disease process and treatment plan
- Respiratory management: oxygen, equipment, suctioning, signs of respiratory distress
- Medication administrations
- Feeding techniques
- Infection prevention, effect of passive smoke exposure
- Signs of overhydration and dehydration
- Developmental stimulation
- Importance of regular health monitoring and immunizations
- Accessing early intervention services
- Availability of parent support group
- Basic Life Support class

Outcomes and Follow-up

- The child will maintain respiratory competence.
- The child will meet growth expectations.
- The child will receive regular health monitoring and immunizations.
- The child will reach developmental milestones for age, adjusted for prematurity.
- The family will demonstrate respiratory management, medication administration, and feeding techniques.
- The family will verbalize an understanding of disease process and treatment plan.
- The family will access available services, support groups, and education opportunities.

CYSTIC FIBROSIS (CF)

Description

CF is an autosomal recessive disorder. About 1,500 possible mutations of the responsible gene result in a variety of disease presentations involving the lungs, gastrointestinal system, pancreas, and hepatobiliary system. Respiratory disease is characterized by impaired mucociliary clearance, hyperactive airway inflammatory response, and chronic bacterial infection. Possible gastrointestinal manifestations include gastroesophageal reflux, meconium ileus, distal obstruction, constipation, and rectal prolapse. Deficiency of pancreatic enzymes leads to malabsorption of fat and protein resulting in growth failure (failure to thrive) and deficiencies of fat-soluble vitamins A, D, E, and K. Other possibilities are CF-related diabetes, biliary cirrhosis, progressive liver disease, and cholelithiasis.

Etiology

The disease is caused by a defect in the cystic fibrosis transmembrane conductance regulator (CFTR) gene found on the long arm of chromosome 7. When this gene that controls movement in and out of body cells is not functioning correctly, chloride secretion is decreased and sodium reabsorption is increased. This limits water movement, causing the production of abnormally thick mucus and secretions.

Incidence and Demographics

CF affects approximately 30,000 people in the United States. About 1,000 new cases are diagnosed each year and, of those, more than 70% are diagnosed in children age 2 years or younger. The median predicted survival age is 37 years. The main cause of death is respiratory failure. 1 in 29 Whites are symptom-free carriers and the incidence of CF is 1 in 3,500 live births. The incidence in Hispanics is 1 in 9,2000; in Native Americans, 1 in 10,900; in Blacks, 1 in 15,000; and in Asian Americans, 1 in 31,000.

Risk Factors

- Specific gene mutation
- Exposure to passive tobacco smoke increases risk for respiratory disease

Prevention and Screening

- No prevention
- Newborn screening

Assessment

History

- Meconium ileus
- Salty taste when kissed
- Growth failure (failure to thrive)
- Delayed puberty
- Chronic cough and sputum production
- Frequent lung or sinus infections, or both
- Nasal polyps
- Rectal prolapse
- Small bowel obstruction
- Large, bulky, frothy, foul-smelling stools

Physical Exam

- Adventitious lung sounds such as wheezing, rhonchi, crackles
- Productive cough
- Dyspnea
- Clubbing of fingers and toes
- Hyperinflated, barrel-shaped chest
- Abdominal pain, nausea, vomiting

Diagnostic Studies

- Newborn screening: elevated blood immunoreactive trypsin (IRT)
- Pilocarpine iontophoresis (sweat chloride test): positive for CF with chloride level at or above 60 mmol/L
- DNA analysis: gene mutation
- Nasal potential difference measurements: CFTR dysfunction
- Chest radiography
- Pulmonary function tests: obstructive airway disease
- Sputum cultures: most common organisms in lungs are *Staphylococcus aureus* and *Haemophilus influenzae* in younger children and *Pseudomonas aeruginosa* later in life
- Fecal elastase testing: pancreatic insufficiency

Management

Invasive Treatment

- Possible heart and/or lung transplantation

Nonpharmacologic Treatment

- Flutter mucus clearance device
- Manual chest physiotherapy
- High-frequency chest compression (mechanical vest)
- Supplemental oxygen as required
- High-calorie, high-protein, unrestricted-fat diet
- Oral or enteral nutritional supplements as needed
- Physical activity and aerobic exercise
- Infection transmission precautions during hospitalization
- Psychosocial support for high-maintenance, chronic, and incurable disease

Pharmacologic Treatment

- Antibiotics for acute infections
- Azithromycin for those at least 6 years of age with chronic airway inflammation
- Inhaled antibiotics: tobramycin (TOBI), aztreonam (Cayston) for chronic *Pseudomonas aeruginosa*
- Chronic treatment with nebulized hypertonic saline
- Hydrator therapies: Dornase alpha (DNAse, Pulmozyme) to liquefy bronchial mucus
- Antiinflammatory agents: ibuprofen to slow progression of pulmonary disease
- CFTR modulator: ivacaftor (VX-770) for those at least 6 years of age with one specific mutation
- Pancreatic enzyme replacement therapy
- Water-soluble multivitamin therapy

Patient and Family Education

- Disease process and treatment
- Diagnostic studies for diagnosis and disease monitoring
- Medication administration
- Nutritional support
- Chest physiotherapy
- Potential long-term complications and prevention strategies

- Importance of regular health care
- Reasons to contact healthcare provider
- Available resources such as counseling, support groups, advocacy organizations (CF Foundation)
- Transition to adult care

Outcomes and Follow-up

- The child will receive daily therapies to maximize quality of life.
- The child will achieve growth measurements appropriate for age.
- The child will receive regular healthcare monitoring and immunizations:
    - Immunizations and annual influenza vaccine
    - Growth and development assessment
    - Nutritional and bone density assessment
    - Testing for CF-related diabetes
- The child will experience minimal exacerbations and hospitalizations.
- The adolescent will receive counseling for possible delayed puberty and long-term infertility.
- The family will demonstrate chest physiotherapy interventions.
- The family will demonstrate medication administration.
- The family will immediately notify provider of changes in mucus, decreased energy or appetite, severe constipation or diarrhea, severe abdominal pain, dark or green vomitus, or fever.
- The child and family will verbalize an understanding of educational content.
- The child and family will receive genetic counseling.
- The child and family will receive information about long-term treatment options.
- The child and family will access available resources.

TUBERCULOSIS (TB)

Description

TB is an infectious disease primarily affecting the respiratory system.

Etiology

Infection is caused by *Mycobacterium tuberculosis,* transmitted via inhaled droplets. The bacilli are deposited in the lungs but may be carried by the lymphatic system to bones, kidneys, or brain, becoming extrapulmonary TB. The bacilli may lie dormant in the lungs, not causing symptoms or being transmitted, and classified as latent TB disease. The disease may progress to active TB disease with reactivation of the infection.

Incidence and Demographics

In 2010, the rate of TB occurrence was 3.6 cases per 100,000 persons, the lowest rate ever reported in the United States. The rate among foreign-born persons was 11 times higher than among those born in the United States. The rate for Asians was 22.4 cases per 100,00 persons, 20.8 for Native Hawaiians and other Pacific Islanders, 7.0 for Blacks, 6.5 for Hispanics or Latinos, 6.4 for American Indians or Alaska Natives, and 0.9 for Whites.

Risk Factors

- Exposure to adults at high risk
  - Residents of nursing homes, homeless shelters, correctional facilities
  - Intravenous substance abuse
  - Homelessness
  - Healthcare workers who work with those at high risk
- Birth in countries with high prevalence
- Travel to countries with high prevalence
- Immunocompromised status
  - HIV, measles, pertussis
  - Corticosteroids or chemotherapy
- Poor nutritional state
- Stress

Prevention and Screening

- Avoid contact
- Maintain healthy nutritional status

- Avoid unpasteurized milk
- Fit tested respirators for healthcare workers caring for patients with TB
- Targeted tuberculin skin testing for those at high risk for contracting disease and for those at risk for progression to active TB disease (immunocompromised, diabetes, renal failure)

Assessment

History

- Exposure to infected person
- Anorexia
- Weight loss or growth failure
- Fatigue
- Night sweats

Physical Exam

- Fever
- Cough
- Crackles
- Chest pain or tightness
- Diminished breath sounds
- Children may be asymptomatic

Diagnostic Studies

- Tuberculin skin testing
  - 2–10 weeks between exposure and positive test
  - Induration, not just erythema, indicates infection
- Chest radiography: pulmonary involvement
- Culture of induced sputum and gastric lavage sputum specimens for *M. tuberculosis*

Management

Invasive Treatment

- Bronchoscopic removal of polyps
- Resection of diseased lung portion

Nonpharmacologic Treatment

- Nutritional support

- Unrestricted activity (school, daycare) if asymptomatic
- Avoid strenuous activity and competitive games or sports during active stage
- Maintain immunization status

Pharmacologic Treatment

- Bacteriocidal: isoniazid, rifampin
- Antituberculous agent: pyrazinamide (Rifater), ethambutol (Myambutol)
    - Those taking ethambutol need monthly screening of visual acuity and red-green color discrimination because of potential optic nerve neuritis
- Observed medication administration is recommended

Patient and Family Education

- Disease process and treatment plan
- Medication compliance
- Strategies to support healthy nutrition

Outcomes and Follow-up

- The child will receive all medications as scheduled.
- The child will experience symptom relief.
- The child will receive routine health care and immunizations.
- The child will experience minimal disruption of usual activities.
- The child will attain growth measurements appropriate for age.
- The family will verbalize an understanding of education content.
- The family and contacts will be screened for infection.

ASTHMA

Description

Asthma is a chronic inflammatory lung disease characterized by airway narrowing and increased responsiveness to a variety of triggers. Chronic inflammation results in airway remodeling. Status asthmaticus is a life-threatening emergency that can lead to respiratory failure.

Etiology

Inflammation leads to smooth muscle constriction, airway edema, increased mucus production, inflammatory cell infiltration of the submucosa, and thickening of the basement membrane, causing airway obstruction.

Incidence and Demographics

Prevalence of asthma in children under 18 years of age is 9.6%. Prevalence is increased among children from families of lower socioeconomic status and in urban areas. It is more common in boys, but the incidence in girls begins to rise at puberty. 25.7% of Puerto Ricans have asthma, 12.7% of Blacks, 8.8% of Whites, and 6.6% of Hispanics.

Risk Factors

- Four or more wheezing episodes in the past year
- Wheezing unrelated to infection
- Atopic dermatitis
- Food sensitivity
- Family history
- Exposure to passive tobacco smoke
- Exposure to environmental pollution
- High percentage of body fat

Prevention and Screening

Although there is no prevention or screening for asthma, exacerbations may be prevented by the use of controller medications, peak flow monitoring, timely use of quick-relief inhalers, infection prevention, and avoidance of known triggers.

Assessment

History

- Risk factors
- Viral upper respiratory illness
- Exposure to known triggers
- Exercise-induced bronchospasm
- Cough: seasonal, nocturnal, lasting longer than 3 weeks

Physical Exam

- Dry, hacking cough
- Wheeze
- Chest tightness
- Tachypnea
- Accessory muscle use

- Retractions
- Shortness of breath
- Prolonged expiratory phase
- Increased anterior-posterior diameter of chest
- Transverse nasal crease (allergic salute)

Diagnostic Studies

- Spirometry: airway obstruction
- Pulmonary function testing
- Chest radiography
- Skin testing for allergies
- Atopy: having IgE antibodies to specific allergens
- Complete blood count
  - Elevated white blood cell count with infection
  - Elevated eosinophile count with allergic or inflammatory disorder

Management

Invasive Treatment

- Not indicated

Nonpharmacologic Treatment

- Peak flow monitoring
- Maintain immunization status and annual influenza vaccine
- Supplemental oxygen or heliox as needed

Pharmacologic Treatment

- As needed quick-relief, short-acting beta$_2$-agonist (SABA)
  - Albuterol
  - Levalbuterol
- Inhaled corticosteroids; rinse mouth after use to prevent fungal infection
  - Budesonide (Pulmicort)
  - Fluticasone (Veramyst)
- Anti-asthma medication: cromolyn sodium (Intal)
- Long-acting beta 2-agonist (LABA)
  - Salmeterol (Serevent)
  - Formoterol (Foradil Aerolizer, Perforomist)

- Leukotriene-receptor antagonist (LTRA)
  - Montelukast (Singulair)
  - Zafirlukast (Accolate)
- Oral systemic corticosteroids
- Immunomodulators: omalizumab (Xolair), anti-IgE
- Methylxanthine: sustained release theophylline, bronchodilator
- Anticholinergic: ipratropium bromide (Atrovent)
- Magnesium sulfate: potent muscle relaxant to decrease inflammation in emergency department
- Epinephrine: status asthmaticus

Patient and Family Education

- Disease process and treatment plan
- Medication administration
- Inhaler, spacer, MDI, nebulizer technique
- Peak flow monitoring
- Environmental control strategies
- Available resources such as support groups, asthma camps

Outcomes and Follow-up

- The child will experience minimal acute episodes.
- The child will exhibit well-controlled status with lung function greater than 80% of predicted or personal best.
- The child will exhibit physical activity levels appropriate for age.
- The child will receive regular health care and immunizations.
- The child will receive regular monitoring of respiratory status.
- The child will have a written management plan for home and school.
- The child and family will demonstrate use of the medication delivery method.
- The child and family will identify triggers.
- The child and family will verbalize an understanding of education content.
- The child and family will access available resources.

SUDDEN INFANT DEATH SYNDROME (SIDS)

Description

Sudden death of an infant (younger than 1 year of age) with unidentified explanation after autopsy, investigation of death scene, and review of case history.

Etiology

The cause is unknown.

Incidence and Demographics

SIDS is the third leading cause of infant deaths between the ages of birth and 12 months. Incidence is higher in boys, Native Americans, and Blacks.

Risk Factors

- Maternal smoking during pregnancy
- Low birth weight
- Low Apgar scores
- Recent viral illness
- Prone or side sleeping
- Soft or loose bedding
- Overheating
- Co-sleeping with adult or older child
- Sibling of two or more SIDS victims

Prevention and Screening

- No screening
- Protective factors
    - Education on risk factors
    - Back-only sleeping
    - Avoidance of soft or loose bedding and objects in bed
    - Avoidance of co-sleeping
    - Breastfeeding
    - Complete immunization status
    - Sleeping in room with adult
    - Pacifier use at nap and bedtime

Management

- Allow family time and privacy to say goodbye.
- Assist with mementos such as footprints, handprints, or lock of hair.
- Refer family members to grief counselor and support groups.

Patient and Family Education

- Risk factors and protective factors
- Supervised, awake tummy time to prevent occipital flattening

Outcomes and Follow-up

- The family will verbalize an understanding that cause of infant's death is unknown.
- The family will experience sufficient time with deceased infant.
- The family will have mementos of infant.
- The family will receive emotional support from healthcare providers.
- The family will access available resources.

REFERENCES

American Academy of Pediatrics. (2011). *Pediatric clinical practice guidelines & policies: A compendium of evidence-based research for pediatric patients* (11th ed.). Elk Grove Village, IL: American Academy of Pediatrics.

American Heart Association and American Academy of Pediatrics. (2011). *Pediatric advanced life support provider manual.* Dallas: American Heart Association.

Baker, R. D., Coburn-Miller, C., & Baker, S. S. (2011). Cystic fibrosis: Nutritional issues. *UpToDate.* Retrieved from http://www.uptodate.com/contents/cystic-fibrosis-nutritional-issues?source=search_result&search=cystic+fibrosis+children&selectedTitle=4%7E150

Barson, W. J. (2011). Epidemiology, pathogenesis, and etiology of pneumonia in children. *UpToDate.* Retrieved from http://www.uptodate.com/contents/epidemiology-pathogenesis-and-etiology-of-pneumonia-in-children?source=search_result&search=risk+factors+for+community+acquired+pneumonia+in+children&selectedTitle=1%7E150

Barson, W. J. (2012). Inpatient treatment of pneumonia in children. *UpToDate.* Retrieved from http://www.uptodate.com/contents/inpatient-treatment-of-pneumonia-in-children?source=search_result&search=pneumonia+treatment+children&selectedTitle=1%7E150

Barson, W. J. (2012). Outpatient treatment of community-acquired pneumonia in children. *UpToDate.* Retrieved from http://www.uptodate.com/contents/outpatient-treatment-of-community-acquired-pneumonia-in-children?source=search_result&search=pneumonia+treatment+children&selectedTitle=2%7E150

Centers for Disease Control and Prevention. (2010). *National health interview survey.* Retrieved from http://www.cdc.gov/asthma/nhis/2010/table2-1.htm

Centers for Disease Control and Prevention. (2011). *Trends in tuberculosis, 2010.* Retrieved from www.cdc.gov/tb

Committee on Infectious Disease. (2009). *Red Book®: 2009 report of the Committee on Infectious Diseases* (28th ed.). Elk Grove Village, IL: American Academy of Pediatrics.

Hitt, E., & Murata, P. (2011). *First-ever guidelines issued for CAP in infants and children.* Retrieved from http://medscape.org/viewarticle/749312?src=cmemp

Hockenberry, M. J., & Wilson, D. (2011). *Wong's nursing care of infants and children* (9th ed.). St. Louis, MO: Elsevier Mosby.

Jones, C. S., & Arney, T. D. (2011). *Guideline assessment of severity, control, and treatment selection in asthma.* Retrieved from http://www.medscape.org/viewarticle/740611

Katkin, J. P. (2012). Cystic fibrosis: Clinical manifestations and diagnosis. *UpToDate.* Retrieved from http://www.uptodate.com/contents/cystic-fibrosis-clinical-manifestations-and-diagnosis?source=search_result&search=cystic+fibrosis+children&selectedTitle=5%7E150

Katkin, J. P., Baker, R.D., & Baker, S. S. (2010). Cystic fibrosis: Assessment and management of pancreatic insufficiency. *UpToDate.* Retrieved from http://www.uptodate.com/contents/cystic-fibrosis-assessment-and-management-of-pancreatic-insufficiency?source=see_link

Katkin, J. P., & Schultz, K. (2011). Cystic fibrosis: Overview of gastrointestinal disease. *UpToDate.* Retrieved from http://www.uptodate.com/contents/cystic-fibrosis-overview-of-gastrointestinal-disease?source=search_result&search=cystic+fibrosis+children&selectedTitle=1%7E150

Litonjua, A. A., & Weiss, S. T. (2012). Risk factors for asthma. *UpToDate.* Retrievedfrom http://www.uptodate.com/contents/risk-factors-for-asthma?source=see_link

Narasimhan, M., & Cohen, R. (2011). New and investigational treatments in cystic fibrosis. *Therapeutic Advances in Respiratory Disease, 5*(4), 275–282. Retrieved from http://www.medscape.com/viewarticle/746221?src=mp&spon=9

National Asthma Education and Prevention Program Expert Panel. (2007). *Guidelines for the diagnosis and management of asthma.* National Institutes of Health. Retrieved from http://www.nhlbi.nih.gov/guidelines/asthma/asthma.summ.pdf

National Heart, Lung, and Blood Institute. (2011). *Explore cystic fibrosis.* Retrieved from http://www.nhlbi.nih.gov/health/health-topics/topics/cf/

National Heart, Lung, and Blood Institute. (2012). *Explore bronchopulmonary dysplasia.* Retrieved from http://www.nhlbi.nih.gov/health/health-topics/topics/bpd/

Paksu, S., Paksu, M. S., Kilic, M., Guner, S. N., Baysal, K., Sancak, R., & Ozturk, F. (2012). Foreign body aspiration in childhood: Evaluation of diagnostic parameters. *Pediatric Emergency Care, 28*(3), 259–264.

Potts, N. L., & Mandleco, B. L. (2012). *Pediatric nursing: Caring for children and their families* (3rd ed.). New York: Thomson Delmar Learning.

Sawicki, G., & Haver, K. (2011). Chronic asthma in children younger than 12 years: Definition, epidemiology, and pathophysiology. *UpToDate.* Retrieved from http://www.uptodate.com/contents/chronic-asthma-in-children-younger-than-12-years-definition-epidemiology-and-pathophysiology?source=search_result&search=pediatric+asthma+children&selectedTitle=14%7E150

Sawicki, G., & Haver, K. (2011). Chronic asthma in children younger than 12 years: Evaluation and diagnosis. *UpToDate.* Retrieved from http://www.uptodate.com/contents/chronic-asthma-in-children-younger-than-12-years-evaluation-and-diagnosis?source=search_result&search=pediatric+asthma+children&selectedTitle=4%7E150

Simon, R. H. (2012). Cystic fibrosis: Overview of the treatment of lung disease. *UpToDate.* Retrieved from http://www.uptodate.com/contents/cystic-fibrosis-overview-of-the-treatment-of-lung-disease?source=search_result&search=cystic+fibrosis+children&selectedTitle=2%7E150

Task Force on Sudden Infant Death Syndrome. (2011). SIDS and other sleep-related infant deaths: Expansion on recommendations for a safe infant sleeping environment. *Pediatrics.* Retrieved from http://pediatrics.aappublications.org/content/128/5/e1341.full.pdf+html?sid=6a0452c2-fd89-4554-9bf3-6cba7ff91423

Woods, C. R. (2011). Approach to the management of croup. *UpToDate.* Retrieved from http://www.uptodate.com/contents/approach-to-the-management-of-croup?source= search_result&search=laryngotracheobronchitis&selectedTitle=2%7E26#H8

Woods, C. R. (2011). Clinical features, evaluation, and diagnosis of croup. *UpToDate.* Retrieved from http://www.uptodate.com/contents/clinical-features-evaluation-and-diagnosis-of-croup?source=search_result&search=laryngotracheobronchitis&selectedTitle=1%7E26

Woods, C. R. (2011). Epiglottitis (supraglottitis): Clinical features and diagnosis. *UpToDate.* Retrieved from http://www.uptodate.com/contents/epiglottitis-supraglottitis-clinical-features-and-diagnosis?source=search_result&search=epiglottitis+in+children&selectedTitle=1%7E45

Woods, C. R. (2011). Epiglottitis (supraglottitis): Treatment and prevention. *UpToDate.* Retrieved from http://www.uptodate.com/contents/epiglottitis-supraglottitis-treatment-and-prevention?source=search_result&search=epiglottitis+in+children&selectedTitle=2%7E45

CHAPTER 10

CARDIOVASCULAR DISORDERS

Mary Jo Gilmer, PhD, MBA, RN-BC, FAAN, and
Karen Corlett, MSN, RN-BC, CPNP-AC/PC, PNP-BC

PEDIATRIC VARIATIONS FROM THE ADULT

- Changes from fetal to postnatal circulation
  - Closure of foramen ovale (without closure may lead to atrial septal defect [ASD])
  - Closure of ductus arteriosus (without closure may lead to patent ductus arteriosus [PDA])
  - Closure of ductus venosus
- Smaller reserve capacity and volume
- Low vascular resistance and low blood pressure
- Heart very sensitive to volume and pressure overload (congestive heart failure)

CONGESTIVE HEART FAILURE (CHF)

Description

Inadequate cardiac output to meet demands of the body

Etiology

- From structural heart disease
  - Extra blood flow to lungs steals blood flow from systemic circulation
  - Obstruction to systemic outflow
- From acquired heart disease
  - Coronary artery disease
  - Cardiomyopathy
  - Myocarditis
- Dysrhythmias
  - Inadequate pumping or inadequate filling

Incidence and Demographics

- 10%–34% of all cardiac admission to the hospital
- 12,000–35,000 children < 19 years each year
- Primarily affects children with congenital heart disease or cardomyopathics

Risk Factors

- Structural heart disease
- Infections causing cardiomyopathy or myocarditis
- Accidental toxic ingestion of substances causing dysrhythmia (e.g., antihistamines, nonsteroidal antiinflammatory drugs [NSAIDs], antidepressants)
- Previous dysrhythmia causing CHF

Assessment

History

- Recent viral illness or ill contacts
- Duration of symptoms

Physical Exam

- Cardiac
  - Tachycardia

    - Decreased peripheral pulses
    - Periorbital, peripheral, or dependent edema, or a combination
    - Cool extremities
    - Delayed capillary refill
    - Hypotension a late sign
    - Cardiogenic shock in severe cases
- Pulmonary
    - Tachypnea
    - Increased work of breathing
        - Flaring, grunting, retracting
- Associated symptoms
    - Altered mental status if severe compromise
    - Decreased activity, increased sleep
    - Fussiness or irritability
    - Nausea, vomiting
        - Sweating with feeding in infants

Diagnostic Studies

- For causation
    - Congenital heart disease
        - Electrocardiogram (ECG)
        - Cardiac ultrasonography
        - Rarely cardiac catheterization
    - Cardiomyopathy or myocarditis
        - Cardiac ultrasonography for function
        - ECG for associated dysrhythmias

Management

Invasive Treatment

- Surgical correction of structural heart defects
    - Cardiac transplantation if myopathy or myocarditis causes permanent heart muscle damage

Nonpharmacologic Treatment

- Prioritize nursing diagnoses and problem as above

- Nutritional
  - Hypercaloric formulas in infants
    - Consider tube feeding if patient unable to take adequate volumes
  - Careful monitoring for weight gain
  - Rarely need to restrict fluid or sodium intake
  - Education of parents regarding potassium-rich foods if patient is on potassium-depleting diuretic therapy

Pharmacologic Treatment

- Digoxin
  - For improved cardiac contractility and for some dysrhythmias
  - Can load over 24 hours to speed accumulation of effective drug level
  - Then dose orally twice daily for children, once daily for teens and adults
  - Side effects
    - Bradycardia
    - Prolongation of PR interval
  - Monitoring
    - Apical heart rate before dosing
    - Serum electrolytes: potassium, magnesium, calcium
    - Blood urea nitrogen (BUN), creatinine to evaluate for need of dosing adjustments in renal insufficiency
    - For digoxin toxicity
      - Anorexia, nausea, vomiting, dizziness, bradycardia, heart block
- Diuretics
  - To promote water loss and appropriate fluid balance
  - Many can be dosed enterally or intravenously
  - Loop diuretics
    - Affect sodium, potassium, and chloride transport
    - Biggest effect in the ascending limb of the loop of Henle
    - Examples: furosemide, ethacrynic acid, bumetanide, torsemide
  - Thiazide diuretics
    - Inhibit reabsorption of sodium and water in the distal convoluted tubules
    - Example: chlorothiazide
  - Potassium-sparing diuretics
    - Inhibit action of aldosterone in the cortical collecting ducts

            - Example: chlorothiazide
        - Monitoring
            - Serum electrolytes for losses with increased urine flow
            - Hyperkalemia a risk with potassium-sparing diuretics
            - Strict intake and output, daily weights
            - Hypotension or postural hypotension if large fluid shifts
- Afterload reducers
    - Dilate peripheral vessels
        - Makes it easy for a poorly functioning heart to pump out systemically
        - Decreased peripheral vascular resistance favors more systemic outflow in patients with predominant left-to-right intracardiac shunting
        - Examples: enalapril, lisinopril (i.e., ACE inhibitors)
    - Vastly different intravenous and oral dosage
    - Monitoring
        - Hypotension with administration
        - Chronic cough
        - Renal function for dosing adjustments
- Intensive care monitoring and therapy if poor cardiac output, shock, or respiratory failure occurs

Patient and Family Education

- Signs and symptoms of worsening congestive heart failure; symptoms as above
- When to seek care
- Appropriate preparation of hypercaloric formulas
    - Tube feedings at home if ordered
- Medication administration
    - Medication safety—digoxin is quite toxic if ingested in inappropriate amounts
    - Signs and symptoms of digoxin toxicity as above
    - Use of reminders and incentives to facilitate compliance

Outcomes and Follow-up

- Goal is restoration of structure and function of heart muscle
- Normal cardiac output, organ, and peripheral perfusion
- Normal growth patterns
    - Height, weight, and development

- Close follow-up with pediatric cardiologist re: adjustment of medications
- Close follow-up with primary care provider re: growth and development
- Evaluation for any associated genetic abnormalities if patient has congenital heart disease
    - Genetic counseling for families

CONGENITAL HEART DISEASE

Description

Structural abnormalities of the heart

- Acyanotic congenital heart disease
    - Patent ductus arteriosus (PDA)
        - Persistence of ductus arteriosus
            - A normal prenatal structure connecting the aorta and the pulmonary artery
            - Allows for bypass of the lung circulation in prenatal life when oxygenation is accomplished by the mother
            - Impetus for ductus to close is increase in oxygen tension
                - Also substances released from the lungs
                - Lack of exposure to maternal circulating prostaglandins
        - More common in premature infants
            - And others with pulmonary issues
        - Causes left-to-right shunting
            - From high-pressure aorta to lower-pressure pulmonary artery
            - Pulmonary overcirculation
                - Steals from systemic circulation
            - Congestive heart failure
        - Continuous murmur that radiates throughout chest
    - Atrial septal defect (ASD)
        - Hole or persistence of opening in the atrial septum
            - Connection between the right and left atria
            - Atria have low pressure, fairly equal between right and left side
        - Some left-to-right shunting
            - Mild pulmonary overcirculation
            - Rarely causes significant congestive heart failure

        - Murmur often absent or soft
            - Fixed split of S2 due to extra and constant flow across pulmonary valve
    - Ventricular septal defect (VSD)
        - Hole in ventricular septum
            - Connection between the lower pumping chambers
            - After the newborn period, the right ventricular pressure only 20%–25% of left ventricular pressure
        - Significant left-to-right shunting
            - Dependent upon size of hole
            - Can cause significant pulmonary overcirculation and steal from systemic circulation
            - Significant congestive heart failure in many cases
        - Harsh, loud systolic murmur best heard at left lower sternal border
    - Atrioventricular canal defect (AVC)
        - Classified as an endocardial cushion defect
            - Failure of endocardial cushions to meet
                - Failure of migration of atrial and ventricular septum as well as abnormalities in formation of mitral and tricuspid valve tissue
                - More common in infants with trisomy 21 (Down syndrome)
            - Range from tiny ASD with mitral valve abnormality and mild regurgitation to large ASD/VSD and essentially single valve separating atria from ventricles with significant regurgitation
        - Predominant left-to-right shunting
            - Direction of shunting can be quite variable in large defects with multiple pathways for left-to-right shunting
            - Symptoms depend on size of holes and severity of valve involvement
            - Congestive heart failure common
        - Harsh systolic murmur of VSD, systolic murmurs of tricuspid, mitral valve regurgitation, or a combination of these
- Cyanotic congenital heart disease
    - Tetralogy of Fallot
        - Four "separate" defects arising from an abnormality in cardiac development
            - Ventricular septal defect
            - Pulmonary stenosis
                - At, below, or slightly above the pulmonary valve
            - Rightward malposition of the aorta

            - Right ventricular hypertrophy
                - Due to increased workload from pulmonary stenosis
        - Cyanosis is predominant feature
            - Due to restriction of pulmonary blood flow
            - Deoxygenated blood in the right ventricle that can't get out across stenotic pulmonary valve crosses the VSD into the left ventricle and exits as deoxygenated blood into the systemic circulation via the aorta
        - Systolic ejection murmur from turbulence across stenotic pulmonary valve
    - Transposition of the great arteries (TGA)
        - Also known as "simple transposition"
            - The aorta arises from the right ventricle and the pulmonary artery arises from the left ventricle
        - Creates two "separate" rather than "in series" circulations
            - Deoxygenated blood travels from inferior and superior vena cava, to right atrium, to right ventricle, to the aorta, to the lungs
            - Oxygenated blood returns from the lungs via the pulmonary veins to the left atrium, to left ventricle, and back to the pulmonary artery to the lungs
            - Potential connection points to mix the blue and red blood are the PDA and the persistence of the prenatally present foramen ovale connecting the right and left atria
        - Mandatory cyanosis
            - Can have pulmonary overcirculation as well
        - Murmur may be unimpressive
            - Only turbulent blood flow is across PDA, ASD, or both
    - Truncus arteriosus
        - Single common "trunk" exits the heart
            - "Trunk" continues out and becomes aorta, gives rise to the pulmonary arteries
                - Classified by how the pulmonary arteries come off of main trunk
            - Implies ventricular septal defect as well
                - "Trunk" originates over the VSD
            - Valve to truncal vessel has components of aortic and pulmonary valves and can be malformed as well
        - Causes pulmonary overcirculation and cyanosis
            - Deoxygenated blood from the right side of the heart and oxygenated blood from the left side mix completely together at the VSD and exit the truncal vessel

- This mixed blood then follows the path of least resistance:
    - Some will go to the pulmonary artery connection back to the lungs
    - The remainder will continue out the aorta to give cardiac output to the body
- As the pulmonary artery pressures of a newborn drop, more blood will travel to the lower-pressure pulmonary arteries

- Congestive heart failure, cyanosis, and low cardiac output can coexist

- Murmur varies
    - Of stenosis or regurgitation across truncal valve
    - Right and left ventricles are fairly equal in pressure, so not a lot of turbulent blood flow across the VSD

- Tricuspid atresia
    - Tricuspid valve never formed
        - No opening between right atrium and right ventricle
        - Typically small, underdeveloped hypoplastic right ventricle
        - May also have VSD, pulmonary stenosis, or both
        - Right ventricle will never be usable as a pump
            - This is a type of single ventricle
    - Cyanosis
        - No blood flow into right ventricle, so no blood flow through pulmonary valve into pulmonary artery and to lungs
    - Murmur may not be impressive—mostly from PDA and ASD unless other anomalies
- Total anomalous pulmonary venous return (TAPVR)
    - The pulmonary veins end up in the wrong place
        - Pulmonary veins bring highly oxygenated blood back from the lungs
        - Should enter as four separate vessels into the back of the left atrium
        - In TAPVR, the vessels typically come together behind the left atrium, then travel through an abnormal vessel to somewhere in the right heart
            - Categorized by the course or entrance point of the pulmonary veins back into the heart, or by both
        - Implies an ASD
    - Pulmonary circulation and cyanosis of varying degrees
        - Recirculation of oxygenated blood back through the right side causes pulmonary overcirculation

      - Because no blood is coming back to the left atrium, there is a mandatory right-to-left shunt at the atrial level
        - Provides blood flow to the left ventricle for cardiac output
        - Deoxygenated blood from the right atrium enters into the systemic circulation
      - If there is narrowing or obstruction of the pulmonary veins on their course back to the heart, infants will present in cyanosis and shock
      - TAPVR may be an isolated condition, or may be just a portion of a complex congenital heart deformity
    - Not an impressive murmur

- Obstructive lesions
  - Pulmonary stenosis
    - Isolated stenosis of the pulmonary valve
    - Limits pulmonary blood flow
    - Increased pressure, workload, and thickness of right ventricle
    - Rarely causes cyanosis
    - Systolic ejection murmur from turbulent flow across pulmonary valve
  - Aortic stenosis
    - Isolated stenosis or narrowing of the aortic valve
    - Can limit blood flow out to the body
    - Increased pressure, workload, and thickness of the left ventricle
    - Can cause poor cardiac output
    - Systolic ejection murmur from turbulent flow across narrowed aortic valve
  - Coarctation of the aorta
    - Narrowing of the aorta
      - Typically just across from the left subclavian artery
    - Newborns present in shock
    - Older children present with some or no symptoms
      - Hypertension on routine blood pressure checks
        - High right arm pressure before obstruction, lower or normal blood pressure of left arm or legs
      - Leg cramps
    - Increased pressure, workload, and thickness of left ventricle
    - May have no murmur
  - Hypoplastic left heart syndrome (HLHS)

- All left-sided structures are small or atretic
  - Mitral valve, left ventricle, aortic valve, and ascending aorta
  - Left side is unusable as a pump for systemic circulation
    - Ascending aorta is inadequate for systemic outflow
  - Oxygenated blood returning to left atrium crosses from the left atrium to the right atrium, then joins the deoxygenated blood returning from the body; this mixed blood enters the right ventricle and is pumped out the pulmonary valve into the pulmonary artery
    - The blood then:
      - Can go through the PDA to the aorta to supply the body with blood flow
      - Can continue out the right and left pulmonary artery and go to the lungs to become fully saturated and return to the left atrium
    - Constant balance between the amount of pulmonary versus systemic blood flow
- Is a type of single ventricle
- Requires a connection between the right and left atrium so the blood returning from the lungs can cross to the right side
- Requires the ductus arteriosus to stay open to provide systemic blood flow
- Minimal to no murmur despite severity of disease

Etiology

- As yet, no clearly defined environmental and genetic factors
- Maternal infections during pregnancy (e.g., rubella)
- Teratogenic drugs (alcohol, lithium, phenobarbital, angiotensin-converting-enzyme [ACE] inhibitors)

Incidence and Demographics

- 0.7 per 1,000 live births
- ~35,000 infants each year born in the United States with congenital heart disease
- Largest cause of infant death compared to all other birth defects

Risk Factors

- Intrauterine exposure to drugs, alcohol, or infections
- Previous child with congenital heart disease
- Parent with congenital heart disease
- Associated genetic syndromes

- Down syndrome
- Williams syndrome
- Turner syndrome
- Noonan syndrome
- Trisomy 13 and 18

Prevention and Screening

- No prevention or screening indicated

Assessment

Physical Exam

- Cardiac exam
  - Heart rate vs. normal for age and condition
    - Higher if febrile, crying, active, or dehydrated
  - Heart rhythm
  - Presence of murmur
    - Grade or loudness (I through VI scale)
      - Grade I: softer than heart tones
      - Grade II: equal in intensity to heart tones
      - Grade III: louder than heart tones
      - Grade IV: louder than heart tones and there is a palpable thrill
      - Grade V: Grade IV criteria and heard with stethoscope partially off chest
      - Grade VI: Grade IV criteria and heard with stethoscope off chest
    - Location best heard
      - In relation to
        - Sternum
        - Clavicle
        - Axillae
        - Intercostal spaces
    - Quality
      - Harsh, blowing, machinery, soft, click
    - Timing
      - During systole
      - During diastole

        - Additional sounds
            - Pericardial rub
                - From pericardial inflammation, fluid accumulation, or both
    - Evaluation of peripheral perfusion
        - Central and peripheral pulses
        - Peripheral warmth
        - Central and peripheral color
            - Cyanosis or pallor
        - Capillary refill time
        - Sweating
    - Evaluation of cardiopulmonary interactions
        - Hepatomegaly
        - Respiratory rate and effort
        - Pulmonary edema
    - Presence of edema
        - Periorbital
        - Peripheral
        - Dependent
        - Pulmonary
        - Strict intake vs. output measurements
    - Point of maximal impulse
    - Jugular venous distention
- Cyanosis
    - Central and peripheral
    - Noninvasive pulse oximetry
    - Invasive arterial blood gas
- Pulmonary overcirculation
    - Respiratory exam
    - Chest radiography
- Impact on other systems
    - Fatigability
        - Sleeping and eating in infants
        - Endurance in older children
    - Growth

        - Decreased intake due to rapid fatigue
        - Increased caloric requirements due to increased workload on heart
    - Development
        - Delayed developmental milestones caused by fatigue from:
            - Increased work of breathing
            - Increased cardiac workload
            - Poor caloric intake
    - Other organ systems
        - Decreased perfusion from inadequate cardiac output can affect the functioning of any other organ system.
            - Central nervous system: confusion, sleepiness, lethargy
            - Renal: increased BUN/creatinine, decreased urinary output
            - Hepatic: decreased hepatic function, increased laboratory parameters (liver enzymes and coagulation studies)
            - Gastrointestinal: edematous, boggy intestinal walls with poor absorption
    - Evaluation of congenital heart defects
        - ECG and cardiac exam point to problem
        - Cardiac echocardiography
            - Noninvasive test to look at structure and function of heart
            - Requires sedation or distraction for infants and young children to cooperate
        - Cardiac catheterization
            - Typically via femoral artery, vein, or both
            - Catheters advanced and contrast injected into bloodstream
                - Look at structure and function
                - Direct measurements of pressures and oxygen saturations within the heart
            - Typically receive sedation or anesthesia for procedure
        - Cardiac magnetic resonance imaging (MRI)
            - Noninvasive study to look at cardiac structures
            - Infants and young or uncooperative children need sedation or anesthesia to accomplish study

Management

- Prioritize nursing diagnosis and problem list as above
- Management of congestive heart failure

  - Optimize cardiac output
  - Optimize balance between pulmonary and systemic circulations
  - Optimize nutrition and growth
  - Avoid intercurrent infections
- Surgical repairs
  - Some defects now treated with cardiac catheterization
    - PDA closures
      - In all but neonates
      - Coils delivered by catheter and placed in PDA
    - ASD closure
      - Device placed by catheter in the ASD
      - Patient must be big enough for safe placement of large catheter to deliver device
    - Opening of stenotic pulmonary or aortic valves
      - Catheter passed across valve and balloon blown up to widen outflow
    - Postprocedure monitoring
      - Bleeding from catheter entry points
        - Extremity straight and still as ordered postprocedure
      - Perfusion distal to catheter entry points
      - Signs and symptoms of infection at catheter entry points
  - Most require cardiopulmonary bypass (CPB)
    - The heart can be stopped, opened, and worked on with maintenance of oxygenation and blood flow to the tissues
      - The heart itself does not receive blood flow
    - Avoids entry of air into the circulation when heart opened
    - Requires blood thinner to limit clotting in the bypass circuit
    - PDA and coarctation of aorta do not require cardiopulmonary bypass
    - CPB initiates a systemic inflammatory response (to the artificial tubing and machinery)
  - Most repairs via midline sternotomy incision
    - Chest tubes for postoperative drainage of thorax
      - Maintenance of suction, water seal, or both
      - Avoidance of leaks in system
      - Careful record of amount and consistency of drainage
    - Dressing changes as ordered

        - Early identification and treatment of local and deep infections
        - 4–6 weeks of limited activities to avoid injury or reinjury to healing sternum
            - May have temporary pacing wires in place in case of dysrhythmia
        - Promote coughing, deep breathing, walking for pulmonary toilet once off mechanical ventilator
        - PDA and coarctation most often via lateral thoracotomy
    - Single-stage repairs
        - Full repair with one surgery
    - Palliations with multistage repairs
        - Shunts or bands to augment or limit pulmonary blood flow
            - May not have normal oxygen saturations after palliations
        - Later full repair or continuation of staged repairs
        - Many complex congenital heart defects can never be fully repaired
            - Goal is to minimize workload on heart
                - Achieve near-normal systemic saturations
                - Create best repair that is surgically possible
        - Cardiac transplantation may be an option

Outcomes and Follow-up

- Failure of medical management of CHF
    - Points to timing for surgical repair
- Surgical morbidity and mortality
    - Highly dependent on age of child, condition, congenital defect, associated anomalies
    - Reoperations required for some
        - Replacement of nongrowing tissues
        - Readdressing narrowed or regurgitant valves
        - Residual holes
- Postoperative infections
    - Rare but can be additional cause of morbidity and mortality
- Lifelong follow-up with cardiologist
    - Even if uncomplicated full repair
- Routine follow-up with primary care provider

- Bacterial endocarditis prophylaxis
  - For those with significant residual heart disease or implanted artificial material
  - Antibiotics immediately before and after procedures that create high risk of introducing bacteria into the bloodstream (e.g., dental work)

KAWASAKI DISEASE

Description

- An acute, systemic vasculitis in children
- Characterized by
  - Fever
  - Rash
  - Conjunctivitis
  - Inflammation of the mucous membranes
  - Swollen lymph glands in the neck
  - Inflammation of arteries

Etiology

- Not well understood
- Likely genetic predisposition and environmental trigger
  - May be postinfectious, but mechanism not well delineated

Incidence and Demographics

- About 4,000 cases in the United States each year
- 80% of patients < 5 years of age
- More common in boys than girls

Risk Factors

- Asian ancestry at higher risk

Prevention and Screening

- No prevention or screening indicated

Assessment

Physical Exam

- Classic symptoms
  - High fever
  - Rash
  - Swollen hands and feet with peeling of palms and soles
  - Conjunctivitis: irritation and redness of sclera
  - Swollen lymph glands in the neck
  - Swollen, red, dry, cracked, and peeling lips
  - Red, coated, pitted, inflamed tongue ("strawberry" tongue)
- May have new murmur, but this is rare

Diagnostic Studies

- Cardiac echocardiography to evaluate coronary arteries
  - Coronary aneurysms can develop
  - Typically develop over time, not often present at beginning of illness
- Evaluation for other cause of illness
  - Blood and urine cultures sent for differential diagnosis

Management

Nonpharmacological Treatment

- Identification of disease as above
  - Cardiology and infectious disease specialists often involved
- Education of family about disease process and treatments
- Continued surveillance with echocardiogram for development of coronary artery aneurysms

Pharmacological Treatment

- Intravenous immunoglobulin
  - Pretreatment with acetaminophen, diphenhydramine, or both, as ordered
  - Administer per hospital policy
  - Careful titration of rate of infusion as per hospital policy
    - Large volume to infuse; monitor intake vs. output, urine output, and cardiorespiratory exams closely during infusion

- Aspirin
  - For antiinflammatory effects
  - Education of family to not use aspirin for routine fever or pain management because of risk of Reye's syndrome

Outcomes and Follow-up

- Mortality < 1%
- Recurrence rare (< 2%)
- 15%–25% with coronary sequelae
  - Continued aspirin therapy if coronary artery aneurysms present
- Emphasize importance of lifelong specialty care follow-up

RHEUMATIC FEVER

Description

- Acute, inflammatory, autoimmune complication of Group A beta-hemolytic streptococcal (GABHS) infection
- Characterized by joint pain, chorea, attack of the heart valves, skin nodules

Etiology

- Autoimmune response
- Post-GABHS infection—classically "strep throat"
  - Often untreated or incompletely treated GABHS infection

Incidence and Demographics

- Highest incidence among 5- to 15-year-olds
  - Higher rates of GABHS infection
- No currently available statistics for rates of attack
- Much more common in developing countries

Risk Factors

- Untreated or undertreated GABHS infection
- Previous occurrence of rheumatic fever

Prevention and Screening

- No prevention or screening indicated

Assessment

Physical Exam

- Typical physical findings:
    - Red, cracked, dry, inflamed, peeling lips
    - Conjunctival injection
    - Strawberry tongue
    - Tender joints
        - May be unwilling to walk
        - Multiple joints involved
        - Affected joints can change daily
    - Swollen, inflamed hands and feet with peeling of soles and palms
    - Chorea: random gyrating movements of body
        - Late symptom but on occasion is only symptom
    - New murmur
        - Or acquired heart disease on cardiac echocardiography

Diagnostic Studies

- ECG changes
    - Prolonged PR interval most common abnormality
- Evidence of inflammation
    - Elevated erythrocyte sedimentation rate (ESR) or C-reactive protein (CRP)
- Evidence of recent streptococcal infection
    - Positive throat culture
        - Rapid test not enough
    - Rising antistreptolysin titer (ASO)
- Evaluation for other causes
    - Infections
    - Autoimmune diseases such as juvenile rheumatoid arthritis

Management

Nonpharmacologic Treatment

- Bed rest until resolution of acute inflammation

Pharmacologic Treatment

- Antibiotics to eradicate the streptococcal infection

- Aspirin as antiinflammatory
    - Rapid improvement with initiation of aspirin
- Antacids for stomach protection

Outcome and Follow-up

- Rheumatic heart disease and rheumatic fever caused > 3,200 deaths in 2004—all ages
- Activity limitations depend on degree of heart damage
    - Attack is usually to the valves
    - Mitral and aortic valves most susceptible
    - Risk of further valve disease with repeated attacks of rheumatic fever
- High incidence of recurrent attacks
    - Secondary prophylaxis
        - Continued therapy with penicillin
        - For at least 10 years since last attack *and* at least until 21 years of age
- In-depth education and discussion re: importance of penicillin regimen and risk of recurrent attack
- Difficult to maintain daily drug therapy when child is well and feels fine
    - Daily oral medication or monthly depot injections
        - May try different forms at different ages and developmental stages
        - Advantage of thinking about therapy only once monthly vs. pain of injection
- Continued follow-up with pediatric cardiologist, then transition to adult cardiology care providers

REFERENCES

Ball, J. W., Bindler, R. C., & Cowen, K. J. (2010). *Child health nursing: Partnering with children and families* (2nd ed.). East Rutherford, NJ: Prentice Hall.

Bowden, V. R., & Greenberg, C. S. (2010). *Children and their families: The continuum of care* (2nd ed.). Philadelphia: Lippincott Williams & Wilkins.

Fischbach, F., & Dunning, M. B. (2009). *A manual of laboratory and diagnostic tests* (8th ed.). Philadelphia: Lippincott Williams & Wilkins.

Hagan, J. F., Shaw, J. S., & Duncan, P. M. (Eds.). (2007). *Bright futures: Guidelines for health supervision of infants, children, and adolescents* (3rd ed.). Elk Grove Village, IL: American Academy of Pediatrics.

Hazinski, M. F. (Ed.). (2012). *Nursing care of the critically ill child* (4th ed.). Philadelphia: Mosby.

Hockenberry, M. J., & Wilson, D. (2011). *Wong's nursing care of infants and children* (9th ed.). St. Louis, MO: Elsevier/Mosby.

Joint Commission, The. (2010). *Meeting the Joint Commission's 2011 national patient safety goals.* Oakbrook Terrace, IL: Joint Commission Resources.

National Association of Pediatric Nurse Practitioners, Society of Pediatric Nurses, American Nurses Association. (2008). *Pediatric nursing: Scope and standards of practice.* Silver Spring, MD: Nursesbooks.org.

Park, M. K. (Ed.). (2008). *Pediatric cardiology for practitioners.* Philadelphia: Mosby Elsevier.

Pillitteri, A. (2010). *Maternal & child health nursing: Care of the childbearing and childrearing family* (6th ed.). Philadelphia: Lippincott Williams & Wilkins.

Tschudy, M. M., Arcara, K. M., Johns Hopkins Hospital, & Children's Medical and Surgical Center. (2012). *The Harriet Lane handbook: A manual for pediatric house officers* (19th ed.). Philadelphia: Elsevier Mosby.

Wilson, B. A., Shannon, M. T., & Shields, K. (2012). *Pearson's nurse's drug guide 2012.* New York: Pearson Education.

CHAPTER 11

GASTROINTESTINAL DISORDERS

Clara J. Richardson, MSN, RN-BC

DEVELOPMENTAL CHARACTERISTICS OF THE PEDIATRIC GASTROINTESTINAL SYSTEM

- Swallowing is an automatic reflex until age 3 months.
- Striated muscle of the throat is not voluntarily controlled.
  - Starts developing at about 6 weeks
  - Not completely developed until age 6 months
- Small amount of saliva secreted until age 2–3 months
  - Glands not full size or fully functional until age 2 years
- Extrusion reflex until age 4 months
- Stomach size and shape
  - Faster emptying time
  - Round until age 2 years
  - Adult-like elongated shape by age 7 years
- Liver immature with decreased ability to store glycogen
  - Prone to hypoglycemia

CLEFT LIP AND PALATE

Description

Cleft lip is defined as unilateral or bilateral separation of the upper lip, which may extend into the upper jaw and the upper gum. The external nose, nasal cartilages, and nasal septum may also be affected. Cleft palate is an opening in the roof of the mouth involving just the soft palate or both soft and hard palates.

Etiology

Orofacial clefts are due to lack of cellular growth, failure of fusion during the embryonic period, or both. It is estimated that 3 to 14 genes contribute to cleft lip and palate. Lip formation occurs between the 6th and 8th weeks of gestation, while palate formation takes place between the 7th and 12th weeks.

Incidence and Demographics

The incidence of cleft lip, with or without cleft palate, is 1 in 700 live births and is more common in males. Cleft palate without cleft lip has an incidence of 1 in 2,500 live births and is more common in females.

Cleft lip and palate together occur more frequently in Asians, Native Americans, and Aboriginal Australians. Cleft lip alone occurs more frequently in Africans and those of African descent.

Risk Factors

- Maternal obesity
- Maternal alcohol abuse, especially binge drinking
- Maternal diabetes prior to pregnancy
- Maternal use of corticosteroids during early pregnancy
- Maternal cigarette smoking during pregnancy
- Maternal folic acid deficiency
- Maternal use of phenytoin (Dilantin) or valproic acid (Depakote, Depokene), topiramate (Topamax), methotrexate
- Maternal exposure to solvents such as carbon tetrachloride, tetrachloroethylene, trichloroethylene; triazine herbicide; pollutants such as chloroform, methyl mercury, and hazardous waste products

Prevention and Screening

Prevention is aimed at avoidance of risk factors. Folic acid supplementation should begin pre-pregnancy. Screening involves examination for physical signs in all newborns.

Assessment

History

- Familial history
- Prenatal history

Physical Exam

- Visualization of cleft lip
- Visualization or palpation of cleft palate
- Nasal regurgitation of feeding

Diagnostic Studies

- May be diagnosed in utero on ultrasound by 13–14 weeks gestation

Management

Invasive Treatment

- Timing is controversial
- Cleft lip repair at 6 weeks to 3 months
- Cleft palate commonly repaired at 6–12 months
- May involve several revisions by plastic surgeon to improve physical appearance
- May need myringotomy tube placement because of frequent bouts of otitis media
- May require bone grafts to support teeth and palate revisions to correct hypernasal speech

Nonpharmacologic Treatment

- Orthodontist to realign teeth
- Audiologist to evaluate for hearing defects
- Speech pathologist to treat speech problems
- Mental health professional to support child and family coping
- Lactation consultant for breastfeeding support
- Preoperative care
  - Variation of position for breastfeeding
  - Use of breast pump to initiate let-down
  - Special nipples, bottles, squeezable tubes
  - High-calorie formula
  - Frequent burping
  - Secretion management with bulb syringe

    - Practice with postoperative feeding methods and restraints
    - Weight monitoring
- Postoperative care
    - Avoid prone position with cleft lip repair
    - Possibly elbow restraints to prevent suture irritation
    - Clean lip sutures with saline and rinse mouth after feedings
    - Silicone tape and scar-minimizing gels for several weeks
    - Gentle aspiration of excess secretions
    - Liquid or pureed foods after cleft palate repair
    - Avoid objects in mouth such as pacifiers, straws, spoons after cleft palate repair

Pharmacologic Treatment

- Postoperative pain management
- Possibly postoperative sedation to keep infant calm and prevent strain on lip sutures from crying
- Antibiotic ointment on lip suture line

Patient and Family Education

- Nature of defect and treatment plan
- Feeding techniques
- Signs of dehydration and inadequate nutritional intake
- Postoperative care
- Pain management
- Massage to minimize lip scarring starting at about 2 weeks after surgery
- Available support groups, local and online

Outcomes and Follow-up

- The child will show no signs of dehydration.
- The child will exhibit adequate growth.
- The child will attain normal developmental milestones.
- The child is comfortable and rests quietly with effective pain management.
- The child will heal with minimum scarring.
- The child will receive the services of a multidisciplinary team.
- The family will exhibit attachment behaviors.
- The family will verbalize an understanding of defect and treatment plan.
- The family will demonstrate successful feeding strategies.

- The family will demonstrate postoperative care strategies.
- The family will return for regular follow-up with the craniofacial team.

TRACHEOESOPHAGEAL FISTULA (TEF) AND ESOPHAGEAL ATRESIA (EA)

Description

Tracheoesophageal fistula (TEF) is a congenital malformation consisting of a connection between the trachea and the esophagus. In a related congenital defect, esophageal atresia (EA), the esophagus ends in a blind pouch with no connection to the stomach. These may occur separately, but most often occur in combination.

Etiology

Respiratory and digestive tubes develop into distinct structures between the 4th and 5th weeks of gestation. When this development is disrupted, TEF and/or EA occur.

Incidence and Demographics

The incidence of these defects is 1 in 3,500 live births. Approximately 88% of cases involve both TEF and EA. Isolated EA accounts for 8% of cases and isolated TEF for another 4%. About half of EA/TEF cases occur as a component of VACTERL-associated anomalies (vertebral, anal, cardiac, tracheal, esophageal, rectal, and limb).

Risk Factors

- Prematurity
- Low birth weight
- Maternal diabetes

Prevention and Screening

No specific prevention has been identified. Screening consists of identification of pertinent history and physical signs, preferably before first feeding. An attempt to pass a feeding tube will be unsuccessful, and further diagnostic testing should begin.

Assessment

History

- Maternal history of polyhydramnios, excess amniotic fluid
- Prenatal ultrasound without visualization of stomach

Physical Exam

- Excessive mucus
- Apnea
- Coughing, choking, cyanosis on feeding
- Respiratory distress with crackles
- Inability to pass catheter into stomach with EA

Diagnostic Studies

- Radiography
- Contrast studies
- Bronchoscopy
- 3-dimensional CT scan

Management

Invasive Treatment

- Surgical ligation of TEF fistula and anastomosis of the esophagus with EA
- When the end of the esophagus is too short to connect, anastomosis is delayed until growth occurs
- Temporary cervical esophagostomy allows drainage of secretions, and gastrostomy tube feedings provide nutrition until repair

Nonpharmacologic Treatment

- Preoperative care
- Nothing by mouth
- Intermittent or continuous suction to clear secretion in pouch
- Supine or right-side position at 30°
- Thermoregulation
- Supplemental oxygen as needed
- Airway management as needed
- Skin care with esophagostomy
- Possible gastrostomy
- Postoperative care
- Premeasured and marked catheter for suctioning
- Radiant warmer
- Chest tube
- Nasogastric tube

- Parenteral nutrition
- Nonnutritive sucking
- Progression to oral or gastrostomy feedings
- Monitor for signs of leak at suture line, including respiratory distress or sepsis
- Monitor for signs of esophageal stricture, including coughing, regurgitation, and recurrent aspiration
- Esophageal dilation to treat stricture

Pharmacologic Treatment

- Intravenous fluids to maintain fluid and electrolyte balance
- Preoperative antibiotics to treat or prevent aspiration pneumonia
- Postoperative pain management

Patient and Family Education

- Nature of defect and treatment plan
- Home care, including feeding technique, promotion of normal development
- Strategies for infection prevention
    - Signs of esophageal stricture including failure to thrive, difficulty swallowing
- Dysphagia
- Cardiopulmonary resuscitation and choking relief

Outcomes and Follow-up

- The child will maintain a patent airway with effective respirations.
- The child will maintain effective thermoregulation.
- The child will attain appropriate growth and developmental milestones.
- The child will not experience complications such as leak at anastomosis, esophageal stricture, dysphagia, gastroesophageal reflux disease, tracheomalacia, respiratory compromise, oral hypersensitivity, or feeding aversion.
- The family will verbalize an understanding of the defect and the treatment plan.
- The family will demonstrate home-care strategies.
- The family will identify signs of complications.
- The family will verbalize an understanding of CPR and choking relief.

IMPERFORATE ANUS

Description

Imperforate anus is a congenital anorectal malformation with varying degrees of severity classified as low, intermediate, or high. The rectum may end in a blind pouch, or it may have fistulas to the genitourinary system or to the perineum.

Etiology

This defect is due to abnormal fetal development during the 6th week of gestation when the rectum fails to assume its normal position.

Incidence and Demographics

Imperforate anus occurs in approximately 1 in 4,000–5,000 live births and is slightly more common in males. The defect may occur alone or as a component of VACTERL-associated anomalies (vertebral, anal, cardiac, tracheal, esophageal, rectal, and limb). Approximately 50% of children with intermediate or high imperforate anus will have long-term problems related to soiling, incontinence, or constipation. Many children with repaired low defects have constipation.

Risk Factors

No risk factors have been identified.

Prevention and Screening

There is no prevention. Screening for physical signs is done on all newborns.

Assessment

History

- No specific history

Physical Exam

- Absent or very small anal opening
- Absence of meconium or presence in urine
- Abdominal distention
- Flat perineum
- Absence of midline intergluteal groove

Diagnostic Studies

- Abdominal and pelvic ultrasound show malformation
- IV pyelogram and voiding cystourethrogram may show contact with urinary system
- MRI
- Radiography

Management

Invasive Treatment

- Depends on extent of defect
- Moving perineal fistula opening to sphincter and enlarging rectal opening
- Posterior sagittal anorectoplasty (PSARP)
- Depending on severity, a temporary colostomy
- Closure of other fistulas
- Anoplasty, attaching the rectum to the created anus

Nonpharmacologic Treatment

- Rectal irrigations to prevent contamination of surgical site
- Manual dilation with a metallic dilator
- Enemas to prevent constipation
- Bowel training program for continued bowel incontinence, including daily bowel irrigations, diet modification, and fiber

Pharmacologic Treatment

- Intravenous fluids to maintain fluid and electrolyte balance
- Pain management
- Stool softeners or laxatives

Patient and Family Education

- Defect, surgery, treatment plan, possible complications
- Diagnostic tests
- Postoperative pain management
- Care of wound and peritoneum
- Colostomy care
- Manual dilation and enema administration
- Medication administration
- Bowel training program

Outcomes and Follow-up

- The child will exhibit signs of pain relief.
- The child will not experience complications such as anal stricture, long-term bowel incontinence, recurrent rectourinary fistula, mucosal prolapse.
- The child will have normal bowel pattern without soilage, incontinence, or constipation.
- The family will verbalize an understanding of the defect and the treatment plan.
- The family will demonstrate care of wound, perineum, and colostomy.
- The family will demonstrate manual dilation and enema administration.
- The family will verbalize an understanding of the bowel-training program.

HYPERTROPHIC PYLORIC STENOSIS

Description

Pyloric stenosis is a narrowing and lengthening of the pyloric canal between the stomach and the duodenum that usually develops in the first 2 to 8 weeks of life, causing stomach dilation and hyperperistalsis.

Etiology

The exact cause is unknown. The pylorus muscle becomes thickened, resulting in progressive narrowing and lengthening of the pyloric canal and causing outlet obstruction.

Incidence and Demographics

The incidence is approximately 1 in 500 live births. It is more common in firstborn children, males, and Whites.

Risk Factors

- Family history
- Maternal smoking
- Prone sleeping
- Erythromycin during neonatal period

Prevention and Screening

No specific prevention, but avoidance of risk factors. Screening consists of evaluation of physical signs.

Assessment

History

- Initially infant feeds without difficulty, prior to onset
- Vomiting without bile after feeding, which progresses in frequency and becomes projectile
- Vomiting may be blood-tinged, but without bile
- Hunger and irritability
- Growth failure
- Weight loss

Physical Exam

- Hard, mobile, nontender, olive-shaped mass just right of umbilicus
- Visible peristaltic waves moving from left to right
- Signs of dehydration

Diagnostic Studies

- Abdominal ultrasound will show the enlarged pylorus
- Radiography will show gastric distention
- Upper GI will demonstrate delayed gastric emptying and narrow pyloric channel
- Blood studies show:
    - Decreased sodium, potassium, and chloride
    - Elevated pH, bicarbonate, and blood urea nitrogen

Management

Invasive Treatment

- Laparoscopic pyloromyotomy: longitudinal incision of the pylorus to allow bulge and relieve obstruction

Nonpharmacologic Treatment

- Possibly nasogastric tube before surgery to decompress stomach
- Gradual progression of feeding after surgery
- Frequent burping

Pharmacologic Treatment

- Preoperative and postoperative intravenous therapy to correct fluid and electrolyte imbalances
- Pain management

Patient and Family Education

- Nature of defect and treatment plan
- Feeding progression
- Pain management
- Some postoperative vomiting is expected for 24–48 hours

Outcomes and Follow-up

- The child's fluid and electrolyte balance will be restored before surgery.
- The child's incision site will show evidence of healing without infection.
- The child will reestablish a normal feeding pattern.
- The child will experience effective pain management.
- The child will show no signs of dehydration.
- The child will regain lost weight and demonstrate adequate growth.
- The family will an verbalize understanding of the defect, treatment plan, feeding progression, and pain management.

GASTROESOPHAGEAL REFLUX

Description

Gastroesophageal reflux (GER) is the physiologic passage of gastric contents into the esophagus. It becomes gastroesophageal reflux disease (GERD) when the reflux causes complications such as esophagitis, recurrent respiratory problems, or growth failure.

Etiology

Gastroesophageal reflux occurs when the lower esophageal sphincter relaxes or when the sphincter tone does not respond to changes in abdominal pressure, allowing gastric contents to pass into the esophagus or the oropharynx.

Incidence and Demographics

Gastroesophageal reflux peaks at approximately 4 months of age, with up to 40% of infants regurgitating more than half of their meals on a daily basis. The majority of these infants outgrow this by 1 year of age. About 5%–10% of older children complain about reflux symptoms on a weekly basis.

Risk Factors

- Family history
- Obesity
- High-fat diet
- Eating quickly
- Marked developmental delay
- Cerebral palsy
- Repaired esophageal atresia
- Cystic fibrosis
- Prematurity
- Bronchopulmonary dysplasia
- Smoke exposure may increase acid reflux in infants, along with wheezing or apparent life-threatening events.

Prevention and Screening

Prevention in infants includes avoidance of overfeeding. For older children, weight control and healthy diet are important. Screening consists of feeding history, pattern of vomiting, medical history, family history, and growth measurements.

Assessment

History

- Risk factors
- Growth failure
- Coughing, wheezing, stridor, gagging, choking with feedings
- Recurrent regurgitation, spitting up, vomiting
- Asthma
- Recurrent pneumonia

Physical Exam

- Infants
    - Feeding refusal
    - Arching
    - Irritability
    - Poor weight gain
    - Apnea or apparent life-threatening event (ALTE)

- Older children
  - Heartburn
  - Abdominal or chest pain
  - Dysphagia or feeding refusal
  - Blood-tinged vomiting
  - Wheezing, stridor, cough
  - Hoarseness

Diagnostic Studies

- Diagnosis based on history and physical exam
- Possible esophageal pH monitoring to evaluate effectiveness of treatment
- Possible multiple intraluminal impedance measurement with pH monitoring to show acidic and nonacidic reflux and associated respiratory symptoms

Management

Invasive Treatment

- For chronic relapsing GERD
  - Nissen fundoplication antireflux surgery
  - Proximal portion of stomach wrapped around esophagus
  - Recreates lower esophageal sphincter to prevent reflux

Nonpharmacologic Treatment

- Infants
  - Smaller, more frequent feeding
  - Thickened formula
  - Elevate head of crib
  - Prone position after feeding for infants who are awake
  - Supine position for all sleeping infants to decrease risk for sudden infant death syndrome
- Older children
  - Healthy diet
  - Weight control
  - Elevate head of bed
  - Prone or left-side sleeping
  - Avoid late-night eating
  - Avoid smoking and alcohol

- Avoid NSAIDs

Pharmacologic Treatment

- Histamine$_2$ receptor antagonists (H_2RAs)
  - Ranitidine (Zantac)
  - Famotidine (Pepcid)
- Protein pump inhibitors (PPIs)
  - Lansoprazole (Prevacid)
  - Omeprazole (Prilosec)

Patient and Family Education

- Effects of gastroesophageal reflux and treatment plan
- Nonpharmacologic management
- Medication administration

Outcomes and Follow-up

- The child will not experience further symptoms.
- The child will attain growth measurements appropriate for his or her age.
- The child will not experience complications such as esophagitis, peptic stricture, delayed growth, dental caries, recurrent otitis media, pneumonia, asthma, changes to lining of esophagus, or esophageal cancer.
- The family will verbalize an understanding of the treatment plan, nonpharmacologic management, and medication administration.

HERNIA

Description

A hernia is a protrusion of an organ or organs through an opening. In congenital diaphragmatic hernia (CDH), the opening is in the diaphragm; in umbilical hernia, through the umbilical ring; and in inguinal hernia, through the processus vaginalis in males and through the round ligament in females.

Etiology

- Congenital diaphragmatic hernia happens between 8 and 10 weeks gestation with incomplete fusion of the diaphragm resulting in protrusion of abdominal contents into the chest cavity, causing compression and hypoplasia of the lung, with possible arrested lung growth and pulmonary hypertension.

- Umbilical hernia is due to opening of abdominal muscle at the umbilicus.
- Inguinal hernias occur during the 8th month of gestation when the structures fail to close.

Incidence and Demographics

- Approximately half of children with hernias have chromosomal abnormalities, congenital heart disease, or neural tube defects.
- Congenital diaphragmatic hernias have a reported incidence of 1 in every 2,200 live births, occur more frequently in males, and have an 80%–90% survival rate.
- Umbilical hernias are the most common type and occur in 10%–30% of births. Incidence is higher in Blacks, infants with low birth weight, and preterm infants. Many close spontaneously in the first 12–18 months of life.
- Inguinal hernias occur in 1%–5% of the population, more often in males, and more often on the right side. They usually present within the first year of life.

Risk Factors

- Preterm birth
- Low birth weight
- Ventriculoperitoneal shunts
- Peritoneal dialysis
- Cystic fibrosis
- Hypospadias

Prevention and Screening

No prevention has been identified. Screening for CDH is prenatal ultrasound.

Assessment

History

- Prenatal polyhydramnios with CDH
- Respiratory distress in the first few hours of life with CDH
- Bulge at umbilicus with crying or straining

Physical Exam

- Congenital diaphragmatic hernia
    - Cyanosis with severe respiratory distress
    - Absent breath sounds on affected side
    - Scaphoid abdomen
    - Barrel-shaped chest

    - Heartbeat displaced to right
    - Persistent pulmonary hypertension
- Umbilical hernia presents as a painless umbilical bulge that enlarges with crying or straining.
- Inguinal hernia
    - Painless bulge in the scrotum or the labia that may be reduced into the peritoneal cavity
    - If the hernia is incarcerated, not reducible, the testicle or the intestine may become ischemic. Incarcerated hernia is a medical emergency.

Diagnostic Studies

- Prenatal ultrasound or MRI; for CDH, prenatal MRI
- Chest radiography
- Echocardiogram
- Scrotal ultrasound

Management

Invasive Treatment

- Congenital diaphragmatic hernia
    - A few medical centers do fetal surgery for CDH
    - Surgical repair of diaphragm, moving abdominal contents into the abdominal cavity
- Umbilical hernia may be surgically corrected if it does not resolve spontaneously by 3–5 years of age
- Inguinal hernia
    - Surgical correction to prevent risk of incarceration
    - Incarceration requires immediate surgical repair

Nonpharmacologic Treatment

- Congenital diaphragmatic hernia
    - Possible intubation and ventilation
    - Supplemental oxygen
    - Possible high-frequency ventilation with extracorporeal membrane oxygenation (ECMO)
    - Permissive hypercapnia to reduce lung injury
    - Nasogastric tube for low continuous suction
    - Arterial and central venous lines

- Thermoregulation
- Skin care to avoid breakdown
- Minimize environmental stimulation

- Umbilical hernia
    - Pressure dressing for 48 hours after surgical repair
    - Avoid strenuous activity or play for 2–3 weeks after surgery
- Inguinal hernia
    - Manual reduction before elective repair
    - Keep incision site clean and dry
    - Avoid strenuous activity or play for 2–3 weeks

Pharmacologic Treatment

- Congenital diaphragmatic hernia
    - Sedation and paralysis
    - Blood pressure stabilization with dopamine or dobutamine
    - Intravenous therapy to maintain fluid and electrolyte balance
- Pain management

Patient and Family Education

- Nature of defect and treatment plan
- Signs of incarceration such as irritability, refusal to eat, vomiting, darkening of umbilical hernia, mass that is tense and irreducible
- Measures to reduce inguinal hernia
- Postoperative care

Outcomes and Follow-up

- The child with CDH will maintain open airway and effective respirations.
- The child will not experience complication of CDH such as chronic lung disease, recurrent pulmonary hypertension, growth failure, gastroesophageal reflux disease, cognitive impairment, musculoskeletal deformities, or delayed developmental milestones.
- The child will receive prompt medical attention for incarceration.
- The child's incision site will heal without complications.
- The family will verbalize an understanding of the defect and the treatment plan.
- The family will demonstrate hernia reduction.
- The family will identify signs of incarceration.
- The family will verbalize an understanding of home care.

INTUSSUSCEPTION

Description

Intussusception is the telescoping of one portion of the intestine into the immediately adjacent distal portion. The most common site is the ileocecal valve.

Etiology

Intussusception may be caused by hypertrophy of intestinal tissue after a viral infection. When the invagination occurs, the mesentery is pulled into the lumen, causing vascular compression. This compression may lead to inflammation, edema, necrosis, and perforation.

Incidence and Demographics

Intussusception is seen most frequently in children between 3 months and 6 years of age. Most cases occur before age 1 year, with a peak occurrence at 5–9 months. It is more common in males and has a higher incidence in spring and autumn months.

Risk Factors

- Viral infection
- Abdominal trauma
- Postoperative abdomen
- Cystic fibrosis
- Nephrotic syndrome
- Meckel diverticulum
- Henoch-Schoenlein purpura

Prevention and Screening

No prevention or screening strategies have been identified.

Assessment

History

- Recent viral infection
- Episodes of intermittent, colicky abdominal pain
- Vomiting
- Anorexia
- Weight loss

- Diarrhea or rectal bleeding
- Bloody, mucous stools ("currant jelly stools")

Physical Exam

- Abdominal distention
- Palpable sausage-shaped mass in right upper abdomen
- Lethargy
- Pallor
- Transient hypertension
- Rectal mucus and blood

Diagnostic Studies

- Radiography shows minimal gas in the right abdomen and ascending colon
- Ultrasound and CT scan show alternating intestinal rings
- Intraperitoneal air with bowel perforation

Management

Invasive Treatment

- Manual reduction if nonpharmacologic measures unsuccessful

Nonpharmacologic Treatment

- Radiologist-guided pneumatic air reduction with or without water-soluble contrast media
- Ultrasound-guided hydrostatic saline enema
- Postoperative incisional care

Pharmacologic Treatment

- Intravenous therapy to maintain fluid and electrolyte balance
- Antibiotics to prevent infection or treat peritonitis
- Pain management

Patient and Family Education

- Nature of defect and treatment plan
- Pain management
- Home care after surgery
- Possibility of recurrence

Outcomes and Follow-up

- The child's intussusception will be reduced with enema.
- The child will not experience perforation, peritonitis, or recurrence.
- The child will experience effective pain management.
- The family will verbalize an understanding of the defect and the treatment plan.
- The family will verbalize an understanding of home care and the possibility of recurrence.

GASTROENTERITIS

Description

Gastroenteritis is acute infectious diarrhea.

Etiology

Gastroenteritis is spread by fecal–oral route. Common bacterial causes are *Escherichia coli, Salmonella, Shigella, Campylobacter, Yersinia, Aeromonas, Clostridium difficile*, and *Staphylococcus aureus*. Viral agents include rotavirus, astrovirus, calicivirus, some adenoviruses, and some picornaviruses. *Giardia lamblia, Cryptosporidium, Isospora belli, Microsporida, Strongyloides,* and *Entamoeba histolytica* are parasitic causes.

Incidence and Demographics

Foodborne pathogens include *Escherichia coli, Salmonella, Yersinia, Campylobacter, Clostridium,* and *Staphylococcus.* Children may also contact *Salmonella, Yersinia,* and *Campylobacter* from pets such as dogs, cats, hamsters, turtles, and iguanas. In the United States, gastroenteritis is responsible for more than 1.5 million outpatient visits, 200,000 hospitalizations, and 300 deaths per year.

Risk Factors

- Immunocompromised state
- Poor hygiene
- Poor sanitation
- Lack of clean water
- Lack of refrigeration
- Nutritional deficiency
- Crowded living conditions

Prevention and Screening

- Maintaining good hygiene
- Regular handwashing
- Thorough cooking of food
- Maintaining food at appropriate temperatures
- Healthy diet
- Diaper disposal in occlusive bags
- Rotavirus vaccine, with first dose between 6 and 14 weeks of age

Assessment

History

- Diarrhea
- Vomiting
- Decreased urine output
- No rotavirus vaccine
- Exposure to animals, birds
- Exposure to untreated drinking water
- Consumption of processed meat
- Recent antibiotic therapy
- Recent travel to developing country

Physical Exam

- Fever
- Anorexia
- Headache
- Abdominal cramping
- Muscle aches
- Lethargy
- Dry mucus membranes
- Dark, sunken eyes
- Lack of tearing
- Loss of skin elasticity
- Increased pulse rate
- Decreased capillary refill

- Cold, mottled extremities
- Sunken fontanel

Diagnostic Studies

- Stool culture to identify causative agent with fever or blood or mucus in stool
- Viral antigen stool test
- Urine specific gravity to identify dehydration
- Complete blood count with differential, serum electrolytes, creatinine, blood urea nitrogen

Management

Invasive Treatment

- No invasive management indicated

Nonpharmacologic Treatment

- Oral rehydration therapy (Pedialyte, Enfalyte), starting with small amounts and increasing slowly over a 4-hour period
- Avoid plain water, homemade sugar solution, carbonated beverages, fruit juice, gelatin, meat broth, caffeine
- Avoid the BRAT diet of bananas, rice, applesauce, toast or tea. This diet has proven to be high in carbohydrates and low in electrolytes, so it fails to provide needed nutrition.
- Continue breastfeeding
- If feedings are tolerated without vomiting, resume the age-appropriate diet within 4 hours of rehydration
- Meticulous skin care of diaper area
- Avoid taking rectal temperatures

Pharmacologic Treatment

- Intravenous fluids to replace lost fluid and to maintain fluid and electrolyte balance
- Antibiotics for *Shigella, Campylobacter, Vibrio cholera,* and *Clostridium difficile*
- Antiemetic, ondansetron (Zofran) for vomiting

Patient and Family Education

- Signs of dehydration
- Oral rehydration process
- Resumption of normal diet
- Skin care

- Avoid over-the-counter medications for vomiting or diarrhea.
- Strategies to prevent spread of infection
- Strategies to prevent future episodes

Outcomes and Follow-up

- The child will exhibit no signs of dehydration.
- The child will exhibit decrease in vomiting and diarrhea.
- The child will return to a normal diet as soon as possible.
- The child will maintain skin integrity.
- The family will verbalize an understanding of the education content.

HIRSCHSPRUNG DISEASE

Description

Hirschsprung disease is the absence of ganglion nerve cells in the distal colon, causing a functional bowel obstruction. The section of bowel proximal to the affected area becomes dilated; hence, the disorder is also called *aganglionic megacolon*.

Etiology

Hirschsprung disease is caused by failure of the ganglion cells to move through the neural crest during the 4th to 12th weeks of gestation. As the bowel distends, pressure on the bowel wall increases and blood flow decreases, leading to bacterial growth that can cause enterocolitis, and inflammation of the intestine and ulceration of the bowel wall.

Incidence and Demographics

The incidence of Hirschsprung disease is 1 in 5,000 live births and is higher in boys. The disease is limited to the rectosigmoid area in 80% of cases. The incidence rate of enterocolitis is approximately 30% and usually occurs within the first year after repair.

Risk Factors

- Family history

Prevention and Screening

No prevention. Screen newborns for passage of meconium, and evaluate neonates' bowel patterns.

Assessment

History

- Newborn period
    - Failure to pass meconium until after the first 72 hours of life
    - Feeding refusal
    - Bilious vomiting
- Infancy
    - Growth failure
    - Constipation
    - Diarrhea and vomiting episodes
- Childhood
    - Growth failure
    - Constipation
    - Foul smelling, ribbon-like stools

Physical Exam

- Pale, thin appearance
- Abdominal distention
- Visible peristalsis
- Palpable fecal mass
- Signs of enterocolitis include abdominal distention, explosive diarrhea, fever, and blood in the stool

Diagnostic Studies

- Radiography with contrast enema may show dilated bowel
- Anorectal manometry shows absence of internal anal sphincter relaxation
- Rectal biopsy confirms diagnosis by showing absence of ganglion cells

Management

Invasive Treatment

- Surgical resection of the aganglionic bowel and anastomosis of the proximal normal bowel to the anal canal, called ileoanal pull-through anastomosis
- Possibly surgical correction of anorectal stenosis, a common complication
- With enterocolitis or significantly dilated colon, colostomy to allow bowel to return to normal size
- Surgical pull-through 4 to 6 months after colostomy

Nonpharmacologic Treatment

- Preoperative care
  - Serial rectal saline irrigations to decompress and clean bowel
  - Serial measurement of abdominal circumference
  - Possible nutritional therapy with low-fiber, high-calorie, and high-protein diet or total parenteral nutrition to strengthen child prior to surgery
- Postoperative care
  - Nasogastric tube for suction
  - Intravenous fluids
  - Incisional care
  - Colostomy care
  - Avoid rectal medications and thermometers for 2–3 weeks
  - Manual dilations for several months to prevent stricture

Pharmacologic Treatment

- Antibiotics to prevent or treat infection
- Intravenous fluids to maintain fluid and electrolyte balance
- Pain management

Patient and Family Education

- Nature of disease and treatment plan
- Home care
- Colostomy care
- Manual dilation procedure
- Bowel retraining
- Constipation prevention strategies, including high-fiber diet

Outcomes and Follow-up

- The child will maintain fluid and electrolyte balance.
- The child will resume his or her usual diet.
- The child will show signs of wound healing.
- The child will exhibit normal bowel patterns.
- The child will exhibit growth appropriate for his or her age.
- The child will not experience complications such as constipation, incontinence, or enterocolitis.
- The family will verbalize an understanding of the disease and the treatment plan.

- The family will demonstrate incisional care, colostomy care, and manual dilation.
- The family will verbalize an understanding of constipation prevention.
- The family will verbalize signs of enterocolitis.

MALABSORPTION SYNDROMES

Description

Malabsorption syndromes are digestive disorders characterized by chronic diarrhea and impaired absorption of fluids and nutrients. Two common pediatric syndromes are celiac disease and short-bowel syndrome. Celiac disease, called gluten-sensitive enteropathy or celiac sprue, is an immune-related disorder with intestinal intolerance to dietary wheat gliadin and related proteins found in rye, barley, and oats. Short-bowel syndrome (SBS) is a decrease in the mucosal surface area of the intestine.

Etiology

The child with celiac disease is unable to completely digest the protein gluten. The small intestine absorbs these proteins, which then cause an inflammatory reaction targeting the mucosa. Damage to the mucosa results in villous atrophy and decreased surface area for absorption of fluid, electrolytes, and nutrients.

In infants, short-bowel syndrome is usually caused by necrotizing enterocolitis, volvulus, jejunal atresias, and gastroschisis. In older children, trauma and Crohn's disease may require bowel resection. Extensive resection results in malabsorption caused by decreased surface area.

Incidence and Demographics

The incidence of celiac disease is 1 in 3,000–4,000 people. It is more prevalent in females and in Europe, but rarely seen in Asians or Blacks. The mean age of presentation is 7 years.

The incidence of SBS in children is 245 per 100,000 live births, and survival rates range from 73% to 89%.

Risk Factors

- Celiac disease
  - First-degree relative with the disease
  - Exposure to gluten in the first 3 months of life
  - Down syndrome
  - Rheumatoid arthritis
  - Type 1 diabetes mellitus

- Short-bowel syndrome
  - Prematurity
  - Bowel resection

Prevention and Screening

No specific prevention or screening is indicated, but breastfeeding has been shown to have a protective effect.

Assessment

History

- Celiac disease
  - Constipation or diarrhea
  - Flatulence
  - Steatorrhea
  - Foul-smelling stools
  - Growth failure
  - Irritability
  - Delayed menarche
  - Anorexia, nausea, vomiting
  - Abdominal pain, distension, bloating
- SBS
  - Diarrhea
  - Steatorrhea
  - Fatigue
  - Rectal bleeding
  - Vomiting or regurgitation
  - Abdominal pain, bloating

Physical Exam

- Celiac disease
  - Abdominal distention and pain
  - Pallor
  - Muscle wasting

- SBS
    - Pallor
    - Growth failure

Diagnostic Studies

- Celiac disease
    - IgA tissue transglutaminase (TTG)
    - Antiendomysium (EMA)
    - Endoscopic exam with duodenal biopsy
- SBS
    - Blood studies: anemia, iron deficiency
    - Upper GI
    - Colonoscopy

Management

Invasive treatment

- Celiac disease
    - No invasive treatment indicated
- SBS
    - Feeding tube placement: gastrostomy, gastrojejunal, or jejunostomy
    - Temporary small bowel ostomies
    - Serial transverse enteroplasty procedure (STEP) to lengthen and taper bowel
    - Intestinal transplant for permanent intestinal failure and liver injury resulting from long-term total parenteral nutrition

Nonpharmacologic Treatment

- Celiac disease
    - Gluten-free diet: no wheat, rye, barley, or commercial varieties of oats
    - Temporary lactose-free, low-fiber diet while bowel is inflamed
- SBS
    - Nonnutritive sucking, oral stimulation
    - Small amounts of oral feeding

Pharmacologic Treatment

- Celiac disease
    - Iron, folic acid, and fat-soluble vitamin supplements as needed

- SBS
    - Total parenteral nutrition (TPN) through a central line for a time
    - Gradual introduction of enteral nutrition of an easily absorbed formula administered continuously, rather than in bolus amounts
    - Periodic enteral antibiotics
    - Vitamin and mineral supplements
    - Proton pump inhibitors for increased gastric acid
    - Ursodeoxycholic acid to prevent gallstones with prolonged parenteral nutrition

Patient and Family Education

- Celiac disease
    - Disease process
    - Gluten-free diet
    - Complications of noncompliance
    - Risk of cross-contamination with kitchen utensils
    - Sources of gluten-free alternatives
    - Gluten-free eating at restaurants
    - Reading food labels
    - Available support groups
- SBS
    - Disease and treatment plan
    - Feeding management: TPN, enteral feeding
    - Oral stimulation strategies
    - Medication administration
    - Signs of complications

Outcomes and Follow-up

- Celiac disease
    - The child will experience relief of symptoms with a gluten-free diet.
    - The child will demonstrate healing of intestinal mucosa with increased tolerance of lactose and fiber.
    - The child will demonstrate adequate growth.
    - The family will verbalize an understanding of the disease process.
    - The family will identify sources of gluten and plan a diet to meet nutritional needs.
    - The child and family will receive ongoing nutritional counseling and support.

- SBS
  - The child will not experience complications of long-term TPN.
  - The child's small intestine will increase its tolerance of enteral feedings.
  - The child will demonstrate adequate growth.
  - The family will verbalize an understanding of the disease process and the treatment plan.
  - The family will demonstrate management of central line and enteral feeding.
  - The family will demonstrate effective medication administration.
  - The family will demonstrate oral stimulation techniques.

INGESTIONS AND POISONINGS

Description

Accidental or unintentional ingestion of toxic substances is one of the most common pediatric emergencies.

Etiology

Young children ingest substances because of their normal developmental curiosity and experimentation, imitation behavior, and misidentification of substances that look like familiar beverages or candy. Another cause is therapeutic error resulting in medication overdose.

Incidence and Demographics

Poison control centers report annual calls of more than one million ingestion cases in children younger than 6 years, 150,000–160,000 in 6- to 12-year-olds, and 160,000–175,000 in 13- to 19-year-olds. More than 90% of ingestions occur at home. The majority of cases are unintentional in young children, but about half in the adolescent population are intentional.

Common substances ingested are cosmetics and personal care products, cleaning substances, analgesics, foreign bodies, plants, topical treatments, cough and cold products, pesticides, vitamins, gastrointestinal preparations, antimicrobials, art and craft supplies, antihistamines, hormones, and hydrocarbons.

Risk Factors

- Access to toxic substances
- Lack of child-resistant medication containers
- Impulsiveness
- Young developmental age

- History of previous ingestion
- Lack of age-appropriate supervision
- Environmental change or chaos
- Parental mental illness, depression, social isolation
- Risk taking, peer pressure, and perceived personal crisis of adolescents

Prevention and Screening

- Family education
- Anticipatory guidance
- Household products and medications stored in locked units out of child's sight and reach
- Store substances in original containers
- Child-resistant packaging
- Call it medication, not candy
- Prevent child from seeing adult take medication
- Safe disposal of old or unused medications
- Teach children not to eat or drink anything that they cannot identify
- Evaluation of physical signs

Assessment

History

- History of ingestion or physical signs

Physical Exam

- Gastrointestinal signs
  - Abdominal pain
  - Vomiting
  - Diarrhea
  - Anorexia
- Respiratory and circulatory signs
  - Respirations may be depressed, labored, shallow, or rapid
  - Skin may be cool, clammy, pale, or cyanotic
  - Signs of shock
  - Slow capillary refill
  - Rapid, weak pulse
  - Decreased blood pressure

- Central nervous system signs
    - Seizures
    - Overstimulation or lethargy
    - Dizziness
    - Loss of consciousness
    - Coma
- Signs of corrosive ingestion
    - Edema of the lips, tongue, or pharynx
    - White or ulcerated mucosa
    - Burning in mouth, throat, or stomach
    - Vomiting
    - Blood in saliva
    - Drooling
    - Agitation
    - Signs of shock
- Signs of hydrocarbon ingestion
    - Nausea and vomiting
    - Coughing, gagging
    - Weakness
    - Lethargy
    - Respiratory distress

Diagnostic Studies

- Toxicology screening of blood or urine

Management

Invasive Treatment

- Hemodialysis and hemofiltration in severe cases

Nonpharmacologic Treatment

- Basic life support and resuscitation
- Intubation for child without adequate gag reflex or with altered mental status
- Cardiac monitoring
- Gastric lavage within 1 hour of ingestion with protected airway, possible sedation, and large-diameter tube

Pharmacologic Treatment

- Activated charcoal within 1 hour of ingestion unless child has unprotected airway, altered mental status, altered bowel function, caustic ingestion, hydrocarbon ingestion, foreign body ingestion
- Specific antidotes such as N-acetylcysteine (Mucomyst) for acetaminophen, naloxone for opioids, flumazenil for benzodiazepines
- Intravenous fluids to maintain fluid and electrolyte balance

Patient and Family Education

- Prevention strategies
- Developmental risk factors
- Medication dosing guidelines
- Physical signs of poisoning
- Universal poison control center number (1.800.222.1222)

Outcomes and Follow-up

- The child will recover without complications.
- The child will verbalize an understanding of poison prevention strategies.
- The child will not have future access to toxic substances.
- The child will not experience additional ingestions.
- The family will verbalize an understanding of the treatment plan.
- The family will verbalize an understanding of prevention strategies.
- The family will identify hazards in the home.
- The family will take steps to poison-proof the home.
- The family will identify the physical signs of poisoning.
- The family will post the poison control number near their telephone.

APPENDICITIS

Description

Inflammation of the vermiform appendix

Etiology

Appendicitis results when the lumen of the appendix is obstructed by fecalith (hardened stool), undigested food, swollen lymphatic tissue, or a bend in the lumen. The obstruction causes mucus to increase pressure in the lumen, leading to compression of the blood vessels with progressive inflammation. The process can progress to gangrenous appendicitis. A ruptured or perforated appendix can cause progressive peritonitis.

Incidence and Demographics

Incidence in children younger than 4 years of age is 1–2 per 10,000 children and 19–28 per 10,000 children in those younger than 14 years. The average age of occurrence is 10 years.

Risk Factors

No risk factors have been definitively identified, although individuals consuming diets high in sugars and low in fiber have shown increased incidence of appendicitis.

Prevention and Screening

No prevention has been identified. Children experiencing signs of appendicitis should be evaluated by a surgeon.

Assessment

History

- Anorexia
- Abdominal pain
- Nausea, vomiting
- Diarrhea or constipation

Physical Exam

- Fever
- Lethargy
- Rectal tenderness
- Abdominal distention

- Psoas sign: pain in the right hip
- Pain migrating from the umbilicus to right lower quadrant in about 50%
- Localized abdominal tenderness when hopping or jumping (less traumatic than palpation for rebound tenderness)
- Perforation: sudden temporary relief of pain
- Peritonitis: abdominal distention, tachycardia, rapid and shallow respirations, pallor, chills, irritability and restlessness

Diagnostic Studies

- Ultrasound or CT scan
- Elevated white blood cell count and elevated neutrophils
- Elevated C-reactive protein
- Urinalysis to rule out urinary tract infection
- Serum human chorionic gonadotropin to rule out ectopic pregnancy in adolescent females

Management

Invasive Treatment

- Appendectomy, the surgical removal of appendix via open or laparoscopic incision
- Possible drain placement for peritonitis

Nonpharmacologic Treatment

- Position for comfort
- Cough, turning, and deep breathing
- Progressive ambulation with small pillow to support incision site
- Advance diet as tolerated
- Possibly nasogastric tube for ruptured or gangrenous appendix
- Care of incision

Pharmacologic Treatment

- IV fluids to maintain fluid and electrolyte balance
- Pain management
- Antibiotics to prevent or treat infections

Patient and Family Education

- Diagnostic tests, disease process
- Preparation for surgery

- Postoperative care including ambulation, diet, pain management
- Home care including activity, care of incision, reasons to call healthcare provider

Outcomes and Follow-up

- The child will experience effective pain control.
- The child will show no signs of infection.
- The child will show evidence of wound healing.
- The child will show evidence of adequate hydration and return to his or her usual diet.
- The child will not experience complications such as abscess, paralytic ileus, or bowel obstruction.
- The child and family will verbalize an understanding of the education content.

INFLAMMATORY BOWEL DISEASE

Description

Inflammatory bowel disease (IBD) is chronic inflammation of the intestine. The two major forms are Crohn's disease (CD) and ulcerative colitis (UC). UC involves the mucosal layer and submucosa of the colon and rectum. CD most commonly affects the ileum and involves all of the layers of the bowel wall, but may extend throughout the entire gastrointestinal tract.

Etiology

IBD is an immune disease characterized by exacerbations and remissions, but the cause is not completely understood. The immune system reacts to antigens in bacteria or in food, causing an inflammatory process. In IBD, the intestinal mucosa becomes inflamed with ulceration, bleeding, edema, and decreased absorption of fluid and electrolytes.

Incidence and Demographics

Average age of onset is 12–20 years of age for ulcerative colitis and 15–25 years for Crohn's disease.

Risk Factors

- Family history
- Jewish ethnicity

Prevention and Screening

No prevention or screening is indicated

Assessment

History

- Ulcerative colitis
  - Abdominal pain, cramping
  - Rectal bleeding
  - Bloody diarrhea
  - Painful stool
  - Mucous in stool
  - Fatigue
  - Anorexia
- Crohn's disease
  - Abdominal pain, cramping
  - Diarrhea
  - Weight loss
  - Nausea
  - Burning epigastric pain
  - Fatigue
  - Anorexia

Physical Exam

- Ulcerative colitis
  - Growth failure
  - Joint pain
  - Lymphadenopathy
  - Erythema nodosum: tender, red, raised nodules
- Crohn's disease
  - Fever
  - Pallor
  - Joint pain
  - Growth failure
  - Lymphadenopathy
  - Erythema nodosum: tender, red, raised nodules
  - Perianal skin tags, abscesses, fissures, fistulas
  - Mouth ulcers

    - Delayed puberty
    - Inflammation of the iris, ciliary body, or choroid

Diagnostic Studies

- CBC to assess for anemia
- Elevated white blood cell count, platelets
- Elevated erythrocyte sedimentation rate
- Elevated C-reactive protein
- Liver transaminases
- Upper GI radiography with small bowel follow-through
- Endoscopy with biopsy
- Colonoscopy
- Stool specimen: occult blood, leukocytes
- CT, MRI, ultrasound
- Reduced bone mineral density

Management

Invasive Treatment

- Surgical removal of the colon or part of the small intestine, if unresponsive to pharmacologic treatment, with ileostomy or pull-through
- Surgical treatment for complications of CD including abscess, bowel obstruction, or fistulas between the intestine and skin

Nonpharmacologic Treatment

- Healthy diet including increased fruits, vegetables, water
- Minimal intake of sweetened beverages
- Smaller, more frequent meals
- Identify foods that increase symptoms
- Avoid high-fiber foods such as seeds, popcorn, corn
- Short-term total parenteral nutrition
- Partial enteral nutrition (PEN) or exclusive enteral nutrition (EEN) for CD

Pharmacologic Treatment

- Antiinflammatory medications
    - Prednisone or prednisolone
    - Methylprednisolone (Solu-Medrol)

- Mesalamine (Asacol)
- Sulfasalazine (Azulfidine) with supplemental folic acid

- Gastrointestinal agents
  - Olsalazine (Dipentum)
  - Balsalazide (Colazal)
- Chimeric monoclonal antibodies
  - Infliximab (Remicade)
  - Adalimumab (Humira)
  - Azathioprine (Imuran)
  - Methotrexate
- Antibiotics for infection
  - Metronidazole (Flagyl)
  - Ciprofloxacin (Cipro)
- Pain management and sedation during exacerbations
- Vitamins, iron, folic acid, nutritional supplements for specific deficiencies

Patient and Family Education

- Nature of disease and treatment plan
- Nutritional support
- Nonpharmacologic management
- Medication administration
- Strategies to prevent infection
- Availability of support groups, counseling

Outcomes and Follow-up

- The child will experience relief of diarrhea, rectal bleeding, and abdominal pain.
- The child will attain appropriate growth for its age.
- The child will maintain a healthy diet and avoid foods that cause symptoms.
- The child will have a DXA scan of the spine and total body at diagnosis and every 1 to 2 years to monitor bone mineral density.
- The child will have an annual vitamin D level to monitor bone health.
- The child will experience minimal effects of long-term corticosteroid use such as growth impairment, low bone mineral density, increased incidence of infection, and lack of mucosal healing.
- The child will not exhibit complications such as liver disease, renal or gallstones, or toxic megacolon.

- The child and family will verbalize an understanding of the disease, treatment plan, nonpharmacologic management, and medication administration.
- The child and family will access available support groups and counseling.

REFERENCES

Askew, N. (2010). An overview of infantile hypertrophic pyloric stenosis. *Paediatric Nursing, 22*(8), 27–30.

Bousvaros, A., & Leichtner, A. (2012). Overview of the management of Crohn's disease in children and adolescents. *UpToDate.* Retrieved from http://www.uptodate.com/contents/overview-of-the-management-of-crohns-disease-in-children-and-adolescents?source=search_result&search=pediatric+crohn+disease&selectedTitle=1%7E150

Bousvaros, A., Leichtner, A., & Burpee, T. (2011). Treatment of ulcerative colitis in children and adolescents. *UpToDate.* Retrieved from http://www.uptodate.com/contents/treatment-of-ulcerative-colitis-in-children-and-adolescents?source=search_result&search=pediatric+ulcerative+colitis&selectedTitle=1%7E150<

Critch, J., Day, A. S., Otley, A., King-Moore, C., Teitelbaum, J. E., & Shashidhar, H. (2012). Use of enteral nutrition for the control of intestinal inflammation in pediatric Crohn disease. *Journal of Pediatric Gastroenterology and Nutrition, 54*(2), 298–305.

Duro, D., Kamin, D., & Duggan, C. (2008). Overview of pediatric short bowel syndrome. *Journal of Pediatric Gastroenterology and Nutrition, 47,* S33–S36.

Freedman, S. B., Sivabalasundaram, V., Bohn, V., Powell, E. C., Johnson, D. W., & Boutis, K. (2011). The treatment of pediatric gastroenteritis: A comparative analysis of pediatric emergency physicians' practice patterns. *Academic Emergency Medicine, 18,* 38–45.

Greenberg, L. (2008). Case management implications of celiac disease. *Professional Case Management, 13*(4), 211–217.

Hedrick, H. L., & Adzick, N. S. (2011). Congenital diaphragmatic hernia in the neonate. *UpToDate.* Retrieved from http://www.uptodate.com/contents/congenital-diaphragmatic-hernia-in-the-neonate?source=search_result&search=pediatric+hernia&selectedTitle=2%7E150

Higuchi, L. M., & Bousvaros, A. (2011). Diagnosis of inflammatory bowel disease in children and adolescents. *UpToDate.* Retrieved from http://www.uptodate.com/contents/diagnosis-of-inflammatory-bowel-disease-in-children-and-adolescents?source=see_link

Hockenberry, M. J., & Wilson, D. (2011). *Wong's nursing care of infants and children* (9th ed.). St. Louis, MO: Elsevier Mosby.

Matson, D. O. (2011). Epidemiology, pathogenesis, clinical presentation and diagnosis of viral gastroenteritis in children. *UpToDate.* Retrieved from http://www.uptodate.com/contents/epidemiology-pathogenesis-clinical-presentation-and-diagnosis-of-viral-gastroenteritis-in-children?source=search_result&search=gastroenteritis+children&selectedTitle=2%7E150

Oermann, C. M. (2011). Congenital anomalies of the intrathoracic airways and tracheoesophageal fistula. *UpToDate.* Retrieved from http://www.uptodate.com/contents/congenital-anomalies-of-the-intrathoracic-airways-and-tracheoesophageal-fistula?source=search_result&search=tracheoesophageal+fistula+children&selectedTitle=1%7E61

Pappa, H., Thaya, M., Sylvester, F., Leonard, M., Zemel, B., & Gordon, C. (2011). Skeletal health of children and adolescents with inflammatory bowel disease. *Journal of Pediatric Gastroenterology and Nutrition, 53*(1), 11–25.

Peppercorn, M. A. (2012). Definition of and risk factors for inflammatory bowel disease. *UpToDate.* Retrieved from http://www.uptodate.com/contents/definition-of-and-risk-factors-for-inflammatory-bowel-disease?source=preview&anchor=H7&selectedTitle=3~150#H7

Ramsook, C., & Endon, E. E. (2011). Overview of inguinal hernia in children. *UpToDate.* Retrieved from http://www.uptodate.com/contents/overview-of-inguinal-hernia-in-children?source=search_result&search=pediatric+hernia&selectedTitle=1%7E150

Raphael, B. P., Jiang, H., Hart, K., Kamin, D. S., Jaksic, T., & Duggan, C. (2011). Cisapride improves enteral tolerance in pediatric short-bowel syndrome with dysmotility. *Journal of Pediatric Gastroenterology and Nutrition, 52*(5), 590–594.

Scanlon, S. A., & Murray, J. A. (2011). Update on celiac disease-etiology, differential diagnosis, drug targets, and management advances. *Clinical and Experimental Gastroenterology, 4,* 297–311.

Stone, M. B., Botto, L. D., Feldkamp, M. L., Smith, K. R., Roling, L., Yamashiro, D., & Alder, S. C. (2010). Improving quality of life of children with oral clefts: Perspectives of parents. *The Journal of Craniofacial Surgery, 21*(5), 1358–1364.

Turowski, C., Dingemann, J., & Gillick, J. (2010). Delayed diagnosis of imperforate anus: An unacceptable morbidity. *Pediatric Surgery International, 26,* 1083–1086.

Vandenplas, Y., Rudolph, C. D., DiLorenzo, C., et al. (2009). Pediatric gastroesophageal reflux clinical practice guidelines: Joint recommendations of the North American Society for Pediatric Gastroenterology, Hepatology, and Nutrition (NASPGHAN) and the European Society for Pediatric Gastroenterology, Hepatology, and Nutrition (ESPGHAN). *Journal of Pediatric Gastroenterology and Nutrition, 49*(4), 498–547.

Vanderpol, R. J., Smits, M. J., VanWijk, M. P., Omari, T. I., Tabbers, M. M., & Benninga, M. A. (2011). Efficacy of proton-pump inhibitors in children with gastroesophageal reflux disease: A systematic review. *Pediatrics, 127*(5), 925–935.

Wassem, M., & Rosenberg, H. K. (2008). Intussusception. *Pediatric Emergency Care, 24*(11), 793–800.

Wesson, D. E. (2010). Acute appendicitis in children: Clinical manifestations and diagnosis. *UpToDate.* Retrieved from http://www.uptodate.com/contents/acute-appendicitis-in-children-clinical-manifestations-and-diagnosis?source=search_result&search=pediatric+appendicitis&selectedTitle=1%7E150

Wesson, D. E. (2011). Congenital aganglionic megacolon (Hirschsprung disease). *UpToDate.* Retrieved from http://www.uptodate.com/contents/congenital-aganglionic-megacolon-hirschsprung-disease?source=see_link&anchor=H5#H5

Wesson, D. E. (2012). Acute appendicitis in children. *UpToDate.* Retrieved from http://www.uptodate.com/contents/acute-appendicitis-in-children-management?source=see_link

Wilkins-Haug, L. (2011). Etiology, prenatal diagnosis, obstetrical management, and recurrence of orofacial clefts. *UpToDate,* Retrieved from http://www.uptodate.com/contents/etiology-prenatal-diagnosis-obstetrical-management-and-recurrence-of-orofacial-clefts?source=search_result&search=cleft+lip+and+cleft+palate&selectedTitle=1%7E150

Zwink, N., Jenetzky, E., & Brenner, H. (2011). Parental risk factors and anorectal malformations: Systematic review and meta-analysis. *Orphanet Journal of Rare Diseases.* Retrieved from http://www.ojrd.com/content/6/1/25

CHAPTER 12

GENITOURINARY DISORDERS

Clara J. Richardson, MSN, RN-BC

DEVELOPMENTAL CHARACTERISTICS OF THE PEDIATRIC GENITOURINARY SYSTEM

- Newborns have a lower rate of water, hydrogen ion, and acid secretion, and a low plasma bicarbonate level; therefore, they are more likely to develop metabolic acidosis.
- Infants are less able to adapt to sodium deficiencies and excesses.
- Kidney development continues during infancy and is not completed until age 1 year.
- The infant has full number of the nephrons, but they are immature and less efficient.
- Tubular sections of the kidney continue to develop and glomeruli to enlarge.
- The infant reaches the adult level of tubular absorption at about age 3 months.
- Glomerular filtration rate and absorption rates are low and do not reach adult levels until age 1–2 years.

HYPOSPADIAS

Description

Hypospadias is a congenital malformation with abnormal position of the male urethral opening on the glans penis or on the underside of the penis.

Etiology

The defect occurs when the urethral folds fail to close completely, resulting in abnormal placement of the urethral opening. Exact cause of this interrupted penile development is unknown, but thought to be a combination of genetic and environmental factors.

Incidence and Demographics

The incidence is 1 out of 250–300 live births.

Risk Factors

- Family history
- Maternal intake of estrogenic compound drugs
- Maternal advanced age
- Maternal diabetes
- Maternal exposure to environmental contaminants, pesticides
- Gestational age less than 37 weeks

Prevention and Screening

- No prevention or screening indicated

Assessment

History

- Presence of risk factors

Physical Exam

- Small penis
- Abnormally positioned urethral opening
- Incomplete or redundant foreskin
- Possible chordee, ventral curve of penis
- Possible undescended testes

Diagnostic Studies

- Possible chromosome analysis in cases of ambiguous genitalia
- Possible pelvic ultrasound to examine internal genitalia

Management

Invasive Treatment

- Surgical repositioning of urethral opening with reconstruction to normalize appearance of penis
- Release of chordee
- May be done in one or two stages, depending on severity

Nonpharmacologic Treatment

- Avoid newborn circumcision because foreskin may be used for surgical repair
- Postoperative urinary diversion with stent or feeding tube for 5–10 days

Pharmacologic Treatment

- Possible preoperative testosterone therapy to augment penile growth
- Prophylactic antibiotics with urinary diversion
- Postoperative oxybutynin for bladder spasms
- Antibiotic ointment to surgical site
- Pain management

Patient and Family Education

- Description of defect and treatment plan
- Care of urinary diversion device: no tub bath, double-diapering technique (disposable diaper next to skin with device positioned to drain into second diaper covering the first to minimize urine contact with surgical site)
- Possible complications: pain or straining on urination, abnormal urine stream, infection
- Medication administration

Outcomes and Follow-up

- The child will experience effective pain management.
- The child will exhibit near normal appearance of penis and urine stream.
- The child will establish normal voiding patterns.
- The child will not experience complications such as meatal stenosis, urethral strictures or fistulas, infection.

- The family will verbalize an understanding of the defect, treatment plan, and possible complications.
- The family will demonstrate care of urinary device, medication administration, and infection prevention.

VESICOURETERAL REFLUX

Description

Vesicoureteral reflux (VUR) involves backward flow of urine from the bladder into the ureters. The severity of the condition is defined by the degree of reflux from the bladder into the upper genitourinary tract.

Etiology

Primary VUR is a congenital anomaly involving incompetent or inadequate closure at the ureterovesical junction and possibly an abnormally implanted ureter, which may resolve as the infant grows. Secondary VUR is an acquired condition caused by high bladder pressure that is often associated with dysfunctional voiding or neurogenic bladder. VUR may result in acute pyelonephritis or intravascular renal scarring and injury.

Incidence and Demographics

About 1% of newborns are born with VUR. It is more common in girls, in Whites, and in identical twins.

Risk Factors

- Family history
- Febrile urinary tract infection
- Prenatal hydronephrosis noted on ultrasound

Prevention and Screening

- No prevention
- Possible screening of siblings or those with parental history

Assessment

History

- Presence of risk factors

Physical Exam

- Most children are asymptomatic

Diagnostic Studies

- Voiding cystourethrogram (VCUG)
- Radionuclide cystogram (RNC)
- Serum creatinine to estimate glomerular filtration rate
- Urinalysis and culture

Management

Invasive Treatment

- Surgical repositioning of ureter in bladder wall
- Endoscopic subureteric transurethral injection of dextranomer/hyaluronic acid, a gel-like bulking agent, to prevent retrograde flow of urine

Nonpharmacologic Treatment

- Prompt recognition and treatment of urinary tract infections
- Postoperative urinary diversion with stents or drains

Pharmacologic Treatment

- Prophylactic low-dose antibiotic therapy
- Postoperative pain management
- Postoperative oxybutynin for bladder spasms

Patient and Family Education

- Nature of defect and treatment plan
- Preparation for diagnostic procedures
- Signs of urinary tract infection
- Maintaining hydration
- Medication administration

Outcomes and Follow-up

- The child will receive prompt treatment of urinary tract infections.
- The child will maintain adequate hydration status.
- The child will experience effective pain management.
- The child will not experience complications such as acute pyelonephritis or intravascular renal scarring and injury.

- The family will verbalize an understanding of the condition, treatment, and diagnostic procedures.
- The family will verbalize an understanding of signs of urinary tract infection.
- The family will demonstrate medication administration.

URINARY TRACT INFECTION

Description

Urinary tract infection (UTI) may involve any structure within the genitourinary system. Pyelonephritis is infection of the renal parenchyma, and cystitis is infection of the bladder.

Etiology

Common causative organisms include *Escherichia coli, Klebsiella, Proteus, Enterococcus*, and *Enterobacter*. The organism ascends through the urinary tract.

Incidence and Demographics

UTI is a common childhood illness with a prevalence of 2%–8%. The peak incidence of UTI in children without structural defect is between 2 and 6 years. After the newborn period, UTI is more common in girls, and the rate of recurrence is also higher in girls.

Risk Factors

- Vesicoureteral reflux
- Constipation
- Voiding dysfunction
- Urinary catheters
- Poor hygiene
- Pinworms
- Bubble baths
- Hot tubs

Prevention and Screening

- Prevention consists of avoiding risk factors
- Screening for nitrates with dipstick urine specimen

Assessment

History

- Infants: diarrhea, poor feeding, growth failure, persistent diaper rash, irritability
- Nausea, vomiting, diarrhea, flank pain with pyelonephritis
- Urinary pain, frequency, or hesitation
- Abdominal pain
- Incontinence in toilet-trained child

Physical Exam

- Fever and chills with pyelonephritis
- Strong- or foul-smelling urine
- Cloudy urine with mucus

Diagnostic Studies

- Elevated white blood cell count
- Elevated C-reactive protein
- Clean-catch urine culture for children who are toilet-trained
- Catheter or suprapubic culture for infants and young children
- Urine: white blood cells, bacteria
- Recurrent UTI: voiding cystourethrogram (VCUG), dimercaptosuccinic acid (DMSA) scan, ultrasound

Management

Invasive Treatment

- No invasive therapy indicated

Nonpharmacologic Treatment

- Regular voiding
- Maintain hydration status
- Avoid caffeinated or carbohydrate beverages that may irritate bladder

Pharmacologic Treatment

- Oral antibiotic therapy
    - Trimethoprim-sulfamethoxazole (Bactrim): use sunscreen
    - Nitrofurantoin (Furadantin)

    - Amoxicillin
    - Amoxicillin-clavulanate (Augmentin)
    - Cephalexin (Keflex)
    - Cefixime (Suprax)
    - Cefdinir (Omnicef)
    - Ciprofloxacin (Cipro)
- Parenteral antibiotics
    - Ampicillin
    - Cefotaxime (Claforan)
    - Ceftriaxone (Rocephin)
    - Cefepime (Maxipime)
    - Gentamicin

Patient and Family Education

- Nature of infection and treatment plan
- Signs of urinary tract infection
- Strategies for prevention
- Specimen collection
- Medication administration

Outcomes and Follow-up

- The child will experience relief of symptoms.
- The child will reestablish normal voiding patterns.
- The child will not experience complications such as renal scarring, sepsis, or abscess formation.
- The family will verbalize an understanding of the infection, treatment, signs of UTI, and prevention strategies.
- The family will demonstrate medication administration and specimen collection.

ACUTE GLOMERULONEPHRITIS

Description

Acute glomerulonephritis is a disorder of the renal system that occurs as a primary disorder or as a manifestation of a systemic disorder. The most common type in children is acute poststreptococcal glomerulonephritis (APSGN), an immune complex disease.

Etiology

APSGN is caused by a group A beta-hemolytic streptococcal infection, but the exact mechanism is unclear. The glomerular capillary loops are swollen and infiltrated by polymorphonuclear leukocytes. The capillary lumens are occluded, reducing glomerular filtration rate and leading to accumulation of water and sodium retention.

Incidence and Demographics

APSGN occurs most commonly in children between the ages of 5 and 12 years, and clinical manifestations usually begin 10–14 days after the infection. The acute edematous phase usually lasts 4–10 days, but possibly up to 2–3 weeks.

Risk Factors

- Streptococcal infection

Prevention and Screening

There is no specific screening, but APSGN may be prevented by prompt treatment of streptococcal infections.

Assessment

History

- Group A beta-hemolytic streptococcal infection
- Mild upper respiratory infection
- Decreased urine output
- Painful urination
- Cloudy tea- or cola-colored urine
- Hematuria
- Headache
- Abdominal discomfort

Physical Exam

- Periorbital edema
- Facial puffiness
- Edema of extremities and abdomen
- Anorexia
- Pallor
- Irritability

- Lethargy
- Hypertension
- Increased body weight

Diagnostic Studies

- Hematuria
- Proteinuria
- Increased urine specific gravity
- Elevated blood urea nitrogen
- Elevated creatinine level
- Elevated antistreptolysin O (ASO) titer
- Decreased serum complement level (C3)
- Throat cultures of others in household

Management

Invasive Treatment

- No invasive therapy indicated

Nonpharmacologic Treatment

- Daily weight
- Avoid foods high in sodium
- Frequent rest periods to avoid fatigue
- Sodium and water restriction with significantly reduced urine output

Pharmacologic Treatment

- Diuretic therapy (Lasix) with significant edema
- Possible antihypertensive therapy
- Intravenous therapy to maintain fluid and electrolyte imbalance

Patient and Family Education

- Nature of disease and treatment plan
- Nonpharmacologic management strategies
- Medication administration
- Signs of complications
- Signs of improvement

Outcomes and Follow-up

- The child's blood pressure will return to normal.
- The child's urine output and body weight will return to normal.
- The child's lab values will return to normal.
- The child will not experience complications such as hypertensive encephalopathy, acute cardiac decompensation, or acute renal failure.
- The family will verbalize an understanding of the disease process, treatment plan, nonpharmacologic management, signs of complications, and signs of improvement.
- The family will demonstrate medication administration.

NEPHROTIC SYNDROME

Description

Nephrotic syndrome is a renal disorder characterized by massive proteinuria, hypoalbuminemia, hyperlipidemia, and edema. The most common type in children is minimal change nephrotic syndrome (MCNS).

Etiology

The exact etiology is not completely understood. The glomeruli become more permeable to proteins, especially albumin. The result is decreased osmotic pressure with fluid accumulation in the interstitial spaces and body cavities.

Incidence and Demographics

Nephrotic syndrome occurs in 16 of 100,000 children. The highest incidence is in preschoolers. Approximately half of affected children will experience relapse.

Risk Factors

- No identified risk factors for first episode
- Viral infection may trigger relapse

Prevention and Screening

- No prevention or screening indicated

Assessment

History

- Mild upper respiratory infection
- Weight gain
- Anorexia
- Diarrhea
- Decreased urine output
- Dark, frothy urine
- Fatigue

Physical Exam

- Periorbital edema
- Facial puffiness
- Generalized edema
- Abdominal edema
- Pallor

Diagnostic Studies

- Total protein/creatinine ratio: proteinuria
- Decreased serum albumin
- Elevated serum total cholesterol, triglycerides, and total lipids
- Decreased serum protein
- Elevated serum creatinine
- Elevated urine specific gravity
- Elevated hemoglobin and hematocrit
- Elevated platelet count

Management

Invasive Treatment

- No invasive therapy indicated

Nonpharmacologic Treatment

- Monitor urine protein by dipstick
- Daily weight
- Elevation of edematous body parts

- Skin care: hygiene, separate edematous areas with clothing, antiseptic powder
- Diet without added salt

Pharmacologic Treatment

- Corticosteroid therapy: prednisone for 4–6 weeks

Patient and Family Education

- Nature of disorder and treatment plan
- Medication administration
- Nonpharmacologic management
- Strategies for infection prevention
- Signs of relapse

Outcomes and Follow-up

- The child's urine protein will return to normal.
- The child will return to normal weight.
- The child will not experience acute infection during therapy.
- The child will not experience skin breakdown.
- The child will not experience relapse.
- The family will verbalize an understanding of the disease, treatment plan, nonpharmacologic management, and signs of relapse.
- The family will demonstrate infection prevention strategies.
- The family will recognize signs of relapse and seek treatment.

WILMS TUMOR

Description

Wilms tumor, or nephroblastoma, is a malignant tumor of the kidney.

Etiology

The exact cause is unknown, but molecular studies suggest that the tumor originates in an embryonic renal progenitor stem cell. Wilms tumor may occur alone or with other congenital syndromes. Clinical manifestations are caused by tumor compression of surrounding structures, secondary metabolic alterations, or metastasis.

Incidence and Demographics

Wilms tumor accounts for 6% of all childhood cancers. It is usually unilateral, but bilateral in 5% of cases. The survival rate is up to 90%.

TABLE 12-1.
INCIDENCE OF WILMS TUMOR PER 100,000 CHILDREN

< 1 YEAR	1-4 YEARS	5-9 YEARS
1.56	1.85	0.54

Risk Factors

- ▶ Family history
- ▶ Congenital syndromes such as Beckwith-Wiedemann syndrome or WAGR syndrome (Wilms tumor, aniridia, genitourinary anomalies, cognitive impairment)

Prevention and Screening

- ▶ No prevention or screening indicated

Assessment

History

- ▶ Family history
- ▶ Congenital syndrome

Physical Exam

- ▶ Painless abdominal mass
- ▶ Hematuria
- ▶ Hypertension
- ▶ Fever
- ▶ Weight loss

Diagnostic Studies

- ▶ CT scan, MRI
- ▶ Chest radiography
- ▶ Urinalysis to evaluate kidney function
- ▶ Serum electrolytes to evaluate kidney function
- ▶ Serum creatinine to evaluate glomerular filtration rate
- ▶ Polycythemia if tumor secretes erythropoietin

- Coagulation studies to check for acquired von Willebrand disease, which is present in approximately 8% of children with Wilms tumor
- Liver function test to check for metastasis

Management

Invasive Treatment

- Surgical removal of kidney

Nonpharmacologic Treatment

- Radiation therapy for advanced cases
- Avoid palpation of mass, which may rupture tumor

Pharmacologic Treatment

- Postoperative pain management
- Chemotherapy
    - Vincristine
    - Dactinomycin, doxorubicin

Patient and Family Education

- Description of tumor and treatment plan
- Side effects of chemotherapy and radiation
- Infection prevention
- Postoperative: pain management and incision care

Outcomes and Follow-up

- The child's incision site will heal completely.
- The child will experience minimal side effects of chemotherapy and radiation.
- The child will not experience acute infections during chemotherapy.
- The family will verbalize an understanding of the tumor, treatment, and side effects of treatment.
- The family will demonstrate infection prevention strategies.
- The family will demonstrate postoperative care.

SEXUALLY TRANSMITTED INFECTIONS

Description, Etiology, Incidence, and Demographics

Sexually transmitted infections are those infections passed from person to person by sexual intercourse or genital contact.

Chlamydia

- Symptoms in females: vaginal bleeding or discharge, burning on urination, lower abdominal or back pain, pain during intercourse, nausea, fever
- Symptoms in males: penile discharge, burning on urination
- Many males and females have no symptoms
- Causative organism: *Chlamydia trachomatis*
- May cause pelvic inflammatory disease (PID), infertility, ectopic pregnancy, premature delivery

Genital Herpes

- Symptoms: periodic outbreak of itching, burning, or tingling followed by eruption of painful blister-like sores around genitals or rectum
- Causative organism: herpes simplex viruses type 1 and type 2
- May cause potentially fatal infection in newborns

Human Papillomavirus (HPV; Genital Warts)

- Symptoms: small isolated bumps or groups of bumps in genital area, groin, thighs
- Causative organisms: multiple types of human papillomaviruses
- This chronic, lifelong disease may cause genital, anal, head, cervical, and neck cancer.

Gonorrhea

- Symptoms in females: vaginal discharge or bleeding, burning on urination; most have no symptoms
- Symptoms in males: penile discharge, burning on urination, swollen and painful testicles; some have no symptoms
- Causative organism: *Neisseria gonorrhoeae*
- May cause pelvic inflammatory disease, ectopic pregnancy, infertility in both males and females, and blindness or life-threatening infection in newborns

Syphilis

- Symptoms during primary stage: painless chancre sore

- ▶ Symptoms during secondary stage: nonitching rash on palms and soles, fever, lymphadenopathy, weight loss, fatigue, headache
- ▶ Symptoms during late stage: potentially fatal damage to brain, internal organs, blood vessels, bones
- ▶ Causative organism: *Treponema pallidum*
- ▶ May cause stillbirth, physical deformity, neurologic complications in newborns

Incidence and Demographics

HPV and genital herpes are not mandatory reportable diseases. The Centers for Disease Control and Prevention estimate that approximately 20 million people are infected with HPV, and that about 50% of those are between the ages of 15 and 24 years. The estimated rate of genital herpes is 1 out of 5 women and 1 out of 9 men between the ages of 14 to 49 years.

The other three infections are reported for teenagers ages 15–19 in 2010 in Table 12–2.

TABLE 12–2.
SEXUALLY TRANSMITTED INFECTIONS, MALES AND FEMALES AGES 15–19 YEARS

	MALES 15–19 YRS/100,000	FEMALES 15–19 YRS/100,000
Chlamydia	730 (6% ▯)	3,378 (2.8% ▯)
Gonorrhea	253 (2.1% ▯)	571 (0.9% ▯)
Syphilis	617 (0.4% ▯)	313 (0.3% ▯)

Risk Factors

- ▶ Unprotected sexual contact with infected partner
- ▶ Multiple sexual partners
- ▶ Injected substance abuse
- ▶ Age less than 15 years
- ▶ Reside in detention facilities

Prevention and Screening

- ▶ Prevention by avoidance of risk factors
- ▶ Human papilloma virus vaccine
- ▶ Annual screening of sexually active individuals

Assessment

History

- ▶ History of risk factors or symptoms

Physical Exam

- See symptoms

Diagnostic Studies

- Penis, cervix, rectum, oral swabs for culture of causative organisms

Management

Invasive Treatment

- No invasive therapy indicated

Nonpharmacologic Treatment

- Contact sexual partners for testing and treatment, or offer treatment alone if patient refuses to be tested

Pharmacologic Treatment

- Chlamydia: single-dose oral azithromycin or oral doxycycline for 7 days; for newborn, erythromycin for infection
- Genital herpes: antiviral therapy with acyclovir, valacyclovir (Valtrex), famciclovir (Famvir) for outbreaks
- Human papillomavirus: no treatment indicated
- Gonorrhea: single dose of IM ceftriaxone (Rocephin) or oral cefixime (Suprax); for newborn, ophthalmic neonatorum eye prophylaxis or ceftriaxone for infection
- Syphilis: single-dose IM penicillin G

Patient and Family Education

- Nature of disease and treatment plan
- Importance of treatment for sexual partners
- Strategies to prevent transmission
- Available counseling
- Risk of HIV infection

Outcomes and Follow-up

- The adolescent will verbalize an understanding of the disease and the treatment plan.
- The adolescent will report relief or symptoms.
- The adolescent will contact sexual partners for treatment.
- The adolescent will practice strategies to prevent transmission.
- The adolescent will access available counseling resources.
- The adolescent will receive HIV testing.
- The adolescent will experience minimal long-term complications.

REFERENCES

Baskin, L. S. (2011). Hypospadias. *UpToDate.* Retrieved from http://www.uptodate.com/contents/hypospadias?source=search_result&search=hypospadias+children&selectedTitle=1%7E63

Centers for Disease Control and Prevention. (2007). *United States cancer statistics.* Retrieved from http://apps.nccd.cdc.gov/uscs/childhoodcancerdetailedbyICCC.aspx

Centers for Disease Control and Prevention. (2011). *2010 Sexually transmitted diseases surveillance.* Retrieved from http://www.cdc.gov/std/stats10/

Chintagumpala, M., & Muscal, J. A. (2011). Presentation, diagnosis, and staging of Wilms tumor. *UpToDate.* Retrieved from http://www.uptodate.com/contents/presentation-diagnosis-and-staging-of-wilms-tumor?source=search_result&search=wilms+tumor+children&selectedTitle=2%7E75

Chintagumpala, M., & Muscal, J. A. (2011). Treatment and prognosis of Wilms tumor. *UpToDate.* Retrieved from http://www.uptodate.com/contents/treatment-and-prognosis-of-wilms-tumor?source=search_result&search=wilms+tumor+children&selectedTitle=1%7E75

D'Souza, G., & Dempsey, A. (2011). *The role of HPV in head and neck cancer and review of the HPV vaccine.* Retrieved August 22, 2012 from http://www.ncbi.nlm.nih.gov/pmc/articles/PMC3287051

Gebhart, F. (2011). HIT more effective than STING in treating VUR. *Urology Times, 39*(4), 28.

Hockenberry, M. J., & Wilson, D. (2011). *Wong's nursing care of infants and children* (9th ed.). St. Louis, MO: Elsevier Mosby.

McLorie, G., & Herrin, J. T. (2011). Management of vesicoureteral reflux. *UpToDate.* Retrieved from http://www.uptodate.com/contents/management-of-vesicoureteral-reflux?source=see_link

McLorie, G., & Herrin, J. T. (2011). Presentation, diagnosis, and clinical course of vesicoureteral reflux. *UpToDate.* Retrieved from http://www.uptodate.com/contents/presentation-diagnosis-and-clinical-course-of-vesicoureteral-reflux?source=search_result&search=vesicoureteral+reflux+in+children&selectedTitle=2%7E83

Niaudet, P. (2012). Etiology, clinical manifestations, and diagnosis of nephrotic syndrome in children. *UpToDate.* Retrieved from http://www.uptodate.com/contents/etiology-clinical-manifestations-and-diagnosis-of-nephrotic-syndrome-in-children?source=search_result&search=nephrotic+syndrome+in+children&selectedTitle=3%7E150

Niaudet, P. (2012). Treatment of idiopathic nephrotic syndrome in children. *UpToDate.* Retrieved from http://www.uptodate.com/contents/treatment-of-idiopathic-nephrotic-syndrome-in-children?source=search_result&search=nephrotic+syndrome+in+children&selectedTitle=2%7E150

Passamaneck, M. (2011). The changing paradigm for the management of pediatric vesicoureteral reflux. *Urologic Nursing, 31*(6), 363–366.

Pode-Shakked, N., & Dekel, B. (2011). Wilms tumor—a renal stem cell malignancy. *Pediatric Nephrology, 26,* 1535–1543.

Saadeh, S. A., & Mattoo, T. K. (2011). Managing urinary tract infections. *Pediatric Nephrology, 26,* 1967–1976.

CHAPTER 13

ENDOCRINE DISORDERS

Clara J. Richardson, MSN, RN-BC

DIABETES MELLITUS

Description

Type 1 diabetes is a chronic autoimmune disorder characterized by gradual destruction of the beta cells of the pancreas with accompanying loss of insulin production. Type 2 diabetes is a chronic metabolic disorder with hyperglycemia resulting from a defect in insulin secretion, in insulin action, or both. Maturity onset diabetes of youth (MODY) is a hereditary disorder caused by mutations in an autosomal dominant gene leading to disrupted insulin production.

Etiology

Without insulin, glucose cannot enter cells, so it remains in the blood vessels. Hyperglycemia causes fluid to move from the intracellular space to the interstitial space to the extracellular space. The renal system cannot reabsorb excess glucose, so it spills into the urine and draws in more fluid, increasing urination. The increased fluid loss causes thirst. Without carbohydrates for energy, the body uses protein and fats. Hunger is triggered, and the cycle continues.

Incidence and Demographics

Approximately 0.26% of people younger than 20 years of age have either type 1 or type 2 diabetes. In children younger than 10 years, the rate of newly diagnosed cases of type 1 per year is 19.7 per 100,000 and 0.4 per 100,000 for type 2. In 10- to 19-year-olds, the rate per 100,000 is 18.6 for type 1 and 8.5 for type 2. Initial presentation of type 1 diabetes peaks in children age 4–6 years, and then again in early puberty.

Among children age 10–19 years, the incidence of type 1 diabetes is higher than that of type 2 in Whites. The incidence of each type is similar in Hispanics/Latinos. Asian/Pacific Islander and Native American children have higher incidence of type 2 than type 1.

Risk Factors

- Type 1 diabetes
  - Family history
  - Diseases of the exocrine system such as cystic fibrosis
  - Diseases of the endocrine system such as Cushing syndrome
  - Some glucocorticoids, HIV protease inhibitors
- Type 2 diabetes
  - Family history
  - Obesity
  - Female gender
  - Hypertension
  - High cholesterol
  - Polycystic ovary syndrome

Prevention and Screening

None for type 1 diabetes. For type 2 diabetes, screening every 2 years beginning at age 10 years or at onset of puberty for overweight children who also have family history, or are of high-risk race or ethnicity, or who have acanthosis nigricans.

Assessment

History

- Type 1 diabetes
  - Polyuria, polydipsia, polyphagia
  - Unexplained weight loss
  - Extreme fatigue

    - Irritability
- Type 2 diabetes
    - Polyuria, polydipsia, fatigue, and lethargy
    - Asymptomatic presentation
    - History of risk factors
    - Recurrent vaginal and urinary tract infections, *Candida albicans*

Physical Exam

- Diabetic ketoacidosis (DKA)
- Nausea and vomiting
- Dehydration
- Fruity-smelling breath
- Ketone bodies in urine
- Labored breathing

Diagnostic Studies

- Elevated fasting glucose levels greater than or equal to 126 mg/dL
- Elevated random glucose levels greater than or equal to 200 mg/dL
- 2-hour oral 75 g glucose tolerance test greater than or equal to 200 mg/dL
- Glycated hemoglobin (A1C) equal to or greater than 6.5%
- Metabolic acidosis with DKA
- C-peptide level less than 0.9 with type 1, normal with type 2
- Autoantibodies present with type 1, but not type 2
- GAD 65
- Tyrosine phosphatase (TPA)
- Insulin autoantibodies (IAA)
- Islet cell antibodies (ICA)
- MODY shows mildly elevated blood glucose of 130–250 mg/dL

Management

Invasive Treatment

- No invasive management indicated

Nonpharmacologic Treatment

- Blood glucose monitoring
- Healthy, nutritious diet with three meals per day and snacks between meals

- Physical activity
- Management of hypoglycemia
    - Shakiness, sweating, tachycardia
    - Hunger, headache, double vision
    - Difficulty concentrating
    - Fatigue, behavior changes
    - Blood glucose less than 70 mg/dL
    - 50% of severe hypoglycemia occurs at night with restlessness, nightmares, sleepwalking
    - Give 10–15 g of simple carbohydrate
    - Recheck in 15 minutes and follow with complex carbohydrate
- Sick-day management for insulin users
    - Monitor blood glucose every 1–2 hrs and ketones with voiding
    - Consume carbohydrates and extra fluids
    - Continue long-acting insulin
    - Call healthcare provider for moderate to large ketones

Pharmacologic Treatment

- Oral or injectable antidiabetes medications, or both, for type 2 diabetes
- Insulin replacement via injection or pump for type 1 or type 2
- Glucagon for hypoglycemia if child cannot eat
- DKA management in hospital
    - Normal saline fluid bolus for dehydration
    - Insulin to correct hyperglycemia
    - Cautious fluid management to prevent cerebral edema
    - Intravenous fluids to provide dextrose and correct electrolyte imbalance
    - Reintroduction of regular diet

Patient and Family Education

- Nature of disease and treatment plan
- Insulin administration, action, interaction with food, dosage adjustment
- Blood glucose monitoring
- Diet modifications, carbohydrate counting
- Balancing food, insulin, and exercise
- Signs of hypoglycemia and hyperglycemia

- Treatment of hypoglycemia
- Managing food and insulin with physical activity
- Care during illness
- Communication of plan of care with daycare, school
- Available resources such as support groups, counseling, diabetes camps

Outcomes and Follow-up

- The child's diet, insulin, and exercise will be balanced to maintain blood glucose within normal limits.
- The child will always have a blood glucose monitor, insulin, and snacks readily available.
- The child will attend regular healthcare appointments to monitor diabetes control and assess for complications of chronic disease.
- The child will maintain immunization status, including pneumococcal and influenza vaccines.
- The child will increase participation in self-care as developmental level allows.
- The child and family will verbalize an understanding of the education content.
- The child and family will access available resources.
- The family will demonstrate blood glucose monitoring, ketone testing, and insulin administration.
- The family will recognize and treat episodes of hypoglycemia and hyperglycemia.
- The family will collaborate with daycare providers or school personnel to plan diabetes management.

GROWTH HORMONE DEFICIENCY

Description

Growth hormone deficiency (GHD) is a condition in which the pituitary gland does not produce enough growth hormone.

Etiology

GHD may be congenital or acquired after brain injury, tumor, or radiation. Growth hormone is necessary for normal growth of muscles and bones and fat distribution. Children with a deficiency grow at a slower rate and are much shorter than other children of the same age.

Incidence and Demographics

The estimated incidence of growth hormone deficiency is 1 per 4,000 to 1 per 10,000.

Risk Factors

- Family history
- Brain injury, tumor, or radiation

Prevention and Screening

- No prevention or screening indicated

Assessment

History

- History of risk factors
- Short birth length
- Breech presentation
- Perinatal asphyxia
- Neonatal hypoglycemia, prolonged jaundice
- Deviation from the normal growth curve
- Delayed puberty

Physical Exam

- Younger facial appearance than expected for age
- Short stature, below the 3rd percentile on standardized growth chart
- Small hands and feet
- Poor muscle tone
- Low blood glucose levels in young children
- Small penis

Diagnostic Studies

- Bone radiographs show younger than expected bone age
- Decrease in insulin-like growth factor-1 (IGF-1)
- Decrease in insulin-like growth factor binding protein-3 (IGFBP-3)
- GH stimulation test shows lack of pituitary response
- MRI of pituitary shows abnormal structure

Management

Invasive Treatment

- No invasive management indicated

Nonpharmacologic Treatment

- Monitoring of growth every 3–6 months
- Psychological counseling related to difference from peers

Pharmacologic Treatment

- Daily injections of synthetic growth hormone

Patient and Family Education

- Nature of disorder and treatment plan
- Potential outcomes of treatment
- Medication administration
- Possible side effects of growth hormone

Outcomes and Follow-up

- The child will attain height within 3rd to 97th percentile expected for age.
- The child will report personal satisfaction with growth outcomes.
- The child will not experience side effects of GH therapy such as headaches, muscle or joint pain, swelling of hands and feet, scoliosis, or breast tissue development in males.
- The child will attend regularly scheduled appointments for growth monitoring.
- The child and/or family will demonstrate administration of growth hormone.
- The child and/or family will report any side effects of growth hormone.

CENTRAL DIABETES INSIPIDUS

Description

Central diabetes insipidus, or neurogenic diabetes insipidus, is an abnormal decrease in the secretion of vasopressin, also called antidiuretic hormone (ADH).

Etiology

When damaged, the hypothalamus can no longer secrete adequate amounts of ADH. The stores of ADH in the pituitary are depleted, and water is no longer absorbed from the collecting tubules in the kidney.

Incidence and Demographics

Approximately 45% to 50% of cases are familial or idiopathic. Conditions listed under Risk Factors are secondary causes.

Risk Factors

- Head injury or trauma
- Tumor
- Central nervous system infection
- Neurosurgical procedure near pituitary gland

Prevention and Screening

- No prevention or screening indicated

Assessment

History

- Polyuria
- Bedwetting
- Polydipsia

Physical Exam

- Fever
- Weight loss
- Signs of dehydration
- Signs of hypernatremia
    - Restlessness, agitation
    - Decreased deep tendon reflexes
    - Seizures

Diagnostic Studies

- Urine specific gravity less than 1.002
- Urine osmolality less than 50 mOsm/kg H_2O
- Serum osmolality greater than 295 mOsm/kg H_2O
- Water deprivation test shows increased serum osmolality
- ADH (vasopressin) test verifies increased serum osmolality
- MRI to rule out tumor

Management

Invasive Treatment

- Surgical removal of tumor if indicated

Nonpharmacologic Treatment

- Free access to fluids
- Free access to restroom
- Monitoring of intake and output

Pharmacologic Treatment

- Desmopressin acetate (DDAVP) nasal spray

Patient and Family Education

- Nature of condition and treatment plan
- Diagnostic studies preparation
- Medication administration
- Signs of dehydration
- Signs of hypernatremia

Outcomes and Follow-up

- The child will maintain hydration and electrolyte balance.
- The child will attain age-appropriate nighttime dryness.
- The child will wear medical alert jewelry.
- The child and family will verbalize an understanding of the condition, treatment, and diagnostic studies.
- The child and family will demonstrate medication administration.
- The child and family will recognize and report signs of dehydration or hypernatremia.
- The family will communicate the need for unrestricted restroom use to daycare or school personnel.

HYPOTHYROIDISM

Description

Hypothyroidism is a condition characterized by deficiency in thyroid hormone (TH).

Etiology

Hypothyroidism in children is either congenital or acquired. Congenital hypothyroidism is due to abnormal thyroid development resulting from inborn error of metabolism, anatomical defect, or dysgenesis. Congenital hypothyroidism can cause decreased cognitive function if not treated. Causes of acquired hypothyroidism include surgical removal of the thyroid, radiation therapy, infections, and deficient dietary iodine.

Incidence and Demographics

Hypothyroidism is one of the most common pediatric endocrine disorders. Congenital hypothyroidism occurs in approximately 1 in 2,370 live births. It is more common in Hispanics/Latinos, Asians, Native Hawaiians, and other Pacific Islanders.

Risk Factors

- Radiation therapy
- Family history
- Maternal autoimmune thyroiditis
- Maternal exposure to radioactive iodine
- Maternal iodine deficiency
- Twin gestation
- Birth weight less than 2,000 g or greater than 4,500 g
- Gestational age less than 37 weeks or greater than 40 weeks

Prevention and Screening

- There is no prevention, but newborn screening identifies the congenital type.

Assessment

History

- History of risk factors
- Constipation
- Sleepiness or lethargy
- Decline in cognitive function

Physical Exam

- Dryness and puffiness around eyes
- Low core temperature
- Bradycardia
- Hair sparseness
- Dry skin
- Growth failure
- Delayed puberty
- Weight gain

Diagnostic Studies

- Decreased level of circulating TH
- Elevated thyroid-stimulating hormone (TSH)

Management

Invasive Treatment

- No invasive management indicated

Nonpharmacologic Treatment

- Regular serum TH and TSH to monitor therapy

Pharmacologic Treatment

- Levothyroxine, TH replacement
- Soy-based formulas may decrease absorption of levothyroxine, so dosage may require adjustment

Patient and Family Education

- Nature of condition and treatment plan
- Medication administration
- Monitoring of TH levels
- Strategies to promote normal development
- Referral to early intervention program if indicated

Outcomes and Follow-up

- The child will maintain TH levels within normal range.
- The child will return for regular monitoring of TH levels.
- The child will have neurodevelopmental assessment to identify problems.
- The child will be enrolled in an early intervention program if indicated.
- The child will receive continuing psychometric evaluations during school years.
- The family will verbalize an understanding of the condition and treatment plan.
- The family will utilize strategies to promote normal development.
- The family will demonstrate medication administration.

HYPERTHYROIDISM

Description

Hyperthyroidism in children is due to Graves' disease, a condition involving an enlarged thyroid gland.

Etiology

Hyperthyroidism in Graves' disease is an autoimmune response to TSH receptors, resulting in overstimulation of the thyroid gland. Treatment may lead to remission.

Incidence and Demographics

Incidence of Graves' disease is 1 per 5,000 children, and usually occurs in those between ages 6 and 15 years. The peak incidence is between the ages of 11 and 15 years, and is higher in girls.

Risk Factors

- Family history
- Twin gestation
- Down syndrome

Prevention and Screening

- No prevention or screening indicate

Assessment

History

- Gradual onset of symptoms
- Hyperactivity, short attention span
- Irritability, frequent mood swings
- Increased appetite, but weight loss
- Vomiting, frequent bowel movements
- Blurred vision, loss of acuity
- Sleep difficulty
- Heat intolerance

Physical Exam

- Tachycardia
- Widened pulse pressure

- Systolic heart murmur
- Cardiomegaly
- Warm, moist, flushed skin
- Protruding eyeballs
- Periorbital edema
- Goiter
- Tremor
- Hyperactive deep tendon reflexes
- Accelerated growth rate
- Delayed puberty

Diagnostic Studies

- Elevated thyroid hormone levels
- Decreased TSH
- Elevated thyroid-stimulating immunoglobulin (TSI)

Management

Invasive Treatment

- Subtotal thyroidectomy

Nonpharmacologic Treatment

- Ablation with radioactive iodine
- Restricted activity until TH levels near normal
- Quiet, restful environment
- Balance of rest and activity
- Regular routine
- Attention to hygiene, light clothing, hydration for heat intolerance

Pharmacologic Treatment

- Antithyroid medications such as propylthiouracil (PTU), methimazole (MTZ)
- Severe leukopenia with sore throat and fever is a side effect that requires discontinuing of medication, isolation, and antibiotic therapy
- Possible need for levothyroxine after surgery or ablation

Patient and Family Education

- Nature of condition and treatment plan

- Risks and benefits of treatment options
- Preparation for procedures, surgery
- Signs of hypothyroidism
- Medication administration
- Nonpharmacologic management
- Communication with daycare or school

Outcomes and Follow-up

- The child will experience relief of symptoms with effective treatment.
- The child and family will verbalize an understanding of the condition and treatment.
- The child will experience prompt recognition and treatment of medication side effects.
- The family will demonstrate medication administration.
- The family will incorporate strategies of nonpharmacologic management.
- The family will communicate activity guidelines and psychosocial support needed during recovery period.

REFERENCES

Ackerman, P., & Carlson, M. (2012, February 1, February 8). *Diabetic management for the pediatric and adolescent populations.* Academy Medical Systems. Webcast retrieved http://AcademyMedicalSystem.coursehost.com

Allen, P. J., & Fomenko, S. D. (2011). Congenital hypothyroidism. *Pediatric Nursing, 37*(6), 324–326.

Ferry, R. J. (2010). Short stature. *Medscape Reference.* Retrieved from http://emedicine.medscape.com/article/924411-overview

Hockenberry, M. J., & Wilson, D. (2011). *Wong's nursing care of infants and children* (9th ed.). St. Louis, MO: Elsevier Mosby.

Hormone Foundation. (2011). *Growth hormone deficiency in children.* Retrieved from http://www.hormone.org/Resources/upload/GH-Deficiency-Bilingual-WEB.pdf

Laffel, L., & Svoren, B. (2011). Epidemiology, presentation, and diagnosis of type 2 diabetes mellitus in children and adolescents. *UpToDate.* Retrieved from http://www.uptodate.com/contents/epidemiology-presentation-and-diagnosis-of-type-2-diabetes-mellitus-in-children-and-adolescents?source=search_result&search=diabetes+in+children&selectedTitle=3%7E150

LaFranchi, S. (2011). Clinical manifestations and diagnosis of hyperthyroidism in children and adolescents. *UpToDate.* Retrieved from http://www.uptodate.com/contents/clinical-manifestations-and-diagnosis-of-hyperthyroidism-in-children-and-adolescents?source=search_result&search=hyperthyroidism+children&selectedTitle=1%7E150

Levitsky, L. L., & Misra, M. (2011). Epidemiology, presentation, and diagnosis of type 1 diabetes mellitus in children and adolescents. *UpToDate.* Retrieved from http://www.uptodate.com/contents/epidemiology-presentation-and-diagnosis-of-type-1-diabetes-mellitus-in-children-and-adolescents?source=search_result&search=diabetes+in+children&selectedTitle=1%7E150

National Center for Chronic Disease Prevention and Health Promotion. (2011). *National diabetes fact sheet, 2011.* Retrieved from http://www.cdc.gov/diabetes/pubs/pdf/methods11.pdf

Richmond, E. J., & Rogol, A. D. (2011). Diagnosis of growth hormone deficiency in children. *UpToDate.* Retrieved from http://www.uptodate.com/contents/diagnosis-of-growth-hormone-deficiency-in-children?source=search_result&search=growth+hormone+deficiency+children&selectedTitle=1%7E81

Simmons, S. (2010, January). Flushing out the truth about diabetes insipidus. *Nursing2010.* Retrieved from http://ovidsp.tx.ovid.com.ezproxy.lib.purdue.edu/sp-3.5.1a/ovidweb.cgi?WebLinkFrameset=1&S=GKMIFPGIHLDDKGKKNCALHDGCMHGAAA00&returnUrl=ovidweb.cgi%3f%26TOC%3dS

CHAPTER 14

HEMATOLOGIC DISORDERS

Clara J. Richardson, MSN, RN-BC

NEONATAL SEPSIS

Description

Sepsis, also called septicemia, is defined as the presence of a microorganism in the bloodstream. Early onset sepsis occurs within the first 3 days of life, while late onset sepsis occurs in infants between 4 and 90 days of age.

Etiology

Causative organisms of early onset sepsis include group B streptococcus (GBS), *Escherichia coli,* coagulase-negative staphylococci, and *Listeria monocytogenes*. Transmission from mother occurs across the placenta, ascending from the cervix, or from the birth canal during delivery.

The primary organisms responsible for late onset sepsis include staphylococci, *Klebsiella*, enterococci, *E. coli*, *Pseudomonas*, and *Candida*. Late onset infections are usually acquired by cross-contamination from other infants, hospital personnel, or the environment.

Incidence and Demographics

The incidence of neonatal sepsis has not decreased significantly in recent years, but mortality due to sepsis has decreased. The frequency of sepsis is up to four times greater in high-risk newborns than in normal newborns, and twice as great in males. Males also have a higher mortality rate.

Risk Factors

- Prematurity
- Invasive procedures
- Congenital anomalies
- Meconium staining
- Difficult delivery
- Birth asphyxia
- Apgar score lower than six
- Prolonged rupture of membranes
- Maternal fever at the time of delivery
- Maternal urinary tract infection
- Maternal history of group B streptococcal infection or herpes simplex virus infection during pregnancy
- Incomplete immunization

Prevention and Screening

Sepsis may be prevented by treatment of maternal infections during pregnancy and adherence to immunization schedule. Breastfeeding has been shown to be a protective factor. Screening consists of prenatal screening of mother.

Assessment

History

- History of risk factors
- Apnea
- Changes in skin color, muscle tone, activity, or feeding

Physical Exam

- Hypoxia
- Cyanosis
- Hyper- or hypoventilation
- Hypothermia or, rarely, hyperthermia
- Irritability or lethargy
- Poor muscle tone
- Petechiae, bruising
- Decreased perfusion

- Irregular heartbeat
- Edema
- Pallor, jaundice
- Vomiting, diarrhea, abdominal distention
- Full fontanel
- Abnormal eye movements
- Hepatomegaly, splenomegaly

Diagnostic Studies

- Elevated or decreased white blood cell count
- Elevated or decreased total neutrophils with increase in immature neutrophils
- Decreased hemoglobin and hematocrit, indicating anemia
- Elevated C-reactive protein and interleukins
- Blood culture to identify microorganism
- Urinalysis and culture may reveal urinary origin of infection
- Lumbar puncture may reveal central nervous system infection
- Chest radiography to rule out pneumonia

Management

Invasive Treatment

- No invasive management indicated

Nonpharmacologic Treatment

- Supplemental oxygen
- Circulatory and respiratory support
- Thermoregulation
- Infection control measures

Pharmacologic Treatment

- Antibiotic therapy with gram-positive and gram-negative spectrum coverage initiated immediately after culture obtained
- Antimicrobial therapy adjusted with identification of causative organism
- Acetaminophen or ibuprofen for fever
- Oral nystatin for candidiasis
- Intravenous therapy to maintain fluid and electrolyte balance
- Blood transfusions for anemia

Patient and Family Education

- Nature of disease process and treatment plan
- Medication administration
- Care of child with fever
- Strategies to prevent spread of infection
- Recommended immunization schedule

Outcomes and Follow-up

- The child will receive prompt treatment and recover without complications such as pulmonary hypertension, necrotizing enterocolitis, meningitis, cerebral edema, brain injury.
- The child will maintain fluid and electrolyte balance.
- The child's temperature will return to normal.
- The family will verbalize an understanding of the disease process and treatment plan.
- The family will demonstrate effective medication administration and fever care.
- The family will identify strategies to prevent spread of infection.
- The family will demonstrate compliance with recommended immunization schedule.

IRON DEFICIENCY AND IRON-DEFICIENCY ANEMIA

Description

Iron-deficiency anemia (IDA) is a decreased number of red blood cells, reduced hemoglobin concentration, or both, due to inadequate supply, loss, or impaired absorption of iron. IDA is defined as a hemoglobin concentration of less than 11.0 g/dL for children between 12 and 35 months of age.

Iron deficiency is the state of having insufficient iron to maintain normal physiologic functions, and may occur with or without anemia.

Etiology

The main cause of iron-deficiency anemia in children is nutritional deficit of iron. Iron is transferred from the mother to the fetus during the last trimester of gestation. These stores are adequate for the first 4 months in full-term infants. When iron stores are depleted, the production of hemoglobin is decreased, as is the oxygen-carrying capacity of the blood.

Iron deficiency is caused by inadequate absorption of iron to meet increased requirements needed for growth or by a long-term negative iron balance resulting in low iron stores or in low bone marrow iron content.

Incidence and Demographics

In children between 12 and 36 months of age, the prevalence of iron deficiency is 9.2%, and 2.1% for iron deficiency anemia. Approximately 14% of preterm infants develop iron deficiency between 4 and 8 months of age.

Risk Factors

- Maternal anemia, hypertension, or diabetes during pregnancy
- Preterm birth or low birth weight
- High intake of unfortified cow's milk
- Immigrants from developing countries
- Low socioeconomic level
- Exclusive breastfeeding after 4 months of age without iron supplementation

Prevention and Screening

- Prenatal vitamins for all pregnant women
- Supplemental iron for breastfed preterm infants between the ages of 1 and 12 months, provided by medicinal iron or iron-fortified foods
- Supplemental iron for healthy, full-term newborns beginning at age 4 months
- Iron-fortified formula until age 12 months
- Infants 6–12 months of age require 11 mg of iron per day
- Toddlers 1–3 years of age require 7 mg of iron per day
- Universal screening of hemoglobin is recommended once during infancy (between 9 and 12 months of age), once between ages 1 and 5 years, once between age 5 and 12 years, and once between age 14 and 20 years

Assessment

History

- Inadequate iron intake
- Presence of risk factors
- Early introduction or excessive intake of cow's milk
- Frequent infections
- Irritability
- Fatigue

Physical Exam

- Pallor
- Growth failure
- Glossitis, inflammation of the tongue
- Poor muscle tone
- Edema
- Elevated pulse and respiratory rates
- Heart murmur
- Enlarged liver or spleen
- Concave "spoon" fingernails

Diagnostic Studies

- Iron deficiency anemia
    - Hemoglobin level less than 11.0 g/dL
    - Decreased mean corpuscular volume (MCV) with IDA
    - Decreased mean corpuscular hemoglobin (MCH) with IDA
    - Elevated red cell distribution width (RDW) with IDA
    - Decreased reticulocyte count with IDA
- Both IDA and iron deficiency
    - Decreased serum ferritin (SF)
    - Decreased reticulocyte hemoglobin concentration (CHr)
    - Elevated transferrin saturation
    - Elevated serum transferring receptor 1 (TfR1)

Management

Invasive Treatment

- No invasive management indicated

Nonpharmacologic Treatment

- Iron-fortified diet
- Follow prevention strategies
- Limit milk intake in toddlers to 2–3 cups per day

Pharmacologic Treatment

- Oral iron supplement (Fer-In-Sol)

Patient and Family Education

- Nature of deficiency and treatment plan
- Safe administration of iron supplement
    - Liquid forms may stain teeth and should be given far back in the mouth, with teeth brushed afterwards.
    - Citrus fruit or juice will enhance absorption.
    - Tea or antacids will decrease absorption.
    - Stools will be dark green or black.
- Nonpharmacologic diet recommendations

Outcomes and Follow-up

- The child's lab tests will return to normal.
- The child's hemoglobin will increase within 1 month, and anemia will be resolved within 6 months.
- The child's intake of iron-rich foods will increase.
- The child's intake will reflect recommended dietary allowances.
- The family will verbalize an understanding of the disorder and treatment plan.
- The family will demonstrate effective medication administration.

SICKLE CELL ANEMIA

Description

Sickle cell anemia is the homozygous (HgbSS) and most severe form of sickle cell disease (SCD), an autosomal recessive inherited blood disorder.

Etiology

Children with sickle cell anemia produce hemoglobin S. A structural defect in the β-globin chain of the hemoglobin S molecule causes the red blood cells to become sickle-shaped when exposed to a state of dehydration, hypoxia, acidosis, or temperature elevation. These stiff, curved cells can obstruct the small vessels, causing tissue ischemia and organ damage. Vaso-occlusion involves a complex interaction of sickled cells, platelets, leukocytes, plasma components, and vascular endothelium. Infants with sickle cell anemia are usually asymptomatic for the first 6 months of life because of the presence of HgbF, which has a high affinity for oxygen. Sickle cell anemia is characterized by acute exacerbations called crises. The most common is a vaso-occlusive crisis with an area of obstruction and ischemia. In a sequestration crisis, large amounts of blood pool in the spleen or liver, causing shock. An aplastic crisis, a severe anemia, occurs when there is a decrease in red blood cell production, usually triggered by an infection. A hyperhemolytic crisis, accelerated rate of red blood cell destruction, may be caused by viral infection, transfusion reaction, or glucose-6-phosphate dehydrogenase (G6PD) deficiency. If sickled cells obstruct a major blood vessel in the brain, the child experiences a cerebrovascular accident, or stroke. Repeat episodes of acute chest syndrome, the result of obstruction of the small vessels in the lungs, can cause restrictive lung disease and pulmonary hypertension.

Incidence and Demographics

Sickle cell anemia is most common in families from Africa, South or Central America, Caribbean islands, Mediterranean countries, India, and Saudi Arabia. In the United States, sickle cell anemia occurs in approximately 1 in 500 Black births and 1 in 36,000 Hispanic births.

Risk Factors

- Both parents carriers of sickle cell trait
- Several conditions may precipitate vaso-occlusive crises: fever, dehydration, acidosis, hypoxia, stress, cold, pollutants, alcohol intoxication, menses, pregnancy
- Aplastic crises may be preceded by parvovirus B19 or folic acid deficiency
- Acute chest syndrome has been associated with infection, pain episodes, and asthma

Prevention and Screening

- Prevention of infection and factors that may precipitate sickling
- Screening of all newborns required in all states
- Sickle cell turbidity test (Sickledex)
- Hemoglobin electrophoresis to distinguish trait from disease

Assessment

History

- Paleness
- Fatigue
- Growth failure
- Chronic bone or joint pain
- Chronic anemia
- Delayed puberty

Physical Exam

- Vaso-occlusive crisis
  - Severe pain
  - Hematuria
  - Visual disturbances
  - Priapism (painful penile erection)
  - Dactylitis (painful swelling of hands and feet) in children younger than 2 years
- Sequestration crisis
  - Hepatomegaly
  - Splenomegaly
  - Profound anemia resulting in circulatory collapse
- Aplastic crisis
  - Pallor
  - Fatigue and muscle weakness
  - Shortness of breath
  - Systolic heart murmur
- Hyperhemolytic crisis
  - Anemia
  - Jaundice
  - Increased reticulocyte count
- Cerebrovascular accident (stroke)
  - Behavioral changes
  - Prolonged headache
  - Sudden weakness or numbness
  - Vision or speech changes

- Dizziness or falls
- Vomiting
- Jerking or twitching of face, arms, legs
- Seizures

- Acute chest syndrome
  - Chest, back, or abdominal pain
  - Fever
  - Wheezing
  - Dyspnea or tachypnea
  - Retractions
  - Hypoxia
  - Cough

Diagnostic Studies

- Chest radiography
- Blood and sputum cultures
- Complete blood counts and serum chemistry
  - Decreased hemoglobin, serum haptoglobin (indicator or hemolysis)
  - Elevated reticulocytes, bilirubin, serum lactate dehydrogenase, fetal hemoglobin
  - Elevated white blood cell count and platelets
  - Possible iron deficiency anemia with decreased MCV, MCH, MCHC, serum ferritin; increased RDW, serum transferrin
  - Possible folate deficiency with increased MCV, MCH, RDW
- Hemoglobin S concentration with Hgb electrophoresis pre- and posttransfusion therapy
- Annual evaluation of renal, liver, and pulmonary function
- Chemistry panel and urinalysis every 2 years
- Annual screening of children with sickle cell anemia with transcranial Doppler (TCD) to identify stroke risk
  - Starting at age 2 years
  - Children with transcranial blood-flow velocity (TBV) equal to or greater than 200 cm per second are considered at high risk
- Retinal screening beginning at school age
- Bone density screening starting at age 12 years
- Electrocardiography every 2 years starting at age 15 years

- Screening with transthoracic Doppler echocardiography for pulmonary hypertension in older adolescents and adults

Management

Invasive Treatment

- Hematopoietic stem cell transplant is curative for sickle cell disease, but transplant is still associated with serious risk of mortality and treatment-induced malignancy.
- Splenectomy after splenic sequestration crisis

Nonpharmacologic Treatment

- Supplemental oxygen only when hypoxia present
- Incentive spirometry
- Monitor oxygen saturation
- Increase oral fluid intake
- Warm compresses for painful areas
- Bed rest and passive range of motion during pain crisis

Pharmacologic Treatment

- Oral prophylactic penicillin to prevent infection
- Daily folic acid supplement and multivitamin without iron
- Antihypertensive medications for blood pressure above 95th percentile for age
- Immunization to prevent pneumococcal infections
- Annual influenza immunization for children 6 months and older
- Pain management
  - Acetaminophen or ibuprofen for mild to moderate pain
  - Opioids for more severe pain
- Hydroxyurea to increase HgbF concentration, reducing severe pain episodes and acute chest syndrome
- Intravenous therapy to maintain fluid and electrolyte balance
- Broad-spectrum antibiotics for infection
- Blood transfusion therapy to rapidly reduce the number of circulating sickled cells
- Chelation therapy for iron overload resulting from chronic blood transfusion therapy

Patient and Family Education

- Disease process and treatment plan
- Nutrition and fluid requirements

- Pain management: heat, rest, massage, medication
- Genetic implications
- Signs of crises
- Signs of infection and prevention strategies
- Signs of dehydration and prevention strategies
- Signs of spleen enlargement
- Medication administration
- Immunization protocol
- Screening protocols
- Physical activity guidelines: frequent breaks, no contact sport with enlarged spleen
- Communication with school personnel
- Available support groups, counseling
- Available genetic counseling

Outcomes and Follow-up

- The child will experience prompt treatment for infection or crisis.
- The child will experience effective pain management of acute and chronic pain.
- The child will attain growth appropriate for age.
- The child will maintain hydration and nutritional status.
- The child will demonstrate balanced rest and activity.
- The child will not experience long-term complications such as bone disease, pulmonary hypertension, retinopathy, renal disease, or cardiac complications.
- The child and family will access available resources.
- The family will verbalize an understanding of the disease process and treatment plan.
- The family will verbalize an understanding of the genetic implications of sickle cell disease.
- The family will identify signs of crisis, infection, and dehydration.
- The family will demonstrate strategies to prevent infection and dehydration.
- The family will demonstrate medication administration.
- The family will demonstrate compliance with immunization and screening protocols.

IMMUNE THROMBOCYTOPENIC PURPURA

Description

Immune thrombocytopenic purpura (ITP) is an autoimmune disorder resulting in thrombocytopenia, platelet count less than 150,000/mm^3. By definition, acute ITP lasts less than 6 months, and the chronic form lasts longer than 6 months.

Etiology

The exact etiology of ITP is unknown. Platelet cell membrane proteins stimulate production of autoantibodies that bind to circulating platelets, which are then destroyed by macrophages in the spleen. The autoantibodies also disrupt the production of new platelets, leaving the child vulnerable to serious bleeding.

Incidence and Demographics

The incidence of acute ITP is approximately 3–8 cases per 100,000 children each year, with the peak occurrence between 2 and 5 years of age. Acute ITP is more common in children between the ages of 2 and 10 years. Spontaneous remission may occur months to years after onset, and about 20%–30% of children with the acute form develop chronic ITP.

Risk Factors

There is an increased risk of developing ITP within 6 weeks following MMR (measles, mumps, rubella) vaccination, but the occurrence is rare.

Prevention and Screening

No prevention or screening

Assessment

History

- Prior infection
- Sudden onset of bruising, petechiae, nosebleeds

Physical Exam

- Bruising
- Petechiae, purpura
- Bleeding of nose, gums, mouth
- Hemorrhagic blisters in the mouth, called wet purpura

- Possible gastrointestinal or genitourinary bleeding
- Rarely intracranial hemorrhage

Diagnostic Studies

- Low platelet count
- Platelets larger than normal

Management

Invasive Treatment

- Splenectomy for significant or persistent ITP, or for lack of response to treatment

Nonpharmacologic Treatment

- Avoid contact sports and activities likely to result in falls
- Avoid aspirin, ibuprofen, and other NSAIDS
- Soft toothbrush, lip balm

Pharmacologic Treatment

- Short course of corticosteroids
- Rituximab (Rituxan) for significant ongoing bleeding
- Intravenous immune globulin (IVIG) to increase number of platelets
- Platelet transfusion only for life-threatening hemorrhage
- Possible anti-Rho (D) immune globulin for RhD-positive children

Patient and Family Education

- Nature of disease process and treatment plan
- Strategies to prevent bleeding
- Medication administration

Outcomes and Follow-up

- The child will not experience bleeding episodes.
- The child's platelet level will increase.
- The family will verbalize an understanding of the disease process and treatment plan.
- The family will utilize strategies to prevent bleeding.
- The family will demonstrate effective medication administration.

HEMOPHILIA

Description

Hemophilia is a group of X-chromosome-linked recessive bleeding disorders. The most common forms are hemophilia A, also called factor VIII deficiency or classic hemophilia, and hemophilia B, also called factor IX deficiency or Christmas disease.

Etiology

Both factors are necessary for blood coagulation. Factor VIII is produced in the liver and is required for the formation of thromboplastin. Children with hemophilia bleed for longer periods, not more profusely. Although hemophilia is primarily an inherited disorder, about 30% of affected children have no family history, and the defect was caused by genetic mutation.

Incidence and Demographics

The disease occurs primarily in males, with rare exceptions. Each year, 1 in 5,000 males is born with hemophilia. Nine out of 10 people with hemophilia have hemophilia A and, of those, 7 out of 10 are classified as severe. Hemophilia A is classified by the level of factor VIII activity (Table 14–1).

TABLE 14–1.
HEMOPHILIA A CLASSIFICATION

CLASSIFICATION	FACTOR VIII ACTIVITY	BLEEDING
Mild	5%–30%	With severe trauma or surgery
Moderate	1%–5%	With trauma
Severe	< 1%	Spontaneous, without trauma

Risk Factors

- Maternal carrier status
- Family history

Prevention and Screening

There is no prevention, but genetic screening for the disease and carrier status is possible.

Assessment

History

- Longer-than-normal bleeding episodes with circumcision, heel sticks, loss of umbilical cord, immunizations, loss of teeth, dental procedures, surgery
- Frequent nosebleeds

Physical Exam

- Hemarthrosis: bleeding into the joint
  - Most common and severe manifestation
  - Repeat joint bleeds result in permanent deformity
  - Joint stiffness, tingling, ache, decreased mobility
  - Joint warmth, redness, swelling, severe pain
- Bleeding into mouth, neck, or chest may lead to airway obstruction
- Intracranial hemorrhage
  - Headache
  - Repeated vomiting
  - Neck pain or stiffness
  - Slurred speech
  - Double vision
  - Sudden weakness or clumsiness
  - Seizure
  - Change in behavior
  - Sleepiness
  - Loss of consciousness
- Bleeding in the gastrointestinal tract
  - Black, tarry stools
  - Anemia
- Hematomas of the spine may result in paralysis
- Hematuria
- Bruising

Diagnostic Studies

- Factor activity assays during fetal period or from umbilical cord blood at delivery for children of carrier parents
- Coagulation factor assays to identify specific factor deficiency
- Prolonged partial thromboplastin time (PTT)
- Prolonged activated partial thromboplastin time (APTT)

Management

Invasive Treatment

- No invasive management indicated

Nonpharmacologic Treatment

- Rest, ice, elevation for bleeding
- Elastic wrap or splint for bleeding
- Avoid passive range of motion during acute episode
- Avoid aspirin, ibuprofen, other NSAIDS
- Prevention of injury in toddlers by use of soft helmets, knee pads, softened environment, if not on prophylactic therapy
- Avoid contact sports, trampolines, three-wheelers
- Wear protective equipment appropriate to activity
- Soft toothbrush or water irrigating device
- Electric shavers instead of razors
- Regular visits to hemophilia treatment center for care
- Follow recommended immunization schedule
- Regular exercise to strengthen muscles and joints

Pharmacologic Treatment

- Intravenous plasma-free recombinant factor VIII for prophylaxis and treatment of bleeding episodes
- Intranasal desmopressin acetate (DDAVP) for minor bleeding with mild hemophilia
- Oral aminocaproic acid (Amicar) for nose or mouth bleeds, before dental procedures
- Acetaminophen (Tylenol) for pain
- Alternative treatment for the 20% of those with hemophilia A who form inhibitors to factor VIII that destroy the clotting factor before it works
    - Factor VIII inhibitor bypassing activity anti-inhibitor coagulant complex (FEIBA)
    - Recombinant activated coagulation factor VII (NovoSeven)

Patient and Family Education

- Nature of disease process
- Genetic implications
- Home factor administration
- Medication administration
- Strategies to prevent bleeding
- Exercise and activity plan
- Medical alert jewelry
- Communication with school personnel

- Available support groups, counseling

Outcomes and Follow-up

- The child will experience minimal bleeding episodes and prompt treatment.
- The child will receive recommended immunizations.
- The child will receive care at a hemophilia treatment center.
- The child will engage in appropriate exercise and physical activity.
- The child will not experience long-term disabling joint damage.
- The family will verbalize an understanding of the disease process and genetic implications.
- The family will demonstrate intravenous factor administration.
- The family will demonstrate medication administration.
- The family will identify strategies to prevent bleeding.
- The family will recognize signs of bleeding episodes.
- The family will demonstrate nonpharmacologic management of bleeding episodes.

LEUKEMIA

Description

Acute leukemia is cancer of the bone marrow and lymphatic tissue. The main types of leukemia seen in children are acute lymphoblastic leukemia (ALL) and acute myeloid leukemia (AML).

Etiology

The exact cause remains unknown. In leukemia, the blood-forming tissues produce large numbers of immature white blood cells called blasts. These blast cells infiltrate body tissues, especially highly vascular areas, and crowd out normal cells by competing for nutrients. Infiltration of the bone marrow causes decreased numbers of red blood cells, white blood cells, and platelets. The accompanying increased pressure within the marrow produces bone pain and bone weakening. Infiltration of the lymph glands, spleen, and liver leads to enlargement and fibrosis. With central nervous system infiltration there is increased intracranial pressure and possibly cranial nerve involvement. Additional sites of infiltration are the kidneys, testes, prostate, ovaries, gastrointestinal tract, and lungs.

Incidence and Demographics

TABLE 14-2.
INCIDENCE OF CHILDHOOD LEUKEMIA PER 100,000 BY AGE

	< 1 YEAR	1-4 YEARS	5-9 YEARS	10-14 YEARS	15-19 YEARS
ALL	1.84	7.55	3.24	1.89	1.71
AML	1.44	0.88	0.5	0.74	0.86

Leukemia accounts for about 30% of all childhood malignancies. ALL, with a 5-year survival rate of 85%, is five times more common than AML, with a 5-year survival rate of 50%–70%. The highest incidence is in Hispanics, followed by Whites and then Blacks.

Risk Factors

- Sibling with leukemia
- Environmental radiation, chemicals
- Down syndrome
- Fanconi's anemia
- Li-Fraumeni syndrome
- Neurofibromatosis
- Past chemotherapy

Prevention and Screening

- No prevention or screening indicated

Assessment

History

- Bone pain
- Bleeding gums
- Pallor
- Fever
- Bruising and petechiae
- Fatigue and lethargy
- Anorexia and weight loss
- Frequent infections

Physical Exam

- Swollen lymph glands

- Hepatosplenomegaly
- Stiffness of neck and back
- Chloromas
- Testicular enlargement
- Anterior mediastinal mass
- Signs of increased intracranial pressure

Diagnostic Studies

- Complete blood count: anemia, elevated blast cells, thrombocytopenia
- Variable white blood cell count: an initial count > 50,000/mm^3 places child in a less favorable prognostic category (high risk)
- Flow cytometry, immunohistochemistry tests to identify type of leukemia
- Bone marrow aspiration for definitive diagnosis and treatment monitoring
- Chest radiography or CT scan for enlarged thymus or chest lymphadenopathy
- Possible MRI, ultrasound, or PET scan

Management

Invasive Treatment

- Bone marrow transplant during second ALL remission or during first AML remission

Nonpharmacologic Treatment

- Strategies to deal with side effects of chemotherapy
- Infection prevention
- Balance of rest and activity

Pharmacologic Treatment

- Prophylactic allopurinol or rasburicase to prevent acute uric acid nephropathy related to tumor lysis syndrome
- Prophylactic antibiotics during chemotherapy
- Administer only inactive immunizations during chemotherapy
- Administer make-up immunizations after checking antibody titers 3–6 months after completion of chemotherapy

TABLE 14-3.
CHEMOTHERAPY AGENTS FOR LEUKEMIA

PHASE	CHEMOTHERAPY
Induction of remission ALL: 3-4 weeks AML: 4-6 weeks	Prednisone, prednisolone, dexamethasone Vincristine Asparaginase Doxorubincin Daunorubicin 90% remission rate for ALL 75% remission rate for AML
Central nervous system preventive therapy	Intrathecal methotrexate Cranial radiation only for high-risk patients
Consolidation 4-6 months	Cytarabine Methotrexate Doxorubicin Daunorubicin Cyclophosphamide Ifosfamide Teniposide Etoposide
Maintenance 24-36 months	Oral 6-mercaptopurine Methotrexate Pulse vincristine and corticosteroid therapy

Patient and Family Education

- Nature of disease process and treatment plan
- Preparation for tests and procedures
- Infection prevention
- Rest and activity
- Strategies to deal with side effects of chemotherapy: hair loss, mouth sores, anorexia, diarrhea, fatigue, nausea, and vomiting
- Signs of relapse: fever, malaise, bleeding, bone pain
- Central nervous system relapse: headache, morning vomiting, nuchal rigidity, papilledema
- Available support groups, counseling

Outcomes and Follow-up

- The child will attain and maintain remission.
- The child will experience minimal side effects of chemotherapy.

- The child will maintain a balance of rest and activity.
- The child will attain and maintain recommended immunization status.
- The family will integrate strategies to deal with side effects of chemotherapy.
- The family will practice infection prevention.
- The child and family will access available resources.
- The child will receive monitoring for potential long-term effects of treatment.
  - Testing for cognitive delay
  - Growth monitoring for pituitary dysfunction
  - Monitoring for reproductive dysfunction
  - Complete blood counts to identify secondary neoplasms
  - Electrocardiography or echocardiography to detect cardiomyopathy
  - Liver function studies
  - Bone density screening
  - Dental exams

HODGKIN'S LYMPHOMA

Description

Hodgkin's lymphoma is a cancer that originates in the lymphoid system, involves primarily the lymph nodes, and spreads through the lymphatic system.

Etiology

The specific cause of Hodgkin's lymphoma is unknown, but research suggests that an abnormal immune response to an infectious agent, possibly the Epstein-Barr virus, may have a role in the development of the disease. In most cases, the disease starts in the B lymphocytes. Staging is based on systemic symptoms, number of sites, location of involved lymph nodes above or below diaphragm, and presence of extranodal involvement. Sites of metastasis are spleen, liver, lungs, bone marrow, and mediastinum.

Incidence and Demographics

Hodgkin's lymphoma is responsible for about 7% of all childhood cancers. More than 80% of people with newly diagnosed disease will be long-term survivors.

TABLE 14-4.
INCIDENCE OF HODGKIN'S LYMPHOMA PER 100,000 CHILDREN, BY AGE

5-9 YEARS	10-14 YEARS	15-19 YEARS
0.35	1.19	3.21

Risk Factors

- HIV infection
- Family history
- Epstein-Barr viral infection
- Compromised immune system

Prevention and Screening

- No prevention or screening indicated

Assessment

History

- Fever
- Fatigue
- Weight loss
- Pruritus
- Anorexia
- Nausea
- Nonproductive cough
- Abdominal pain

Physical Exam

- Swollen lymph nodes, commonly the cervical, supraclavicular, and axillary areas
- Nodes are firm and nontender
- Hepatosplenomegaly
- Mediastinal mass

Diagnostic Studies (also used for staging)

- Biopsy of lymph nodes shows Reed-Sternberg cells, an abnormal type of B lymphocytes
- Chest radiography
- CT scan

- Positron emission tomography (PET)
- Complete blood count
- Erythrocyte sedimentation rate
- C-reactive protein
- Alkaline phosphatase
- Renal and liver function tests
- Urinalysis
- Uric acid level
- Bone marrow aspiration
- Bone scan

Management

Invasive Treatment

- Autologous stem cell transplantation (ASCT)

Nonpharmacologic Treatment

- Radiation therapy

Pharmacologic Treatment

- Combination chemotherapy
    - Doxorubicin
    - Vinblastine
    - Methotrexate
    - Etoposide
    - Prednisone

Patient and Family Education

- Nature of disease and treatment plan
- Preparation for diagnostic tests and procedures
- Rest and activity
- Infection prevention
- Strategies to deal with common side effects of treatment (see Leukemia)
- Delayed secondary sexual characteristics, delayed menses, risk of sterility
- Available support groups, counseling

Outcomes and Follow-up

- The child will experience full remission.
- The child will experience minimal side effects of chemotherapy and radiation.
- The child will show evidence of adequate rest during treatment.
- The child and family will verbalize an understanding of the disease process and treatment plan.
- The child and family will verbalize understanding of the education content.
- The family will demonstrate infection prevention strategies.
- The child and family will access available resources.

REFERENCES

American Cancer Society. (2010). *Childhood leukemia.* Retrieved from http://www.cancer.org/acs/groups/cid/documents/webcontent/003095-pdf.pdf

American Society of Hematology. (2011). *Guideline on the evaluation and management of immune thrombocytopenia (ITP).* Retrieved from http://www.hematology.org/Practice/Guidelines/2934.aspx

Anderson-Berry, A. L. (2011). *Neonatal sepsis.* Retrieved from http://emedicine.medscape.com/article/978352-overview

Baker, R. D., & Greer, F. R. (2010). Clinical report – diagnosis and prevention of iron deficiency and iron-deficiency anemia in infants and young children (0–3 years of age). *Pediatrics, 126*(5), 1–11.

Centers for Disease Control and Prevention. (2007). *United States cancer statistics.* Retrieved from http://apps.nccd.cdc.gov/uscs/childhoodcancerdetailedbyICCC.aspx

Field, J. J., Vichinsky, E. P., & DeBaun, M. R. (2011). Overview of the management of sickle cell disease. *UpToDate.* Retrieved from http://www.uptodate.com/contents/overview-of-the-management-of-sickle-cell-disease?source=search_result&search=sickle+cell+disease+in+children&selectedTitle=2%7E150

Gottschalk, S. M., & McClain, K. L. (2011). Overview of Hodgkin lymphoma in children and adolescents. *UpToDate.* Retrieved from http://www.uptodate.com/contents/overview-of-hodgkin-lymphoma-in-children-and-adolescents?source=search_result&search=hodgkin+lymphoma+in+children&selectedTitle=1%7E150

Hockenberry, M. J., & Wilson, D. (2011). *Wong's nursing care of infants and children* (9th ed.). St. Louis, MO: Elsevier Mosby.

Horton, T. M., & Steuber, C. P. (2012). Overview of the presentation and classification of acute lymphoblastic leukemia in children. *UpToDate.* Retrieved from http://www.uptodate.com/contents/overview-of-the-presentation-and-classification-of-acute-lymphoblastic-leukemia-in-children?source=see_link

Horton, T. M., & Steuber, C. P. (2012). Overview of the treatment of acute lymphoblastic leukemia in children. *UpToDate.* Retrieved from http://www.uptodate.com/contents/overview-of-the-treatment-of-acute-lymphoblastic-leukemia-in-children?source=search_result&search=childhood+leukemia&selectedTitle=3%7E150

Khair, K. (2011). Minimizing joint damage: The role of the nurse in promoting adherence to hemophilia treatment. *Orthopaedic Nursing, 29*(3), 193–200.

Khan, S., & Rodgers, G. P. (2011). Hematopoietic cell transplantation in sickle cell disease. *UpToDate.* Retrieved August 20, 2012, from http://www.uptodate.com/contents/hematopoietic-cell-transplantation-in-sickle-cell-disease?source=see_link

Maakaron, J. E., & Taher, A. (2012). Sickle cell anemia. *Medscape Reference Drugs, Diseases, & Procedures.* Retrieved from http://emedicine.medscape.com/article/205926-overview

McCarthy, J., & Mathew, P. (2011). Treatment of hemophilia with inhibitors: An advance in options for pediatric patients. *Journal of Emergency Nursing, 37*(5), 474–476.

National Heart, Lung, and Blood Institute. (2011). *Hemophilia.* Retrieved from http://www.nhlbi.nih.gov/health/health-topics/topics/hemophilia

National Heart, Lung, and Blood Institute. (2011). *Sickle cell anemia.* Retrieved August 20, 2012, from http://www.nhlbi.nih.gov/health/health-topics/topics/sca/

Steuber, C. P. (2011). Treatment and prognosis of immune (idiopathic) thrombocytopenic purpura in children. *UpToDate*. Retrieved from http://www.uptodate.com/contents/treatment-and-prognosis-of-immune-idiopathic-thrombocytopenic-purpura-in-children?source=search_result&search=idiopathic+thrombocytopenic+purpura+children&selectedTitle=1%7E150

Steuber, C. P. (2011). Clinical manifestations and diagnosis of immune (idiopathic) thrombocytopenic purpura in children. *UpToDate*. Retrieved from http://www.uptodate.com/contents/clinical-manifestations-and-diagnosis-of-immune-idiopathic-thrombocytopenic-purpura-in-children?source=search_result&search=idiopathic+thrombocytopenic+purpura+children&selectedTitle=2%7E150

Vichinsky, E. P. (2011). Overview of the clinical manifestations of sickle cell disease. *UpToDate*. Retrieved from http://www.uptodate.com/contents/overview-of-the-clinical-manifestations-of-sickle-cell-disease?source=search_result&search=sickle+cell+disease+in+children&selectedTitle=1%7E150

Wang, C. J., Kavanagh, P. L., Little, A. A., Holliman, J. B., & Sprinz, P. G. (2011). Quality-of-care indicators for children with sickle cell disease. *Pediatrics, 128*(3), 484–493.

CHAPTER 15

IMMUNOLOGIC DISORDERS

Clara J. Richardson, MSN, RN-BC

HIV AND AIDS

Description

Human immunodeficiency virus (HIV) is the organism that causes acquired immunodeficiency syndrome (AIDS), a chronic disease of the immune system.

Etiology

HIV is transmitted by contact with another person's infected blood, body fluids, or secretions. Adolescents acquire HIV through high-risk behaviors. The virus then binds to the CD4 receptor on the cell member of the T lymphocytes. The DNA of the virus joins the T-cell DNA and is reproduced as the T cell replicates, a process called reverse transcription. HIV also causes dysfunction of the B cells, and antigen-presenting cells suppress humoral immunity. The result is suppression of cell-mediated immunity. Immediately after infection, the virus is disseminated throughout the lymphoid organs. The speed of progression from HIV infection to AIDS is variable. As CD4 lymphocytes decrease, physical symptoms appear. The diagnosis of AIDS is based on an extremely low CD4 cell count and development of AIDS-defining illnesses.

Incidence and Demographics

The incidence of HIV/AIDS in children under the age of 13 years is 0.1 per 100,000 in the United States. The occurrence of HIV infection is greatest in Blacks, then in Whites, and then in Hispanics. Perinatal exposure during pregnancy, birth, or breastfeeding is the route of infection for 90% of children with HIV.

TABLE 15-1.
NEWLY DIAGNOSED WITH HIV OR AIDS CHILDREN BY AGE, 2009

AGE (YEARS)	HIV	AIDS
< 13	166	13
13–14	21	58
15–19	2,036	484

Risk Factors

- Maternal HIV infection, IV drug use, sexual relationship with IV drug user
- Human blood product recipient in areas without adequate product screening
- IV drug use, needle sharing
- Sexual partner with HIV infection
- Sexual relationship with IV drug user
- Unprotected vaginal, anal, oral sexual contact
- Multiple sexual partners
- Males having unprotected sex with males

Prevention and Screening

- Prevention by decreasing risk of maternal transmission:
    - Antiretroviral therapy for pregnant women with HIV and prophylaxis therapy for opportunistic infections
    - Cesarean section delivery
    - Limit time between rupture of fetal membranes and delivery to under 4 hours
    - Avoid breastfeeding
- Screening of pregnant women for HIV allows prevention and early treatment for infected infants
- Rapid HIV screening during labor, if not done earlier
- Screening of newborns at risk for maternal transmission

Assessment

History

- Chronic or recurrent diarrhea
- Growth failure
- Frequent infections
- Developmental delay

Physical Exam

- Swollen lymph glands
- Hepatosplenomegaly
- Oral candidiasis
- Dermatitis
- Inflammation of the parotid gland
- AIDS-defining conditions:
    - *Pneumocystis carinii* pneumonia: life-threatening fungal lung infection
    - Lymphoid interstitial pneumonitis: infiltration of alveoli and interstitial spaces with mature lymphocytes
    - Recurrent bacterial infections
    - HIV encephalopathy: impaired brain growth, cognitive impairment, loss of developmental milestones
    - Cytomegalovirus disease: viral infection causing retinitis, death of retinal cells
    - *Mycobacterium avium-intracellulare* complex infection
    - Pulmonary or esophageal candidiasis: yeast infection
    - Herpes simplex disease: viral infection with painful skin eruptions
    - Cryptosporidiosis: parasitic infection causing diarrhea
    - Wasting syndrome: weight loss, muscle wasting, diarrhea, extreme weakness, fever

Diagnostic Studies

- CD4+ (helper T cell) counts and percentages every 3–4 months (< 200 or 14% of lymphocytes indicative of AIDS)
- Repeat positive HIV DNA polymerase chain reaction (PCR) survey every 3–4 months
- Positive HIV RNA assay: monitored every 3–4 months
- Positive viral load test confirmed by repeat test to rule out false positive
- HIV DNA virologic assays to detect HIV in children younger than 18 months of age
- HIV antibody test and Western blot or IFA assay for children 18 months of age or older
- HIV DNA virologic assays for perinatal exposure at ages 14–21 days, 1–2 months, and 4–6 months
- Pharmacologic management monitored for adverse medication effects every 6–12 months by urinalysis, complete blood count with differential, blood chemistries, and lipid panel

Management

Invasive Treatment

- No invasive management indicated

Nonpharmacologic Treatment

- Healthy diet
- Balance of rest and activity

Pharmacologic Treatment

- Age for initiation of treatment depends on CD4, HIV RNA, and severity of symptoms for children 1 year of age and older
- All HIV-positive infants (younger than 12 months of age) should be treated
- Antiretroviral therapy (ART) for children should include at least three drugs in at least two classes
- Nucleoside reverse transcriptase inhibitors (NRTI) to prematurely end DNA replication
    - Abacavir
    - Emtricitabine
    - Didanosine
    - Zidovudine
    - Stavudine
    - Lamivudine for those at least 16 years of age
    - Etravirine for those at least 6 years of age
    - Atazanavir/ritonavir
    - Tenofovir for those at least 12 years of age and Tanner stage 4
- Nonnucleoside reverse transcriptase inhibitors (NNRTI) to reverse transcriptase
    - Efavirenz
    - Nevirapine
- Protease inhibitors (PI) to inhibit viral replication later in process
    - Lopinavir/ritonavir
    - Fosamprenavir

Patient and Family Education

- Disease process and treatment plan
- Transmission and prevention
- Implications of lab results
- Medication regimen and implications of noncompliance, such as multiplying of virus and development of resistant forms of virus
- Nutrition
- Balance of rest and activity
- Prevention and signs of opportunistic infections
- Advocacy: social stigma, rights, communication with school
- Availability of community resources, support groups, counseling
- Contraception and safe sex techniques

Outcomes and Follow-up

- The child will experience balance of rest and activity.
- The child will maintain a healthy diet as evidenced by adequate growth.
- The child will attain age-appropriate developmental milestones.
- The child will receive recommended well-child care.
- The child will not experience social stigma related to HIV status.
- The family will verbalize an understanding of the disease process and treatment plan.
- The family will demonstrate strategies to prevent transmission of HIV.
- The family will verbalize an understanding of the lab results.
- The family will maintain strict adherence to the medication regimen.
- The family will seek prompt treatment for drug-related side effects and toxicity.
- The family will demonstrate strategies to prevent opportunistic infections.
- The family will recognize signs and seek prompt treatment of opportunistic infections.
- The family will actively advocate within the healthcare system, childcare setting, school system, and community to ensure the child's rights.

SYSTEMIC ALLERGIC REACTIONS (ANAPHYLAXIS)

Description

Systemic allergic reaction or anaphylaxis is the body's acute-onset, potentially fatal response to an allergen. This reaction is characterized by severe bronchospasm, laryngeal edema, shock, and cardiovascular collapse.

Etiology

IgE is synthesized upon exposure to an allergen and becomes fixed on mast cells and basophils. Mast cells and basophils release histamine and other mediators of inflammation, causing vasodilation, bronchoconstriction, and increased capillary permeability. Fluid leaks into the interstitial spaces with reduced arterial pressure and rapid onset of symptoms.

Common allergens in children include:

Foods

- Cow's milk
- Eggs
- Peanuts and tree nuts
- Fish and shellfish
- Wheat, soy, or sesame
- Citrus fruits, strawberries
- Chocolate

Medical products

- Drugs
- Contrast media
- Latex
- Blood products

Venom

- Hymenoptera (bees, wasps)
- Snakes
- Jellyfish
- Spiders

Incidence and Demographics

The incidence of anaphylaxis is not known, but several trends have been identified. The incidence seems to be increasing, on the basis of emergency room statistics. Anaphylaxis occurs more commonly in community settings than in healthcare settings, and the largest number of occurrences is in children and adolescents.

Risk Factors

- Positive allergen skin test
- Elevated quantitative allergen-specific IgE level
- Recent insect stings
- Concurrent asthma

Prevention and Screening

- Prevention consists of avoidance of allergen exposure.
- Screening to identify an allergen may be done with allergen skin testing and quantitative allergen-specific IgE levels.

Assessment

History

- Exposure to allergen

Physical Exam

- Skin
    - Itching
    - Flushing
    - Hives
    - Periorbital or perioral edema
- Respiratory
    - Cough
    - Sneezing
    - Dyspnea
    - Hoarseness
    - Stridor
    - Wheezing
- Gastrointestinal
    - Nausea

    - Vomiting
    - Diarrhea
    - Abdominal pain
- Cardiovascular
    - Dizziness
    - Tachycardia
    - Headache
    - Dysrhythmia
    - Loss of consciousness
    - Seizure
    - Hypotension
    - Shock

Diagnostic Studies

- Plasma histamine within 15–60 minutes of onset
- Serum or plasma tryptase within 15–180 minutes of onset

Management

Invasive Treatment

- No invasive management indicated

Nonpharmacologic Treatment

- Establish airway
- Supplemental oxygen
- Elevate head unless hypotensive
- Cardiac monitor
- Basic life support and resuscitation

Pharmacologic Treatment

- Epinephrine for first-line therapy
- Bronchodilator: albuterol
- Antihistamine: diphenhydramine
- Corticosteroid: methylprednisolone

Patient and Family Education

- Description and treatment of anaphylaxis

- Avoidance strategies
- Use of Epi-Pen
- Medical alert jewelry
- Emergency action plan

Outcomes and Follow-up

- The child will receive prompt treatment of anaphylaxis.
- The child will maintain an open airway and adequate circulation.
- The child will experience relief of symptoms.
- The child will wear medical alert jewelry.
- The child will have an Epi-Pen available at all times.
- The child and family will identify allergens.
- The child and family will practice avoidance strategies.
- The family will verbalize an understanding of anaphylaxis.
- The family will demonstrate use of the Epi-Pen.
- The family will develop an emergency action plan for childcare, school, and extracurricular activities.

SYSTEMIC LUPUS ERYTHEMATOSUS

Description

Systemic lupus erythematosus (SLE) is a chronic, autoimmune, inflammatory disease affecting multiple body systems, and is characterized by exacerbations and remissions.

Etiology

The exact mechanism of SLE initial onset is not completely known. It is thought that predisposing factors such as genetic factors and unidentified triggers interact to initiate a disordered immune response. Environmental triggers that are being investigated include exposure to ultraviolet light, estrogen, pregnancy, infections, and drugs. The immune response is characterized by activated helper T cells that stimulate B cells to cause secretion of auto-antibodies and immune complex. The immune complexes are deposited in kidney, brain, heart, spleen, lung, gastrointestinal, skin, and peritoneum tissues. The final result is organ disease and death.

Incidence and Demographics

It is estimated that SLE affects between 5,000 and 10,000 children in the United States. It occurs more commonly in girls. Although it can occur at any age, the incidence increases in children age 5 years and above and then increases again in those age 10 years and above. In children between the ages of 10 and 18 years there are 31 cases per 100,000 female Asian Americans, 20 cases per 100,000 Blacks, 13 cases per 100,000 Hispanics/Latinos, and 4 cases per 100,000 Whites. The 5-year survival rate in children is close to 100% and the 10-year rate close to 90%.

Risk Factors

- Family history of autoimmune diseases

Prevention and Screening

- There is no known prevention and no screening indicated.

Assessment

History

- Recurrent fevers
- Fatigue
- Joint pain
- Anorexia
- Abdominal pain
- Nausea, vomiting
- Headache
- Behavior change
- School performance change
- Weight loss
- Seizure

Physical Exam

- Arthritis
- Hypertension
- Butterfly rash over nose and across cheeks
- Disc-shaped rash: red, scaling patches
- Photosensitivity
- Mouth or nose ulcers
- Alopecia

- Hepatomegaly
- Splenomegaly
- Lymphadenopathy
- Retinopathy
- Pleuritis
- Pericarditis

Diagnostic Studies

- Complete blood count shows hemolytic anemia, leukopenia, thrombocytopenia
- Elevated antinuclear antibody (ANA) titer
- Positive antiphospholipid antibodies (aPL) or lupus anticoagulant (LA)

Management

Invasive Treatment

- No invasive management indicated

Nonpharmacologic Treatment

- Strategies to prevent coronary artery disease
    - Avoid smoking
    - Maintain healthy weight
    - Healthy diet
    - Exercise and physical activity
    - Monitor blood pressure, cholesterol, lipids
- Strategies to prevent infection
- Strategies to prevent osteoporosis
    - Exercise and physical activity
    - Diet fortified with calcium and vitamin D
- Strategies to limit sun exposure to minimize photosensitive rash

Pharmacologic Treatment

- Corticosteroids: prednisone for antiinflammatory and immunosuppressive properties
- Antimalarial drugs: hydroxychloroquine (Plaquenil)
- Low-dose corticosteroids: prednisone
- Immunosuppressive drugs: azathioprine (Imuran), mycophenolate mofetil (CellCept), methotrexate, cyclophosphamide (Cytoxan)
- Calcium and vitamin D supplements to prevent osteoporosis with corticosteroids

- Nonsteroidal antiinflammatory drugs (NSAIDS) for arthritis: naproxen, ibuprofen

Patient and Family Education

- Nature of disease and treatment plan
- Medication administration with strict compliance
- Balance of rest and activity
- Contraceptive (low estrogen) options for adolescents
- Strategies to prevent coronary artery disease, infection, osteoporosis, sun exposure
- Available support groups, counseling

Outcomes and Follow-up

- The child will experience minimal exacerbations of the disease.
- The child will experience minimal side effects of drug therapy.
- The child will experience balanced activity and rest.
- The child will attend school regularly.
- The child will participate in regular physical activity and sports.
- The child and family will verbalize an understanding of the disease process and treatment plan.
- The child and family will integrate strategies to prevent coronary artery disease, infection, osteoporosis, and sun exposure.
- The child and family will access available support groups and counseling.
- The family will demonstrate effective medication administration.

REFERENCES

Centers for Disease Control and Prevention. (2011). *HIV surveillance report, 2009*. Retrieved from http://www.cdc.gov/hiv/topics/surveillance/resources/reports/

Centers for Disease Control and Prevention. (2011). *Lyme disease*. Retrieved from http://www.cdc.gov/lyme/

Hockenberry, M. J., & Wilson, D. (2011). *Wong's nursing care of infants and children* (9th ed.). St. Louis, MO: Elsevier Mosby.

Lehman, T. J. A. (2011). Systemic lupus erythematosus in children. *UpToDate*. Retrieved from http://www.uptodate.com/contents/systemic-lupus-erythematosus-in-children?source=search_result&search=systemic+lupus+erythematosus+children&selectedTitle=1%7E150

Panel on Antiretroviral Therapy and Medical Management of HIV-Infected Children. (2011). *Guidelines for the use of antiretroviral agents in pediatric HIV infection*. Retrieved from http://aidsinfo.nih.gov/ContentFiles/PediatricGuidelines.pdf

Pickering, L. K., Baker, C. J., Kimberlin, D. W., & Long, S. S. (Eds.). (2009). *Red book: 2009 report of the Committee on Infectious Diseases* (28th ed.). Elk Grove Village, IL: American Academy of Pediatrics.

CHAPTER 16

NEUROMUSCULAR DISORDERS

Clara J. Richardson, MSN, RN-BC

DEVELOPMENTAL CHARACTERISTICS OF THE PEDIATRIC NEUROMUSCULAR SYSTEM

- Children experience a rapid growth rate of the nervous system during infancy and early childhood, which slows during late childhood and adolescence.
- Nerve fibers conduct impulses at a slower rate in young children.
- Myelinization of the nerve tracts proceeds from head to toe (cephalocaudal development) and from near to far (proximodistal development).
- Motor skills develop as the nervous system matures.

NEURAL TUBE DEFECTS

Description

Neural tube defects (NTD) are congenital malformations of the spinal cord, brain, and vertebrae. The main NTDs are encephalocele, anencephaly, and spina bifida. Encephalocele is an opening in the skull that allows a portion of the brain to protrude. In anencephaly, there is no brain development above the brainstem. The most common NTD is spina bifida, which takes three forms. Spina bifida occulta is nonvisible separation in the vertebrae. Meningocele is a vertebral defect with a visible protruding sac filled with spinal fluid. The third, more serious, form is myelomeningocele, in which the protruding sac contains portions of spinal cord.

Etiology

The neural groove of the fetus folds to become the neural tube, which develops into the spinal cord and vertebral arches by 28 days. A neural tube defect develops if the groove does not close completely. Although the cause remains uncertain, genetic and environmental factors have been identified.

Incidence and Demographics

Incidence of neural tube defects is 17.96 per 100,000 live births, with females more commonly affected. These defects occur most often in Hispanics, then in Whites, and then in Blacks. Ninety percent of spinal lesions are myelomeningoceles, the focus of this section.

Risk Factors

- Folic acid deficiency
- Some chromosomal disorders
- Increased in maternal age
- Maternal use of certain antiepileptic medications
    - Valproic acid (Depakene, Depakote)
    - Carbamazepine (Tegretol)
    - Phenobarbital
- Maternal exposure to toxic solvents
- Maternal prepregnancy obesity
- Past history of child with NTD

Prevention and Screening

- Enrichment of grain products with folic acid, mandated by the Food and Drug Administration in 1998
- Use of multivitamin containing folic acid for all women of childbearing age
- Screening by measurement of alpha-fetoprotein (AFP) in maternal blood between 15 and 20 weeks' gestation

Assessment

History

- History of risk factors

Physical Exam

- Findings quite variable depending on level and extent of defect
- Neurological

- Motor paralysis and sensory loss below the level of the defect
- Chiari malformation with defect above sacral area
  - Brainstem and part of cerebellum displaced downward toward neck
  - Spinal cord compression causes difficulty swallowing, choking, apnea, stiff arms, opisthotonos position, sleep disorders
- Hydrocephalus
- Seizure disorder
- Strabismus

- Cognitive
  - Mild cognitive disability
  - Learning disability
  - Impaired organizational skill
  - Impaired motor response, memory, hand function
  - Attention-deficit hyperactivity disorder
- Musculoskeletal
  - Delayed rolling over, sitting, walking
  - Joint deformities
  - Pathological fractures
  - Spinal curvatures
- Bowel and bladder
  - Incomplete bladder emptying
  - Urine incontinence
  - Constipation or diarrhea
  - Fecal incontinence
- Skin irritation or decubitus ulcers on weightbearing body surfaces
- Latex allergy highly prevalent as a result of repeated exposure to latex products
- Obesity
- Sexual issues
  - Uncontrolled erections and retrograde ejaculations in males
  - Decreased genital sensation and lubrication in females
  - Precocious puberty in females

Diagnostic Studies

- High-resolution fetal ultrasound to detect specific anomaly
- Amniocentesis to measure AFP for definitive diagnosis

- CT scan, MRI, ultrasound at birth to detect sac contents

Management

Invasive Treatment

- The benefits of prenatal surgical repair have not been proven to outweigh the risks of the procedure
- Delivery by cesarean section to prevent damage of the sac
- Surgical closure of the defect within the first 72 hours of life
- Surgical placement of ventricular shunt to treat hydrocephalus
- Spinal surgery to allow more brainstem room with Chiari malformation
- Vesicostomy to form opening through abdominal wall and into bladder
- Creation of an artificial urinary sphincter to drain urine from bladder
- Enterocystoplasty, bladder augmentation to increase bladder capacity
- Suburethral sling or suburethral injection of collagen to relieve intrinsic sphincter deficiency
- Orthopedic surgery to repair any skeletal deformities of the lower extremities

Nonpharmacologic Treatment

- Preoperative
    - Prone position with hips and legs slightly flexed
    - Cover sac with sterile, saline-moistened, nonadherent dressing
    - Infant warmer
    - Monitor head circumference
    - Meticulous skin care
    - Pressure-relieving mattress
- Postoperative
    - Prone or side position
    - Monitor head circumference
    - Meticulous skin care
    - Pressure-relieving mattress
- Ongoing
    - Early intervention program beginning in infancy
    - Braces, splints, walker, wheelchair for mobility
    - Daily intermittent urinary clean catheterization
    - Bowel training program

- Padding to prevent skin irritation
- Weight control with healthy diet and exercise
- Latex precautions: avoid all contact with products containing latex
- Penile implant, injection, or prostaglandin prior to sexual intercourse
- Vaginal lubrication prior to intercourse

Pharmacologic Treatment

- Antibiotics to treat or prevent central nervous system infection
- Pain management during postoperative period
- Antispasmodic medications to enhance bladder function
  - Oxybutynin chloride (Ditropan)
  - Propantheline (Pro-Banthine)
  - Imipramine (Tofranil)
- Medications to enhance bowel function
  - Laxatives
  - Fiber supplement
  - Enemas

Patient and Family Education

- Nature of defect and treatment plan
- Surgical procedures
- Complications
- Importance of early intervention
- Strategies to promote attainment of developmental skills
- Skin care
- Bowel and bladder training
- Items containing latex
- Nutrition and weight control
- Medication administration

Outcomes and Follow-up

- Preoperative
  - The child will not experience spinal cord infection.
  - The child's exposed spinal cord and nerves will not be physically injured.
  - The child will maintain adequate body temperature.

    - The family will verbalize an understanding of the defect, surgical procedures, and treatment plan.
- Postoperative
    - The child will experience healing of the incision.
    - The child will experience effective pain management.
- Ongoing
    - The child will participate in an early intervention program beginning in infancy.
    - The child will maintain skin integrity.
    - The child will exhibit adequate growth.
    - The child will attain normal developmental milestones.
    - The child will not develop a latex allergy.
    - The child will experience prompt treatment of complications.
    - The child and family will manage adaptive equipment to promote mobility.
    - The child and family will manage equipment for bladder and bowel function.
    - The family will identify signs of complications.
    - The family will demonstrate safe, effective medication administration.

HYDROCEPHALUS

Description

Hydrocephalus is an accumulation of excess cerebrospinal fluid (CSF) in the ventricles of the brain. The disorder is classified as congenital when it is the result of neural tube defect or developmental malformation of the brain. It is classified as acquired when the cause is infection, hemorrhage, or tumor.

Etiology

Excess accumulation of CSF occurs when there is an excess secretion, impaired absorption, or obstruction of CSF pathways. The most common problem is flow obstruction. As fluid accumulates, the ventricles enlarge, the skull expands, and the brain thins and atrophies.

Incidence and Demographics

Incidence of congenital hydrocephalus is 0.48–0.81 per 1,000 births.

Risk Factors

- Neural tube defects

- Meningitis
- Traumatic head injury
- Brain tumor
- Prematurity with intraventricular or subarachnoid hemorrhage
- Prenatal infections such as toxoplasmosis, cytomegalovirus, rubella, or syphilis

Prevention and Screening

- Screening is not indicated
- Prevention includes
  - Folic acid supplements for all women of childbearing age
  - Prompt treatment of meningitis, head injury, brain tumor, complications of prematurity, prenatal infections

Assessment

History

- History of risk factors
- Infants
  - Poor feeding
  - Irritability
  - Lethargy
  - Seizures
- Older children
  - Morning headache
  - Nausea and vomiting
  - Urinary incontinence
  - Seizures
  - Visual disturbances

Physical Exam

- Infants
  - Tense, bulging fontanel
  - Increased head circumference
  - Visibly dilated scalp veins when crying
  - Decreased level of consciousness
  - Slow, unequal pupil response

  - Sunset eyes with sclera visible above iris
  - Lower extremity spasticity
  - Opisthotonos position
  - High-pitched cry
- Older children
  - Ataxia
  - Confusion
  - Decreased level of consciousness

Diagnostic Studies

- Ultrasound in prenatal period or infancy
- CT scan
- MRI

Management

Invasive Treatment

- Surgical placement of ventricular shunt to drain excess CSF
- Shunt revisions due to child's growth, or shunt infection or malfunction
- Endoscopic third ventriculostomy, a small opening made in floor of third ventricle
- Surgical removal of cause of obstruction

Nonpharmacologic Treatment

- Preoperative
  - Elevate head of bed for untreated hydrocephalus
  - Daily head circumference
- Postoperative
  - Flat position on unoperated side
  - Raise head of bed gradually
  - Support head and neck
  - Incision care

Pharmacologic Treatment

- Diuretics such as furosemide (Lasix) and acetazolamide (Diamox) to decrease CSF production
- Pain management after surgical procedures
- Postoperative antibiotic therapy

Patient and Family Education

- Nature of defect and treatment plan
- Preparation for procedures and surgery
- Care of incision after surgical procedure
- Signs of shunt infection
- Signs of shunt malfunction
- Strategies such as helmets to prevent head injury

Outcomes and Follow-up

- The child will experience effective pain management.
- The child will exhibit symptom relief with treatment.
- The child will attain expected developmental milestones.
- The child and family will verbalize an understanding of the procedures and surgery.
- The family will verbalize an understanding of the defect and treatment plan.
- The family will demonstrate incision care after surgical procedure.
- The family will identify and promptly report signs of shunt infection or malfunction:
    - Drainage, odor, tenderness, swelling at incision site
    - Fever
    - Headache with progressive worsening
    - Nausea or vomiting
    - Abdominal pain
    - Behavioral change such as irritability, drowsiness, change in school performance, change in level of consciousness
    - Sunset eyes or visual disturbance
    - Tense, bulging fontanel in infants
    - Loss of developmental milestones

EPILEPSY OR SEIZURE DISORDER

Description

A seizure is an excessive, synchronized discharge of cortical neurons, causing a change in motor, sensory, or cognitive function. Epilepsy, or seizure disorder, is defined as multiple seizures not precipitated by a known cause. The term *status epilepticus* refers to a prolonged seizure lasting at least 30 minutes. Seizures are classified by focus and physical signs.

Etiology

Any insult to the cerebral cortex can cause seizures. Seizures may be caused by acute illness, toxin ingestion, central nervous system infection, or traumatic brain injury. They can arise from any site in the brain.

Incidence and Demographics

Incidence of epilepsy is 6.3 per 1,000 children. The disorder shows no relationship to family structure, race or ethnicity, or parent education level. It is more prevalent in children from low-income families and in boys. Children with seizure disorders have a higher incidence of attention-deficit hyperactivity disorder, learning disability, anxiety disorder, and depression.

Risk Factors

- Cerebral palsy
- Autism spectrum disorder
- Inborn error of metabolism
- Progressive neurologic disorder

Prevention and Screening

No screening is indicated. Prevention strategies include prompt treatment for infections, prevention of head injury, and fever care.

Assessment

History

- Changes in behavior on the previous day
- Unusual sleep pattern on the prior evening or morning
- Exposure to possible precipitating factors such as infection, trauma, drugs, ingested substances

Physical Exam

- See Classification section below

Diagnostic Studies

- Complete blood count and lumbar puncture to rule out infection
- Serum toxin screens for suspected ingestions
- Electroencephalogram (EEG) to classify seizure type
- CT scan or MRI to rule out physical causes

- PET scan to show brain metabolic activity and SPECT scan to map brain blood flow before surgery
- Newer tests include magnetoencephalography (MEG) and functional MRI (fMRI) to show seizure focus and metabolic changes in the brain
- Routine blood studies such as drug levels, complete blood counts, liver function tests to monitor effectiveness of antiepileptic drugs

Classification of Seizures

- Partial seizures account for 60% of seizure disorders in children. They have one focal area and often start with an aura, an abrupt change in behavior, or both.
  - Simple partial seizures may have sensory sensations or local motor symptoms, but no loss of consciousness.
  - Complex partial seizures (previously called psychomotor) involve impaired consciousness, sensory sensations, purposeless movements, amnesia for the event, and sleepiness after the event.
- Absence seizures (petit mal) are characterized by a brief loss of consciousness with minimal alteration in muscle tone; they may be mistaken for "daydreaming."
- Myoclonic seizures involve brief contraction of muscles with or without loss of consciousness.
- Tonic-clonic seizures (grand mal) consist of loss of consciousness, brief muscle rigidity, then jerking of the extremities; the seizure is followed by semiconsciousness, visual and speech difficulty, impaired fine motor movement, confusion, vomiting, headache, and amnesia for event.
- Atonic seizures (akinetic or drop attacks) have momentary loss of muscle tone and consciousness, causing the child to fall.

Management

Invasive Treatment

- Surgical removal of the seizure focus to cure seizure disorder
- Hemispherectomy (removal of one side of the brain) is a more drastic cure
- Corpus callosotomy (cutting the area that connects the two sides of the brain) is a palliative procedure
- Electrical stimulation of the vagus nerve with a subcutaneous device is also palliative

Nonpharmacologic Treatment

- During seizure, position child safely on side, loosen clothing around neck, avoid restraint or inserting anything in mouth
- Ketogenic diet, high in fat and low in carbohydrates, has been shown to be effective in treating intractable seizures without medication
- Regular sleep appropriate for age

- Infection prevention and fever control
- Multivitamin supplement
- Safety precautions depending on type of seizure activity
- Padded side rails for jerking seizures
- Helmet for atonic seizures
- Emergency equipment at bedside for tonic-clonic seizures

Pharmacologic Treatment

- Phenytoin (Dilantin) for tonic-clonic or partial seizures, or status epilepticus
- Phenobarbital (Luminal) for tonic-clonic or partial seizures
- Carbamazepine (Tegretol, Carbatrol) for partial motor or tonic-clonic seizures
- Oxcarbazepine (Trileptal) for partial seizures
- Valproic acid (Depakote, Depakene) for myoclonic, absence, tonic-clonic, and partial seizures
- Ethosuximide (Zarontin) for absence and myoclonic seizures
- Lamotrigine (Lamictal) for absence, atonic, myoclonic, and tonic seizures and infantile spasms
- Topiramate (Topamax) for partial and tonic-clonic seizures
- Gabapentin (Neurontin) for partial seizures
- Levetiracetam (Keppra) for partial seizures
- Primidone (Mysoline) for partial and myoclonic seizures
- Clorazepate (Gen-Xene, Tranxene) for partial seizures
- Clonazepam (Klonopin) for tonic-clonic seizures
- Rectal diazepam for home emergency use
- Buccal midazolam (Versed) for home emergency use

Patient and Family Education

- Nature of condition and treatment options
- Care during seizure
- Basic life support
- Medication administration
- Safety and injury prevention
- Common side effects of antiepileptic drugs such as sleepiness, decreased attention and memory, dysphasia, ataxia, visual disturbance, cognitive impairment
- Potential teratogenic effects of antiepileptic drugs such as valproate, phenytoin, carbamazepine, phenobarbital, and topiramate

- Nonpharmacologic management strategies
- Communication with childcare providers and school personnel
- Available resources such as support groups and counseling

Outcomes and Follow-up

- The child will maintain patent airway status.
- The child will experience reduction in seizures or freedom from seizures.
- The child will experience prompt attention for signs of infection or fever.
- The child will establish a regular sleep pattern and healthy diet.
- The child will experience minimal antiepileptic drug side effects.
- The child will not experience progressive cognitive and behavioral impairments as a result of seizure activity.
- The child will participate in activities appropriate for his or her developmental level, avoiding heavy contact sports or unusually risky activities such as rock climbing.
- The family will demonstrate care during seizure.
- The family will demonstrate safe medication administration.
- The family will identify the side effects of antiepileptic drugs.
- The family will provide supervision with bathing or swimming.
- The family will develop an individualized plan of care with the school nurse.
- The family will investigate state driving restrictions for adolescents with seizures.

CEREBRAL PALSY

Description
Cerebral palsy is a nonprogressive central nervous system disorder of movement and posture.

Etiology
This disorder is the result of a brain insult or injury or a genetically based problem with brain development.

Incidence and Demographics
The prevalence of cerebral palsy is about 2–4 per 1,000 children. Associated problems include cognitive disability, visual impairment, hearing impairment, speech disorders, seizures, feeding and growth failure, behavioral or emotional disorders, chronic pulmonary disease, voiding disorders, osteopenia, and orthopedic disorders.

Risk Factors
- Family history
- Preterm birth
- Low birth weight
- Antepartum hemorrhage
- Birth asphyxia
- Congenital brain malformation
- Coagulation abnormalities, stroke
- Complications of multiple gestation and intrauterine infection
- Kernicterus as a result of hyperbilirubinemia
- Bacterial, viral, or fungal infection
- Near drowning
- Trauma

Prevention and Screening
Prevention strategy includes effective obstetrical care. Ultrasound is useful screening for brain malformations.

Assessment

History

- Delayed motor development
- Uncoordinated movement
- Poor muscle control
- Poor balance
- Weakness
- Easily fatigued
- Frequent respiratory infections
- Constipation
- Hypotonicity during the first few months of life

Physical Exam

- Spastic, hypertonicity
- Exaggerated reflexes
- Persistent primitive reflexes
- Asymmetrical reflex response
- Drooling
- Dental caries
- Atypical, involuntary movements (dyskinesias)
- Slow, writhing movements (chorea)
- Rigid posturing of head and neck (dystonia)
- Wide-based, unsteady gait
- Scissoring of legs or toe-walking position of feet
- Difficulty controlling hand and arm muscles during reaching

Diagnostic Studies

- CT scans and MRI
- Positron emission tomography (PET)
- Single photon emission computed tomography (SPECT)
- Diffusion tensor imaging (DTI)
- Swallowing studies for feeding difficulty

Management

Invasive Treatment

- Selective dorsal rhizotomy to permanently reduce leg spasticity
- Muscle-tendon surgery to increase joint movement
- Stereotactic encephalotomy, cutting specific tracts in basal ganglia

Nonpharmacologic Treatment

- Speech therapy, occupational therapy (OT), and physical therapy (PT)
- Neurodevelopmental therapy focusing on motor function
- Early intervention program beginning in infancy
- Bracing, splinting, standing tables, positioning devices to maintain range of motion, prevent contractures, provide stability, control involuntary movements, and prevent osteoporosis
- Adaptive equipment such as crutches, walkers, canes, wheelchairs to maximize mobility
- Assistive technology such as self-care devices, computers to promote independence

Pharmacologic Treatment

- Botulinum toxin (Botox) to decrease spasticity
- Antispasmodics
  - Dantrolene (Dantrium)
  - Intrathecal Baclofen
- Pain management for muscle spasms

Patient and Family Education

- Disorder and treatment plan
- Therapeutic strategies (PT, OT, speech, etc.)
- Strategies to promote effective eating and swallowing
- Skin care with adaptive equipment, splints, braces, positioning devices
- Assistive technology
- Communication strategies
- Medication administration
- Available resources such as support groups, counseling, early intervention program

Outcomes and Follow-up

- The child will participate in an early intervention program.
- The child will receive prompt intervention for associated problems (hearing, vision, etc.).
- The child will utilize adaptive equipment effectively.

- The child will achieve maximum mobility.
- The child will achieve maximal independence in self-care activities.
- The child will utilize assistive technology.
- The child will develop effective communication.
- The child will maintain intact skin.
- The child will demonstrate adequate growth.
- The child will participate in a variety of environments, including home, school, childcare, neighborhood settings.
- The family will verbalize an understanding of the disorder and treatment plan.
- The family will utilize a variety of professional disciplines to determine a therapy plan.
- The family will demonstrate medication administration.
- The family will access available resources.

DUCHENNE MUSCULAR DYSTROPHY

Description

Duchenne muscular dystrophy is an X-chromosome-linked recessive, progressive skeletal muscle disorder and the most common form of muscular dystrophy in children

Etiology

The disorder is caused by a genetic mutation in the dystrophin gene, which causes an absence of dystrophin, a protein necessary for skeletal and cardiac muscle stability. Without dystrophin, an inflammatory process in the muscles causes progressive necrosis of muscle fibers.

Incidence and Demographics

The incidence is 1 in 3,000 male births. Muscle weakness is usually noticed by age 3–4 years. Affected boys are usually unable to walk by early adolescence. Respiratory failure or cardiomyopathy often causes death in the early to mid-20s. With long-term ventilation, some young men are living into their 30s and 40s.

Risk Factors

- Family history

Prevention and Screening

- No prevention or screening indicated

Assessment

History

- Progressive deterioration
- Family history
- Delayed walking
- Frequent tripping, falls
- Abnormal gait on level surface

Physical Exam

- Muscle weakness starting with hip girdle muscles
- Walking on tiptoes or waddling gait
- Difficulty getting up from supine position on floor
- Hypertrophy of calf muscles
- Contractures
- Spinal curvatures
- Mild cognitive impairment
- Respiratory failure
- Cardiomyopathy

Diagnostic Studies

- Elevated serum creatinine kinase (CPK)
- Muscle biopsy shows decreased dystrophin levels and fatty infiltration
- Electromyography (EMG) shows decreased muscle potential
- Radiography to monitor spinal changes
- Body density monitoring
- Pulmonary function tests twice each year starting at 9–10 years of age
- Echocardiography or cardiac MRI every 1–2 years starting at age 10 years

Management

Invasive Treatment

- Surgical release of contractures
- Spinal surgery to correct scoliosis
- Tracheostomy as pulmonary disease worsens

Nonpharmacologic Treatment

- Physical and occupational therapy
- Range of motion exercises
- Adaptive equipment such as braces, walkers, wheelchairs
- Noninvasive ventilation (NIV) for sleep-related upper airway obstruction and chronic respiratory insufficiency
- Intermittent positive pressure breathing (IPPB), CPAP, mechanical in-exsufflator to mimic cough
- Standing and weightbearing exercises
- Regular gentle exercise such as swimming
- Psychologist or psychiatrist as needed

Pharmacologic Treatment

- Corticosteroid therapy with prednisone to slow progression of muscle weakness
- ACE inhibitor, perindopril (Aceon) to slow progression of cardiomyopathy
- Beta-blocker, carvedilol (Coreg) or metoprolol to slow progression of cardiomyopathy
- Antibiotics to treat infection
- Vitamin and mineral supplements as indicated
- Recommended immunizations, including pneumococcal and annual influenza vaccines

Patient and Family Education

- Disease progression and treatment plan
- Medication administration
- Adaptive equipment
- Use of respiratory devices
- Nutritional modifications
- Exercise program
- Available resources: support groups, counseling, financial assistance
- Care options such as home care, respite care, nursing facility care

Outcomes and Follow-up

- The child will demonstrate the use of adaptive equipment.
- The child will maintain intact skin.
- The child will receive adequate nutrition.
- The child will participate in activity and exercise as tolerated.
- The child will participate in self-care as able.

- The child and family will verbalize an understanding of the disease's progression and the treatment plan.
- The child and family will verbalize satisfaction with the choice of care setting.
- The child and family will discuss quality-of-life concerns and end-of-life care.
- The child and family will not experience social isolation.
- The child and family will utilize a variety of professional disciplines to cope with their physical and emotional needs.
- The child and family will access available resources.
- The family will demonstrate the use of respiratory devices, adaptive devices, and medication administration.

MENINGITIS

Description

Meningitis is inflammation of the arachnoid matter of the meninges and the spinal cord. Suspected meningitis is considered a medical emergency.

Etiology

Meningitis may be caused by bacteria or viruses. The most common causes of bacterial meningitis in infants younger than 3 months of age are group B streptococci, *Streptococcus pneumoniae,* and *Neisseria meningitides.* For children between 3 months and 10 years, *Streptococcus pneumoniae* and *Neisseria meningitides* are the most common cause. In children 10 years of age or older, *Neisseria meningitides* is the most common. Meningitis usually follows invasion of the bloodstream by the causative organism. The organism then penetrates the blood–brain barrier and reaches the subarachnoid space. The progression of symptoms may occur over several days or over several hours.

Incidence and Demographics

Incidence is 80.69 per 100,000 in infants younger than 2 months; 6.91 per 100,000 in children between 2 and 23 months; 0.56 per 100,000 in children between 2 and 10 years; and 0.43 per 100,000 in children between and 17 years.

Risk Factors

- Exposure
- Maternal perinatal infection
- Incomplete immunization status
- Recent infection

- Recent international travel
- Recent neurosurgical procedure
- Cochlear implant device
- Penetrating head trauma
- Skull fracture

Prevention and Screening

Prevention involves immunizations against causative organisms and effective treatment of bacterial infections. Pregnant women should be treated with ampicillin or penicillin for group B streptococcal infection. No widespread screening is indicated.

Assessment

History

- History of risk factors
- Upper respiratory infection
- Fever, chills
- Vomiting
- Severe headache
- Photophobia
- Back or joint pain

Physical Exam

- Nuchal rigidity
- Irritability, confusion, lethargy
- Signs of increased intracranial pressure
- Positive Kernig sign: pain when knee is flexed then extended in supine position
- Positive Brudzinski sign: involuntary hip or knee flexion when head is flexed while lying in supine position
- Petechial or purpuric rash and joint pain with *Neisseria meningitides*
- Infants have more general signs
    - Fever, chills
    - Change in feeding habits
    - Vomiting
    - Seizure
    - Irritability, altered level of consciousness, high-pitched cry

Diagnostic Studies

- Lumbar puncture (LP)

TABLE 16-1.
LUMBAR PUNCTURE RESULTS

	NORMAL CSF	BACTERIAL	VIRAL
Color	Clear	Cloudy	Slightly cloudy or clear
White blood count	0–5	High with increased polys	Slightly high with increased lymphs
Protein	10–30	Elevated	Normal or slightly elevated
Glucose	40–80	Decreased	Normal

- Causative organism may be identified with culture of CSF, blood, urine, or throat

Management

Invasive Treatment

- Possible intracranial pressure monitoring

Nonpharmacologic Treatment

- Basic life support and resuscitation as indicated
- Continued ventilation support as needed
- Droplet isolation for *Neisseria meningitides*
- Isolation for all until 24 hours of antibiotic therapy complete
- Decrease environmental stimuli, specifically noise and lighting
- Position for comfort with head of bed slightly raised
- Possible fluid restriction
- Monitor head circumference of infants and toddlers

Pharmacologic Treatment

- Start antibiotic therapy immediately after LP and cultures drawn
- Younger than 3 months of age: ampicillin and cefotaxime (Claforan)
- 3 months or older: ampicillin and cefotaxime (Claforan), ceftriaxone (Rocephin), or vancomycin
- Possible dexamethasone
- Pain management
- Antipyretics and anticonvulsants as needed
- Intravenous therapy to maintain fluid and electrolyte balance

Patient and Family Education

- Disease process and treatment plan
- Preparation for diagnostic procedures
- Nonpharmacologic management
- Isolation precautions
- Prevention by immunization

Outcomes and Follow-up

- The child will verbalize feeling of comfort in position and environment.
- The child will experience effective pain management.
- The child will receive prompt treatment for fever and seizures.
- The child will show signs of adequate hydration without fluid overload.
- The child will recover without long-term complications such as neurological sequelae.
- The family will verbalize an understanding of the disease and treatment plan.
- The family will provide immunizations to all family members.

VIRAL ENCEPHALITIS

Description

Encephalitis is an inflammatory process of the central nervous system caused by a variety of viruses, bacteria, fungi, and parasites.

Etiology

Viruses are the main causative agent of encephalitis in children. The virus may directly invade the central nervous system or cross the blood–brain barrier from another site of infection. The result is inflammation, edema, and neuronal cell death. The most prevalent cause in children is herpes simplex types 1 and 2 (HSV).

Incidence and Demographics

Herpes simplex encephalitis is uncommon, but children account for 30% of the cases. The mosquito is the most common vector for most viruses, so most cases occur in the summer.

Risk Factors

- Maternal infection during pregnancy
- Exposure to mosquito-infested areas

Prevention and Screening

Prevention includes effective treatment for maternal infection during pregnancy, cesarean delivery if mother has active HSV lesions, and insect control.

Assessment

History

- Nausea and vomiting
- Headache
- Dizziness
- Malaise
- Fever
- Lethargy

Physical Exam

- Altered level of consciousness
- Seizures
- Neck stiffness
- Ataxia or tremors
- Flaccid paralysis
- Speech difficulty
- Infants more likely to present with:
    - Poor feeding
    - Irritability
    - Lethargy
    - Decreased perfusion
    - Fever
    - Seizures

Diagnostic Studies

- CT scan
- MRI
- Culture from CSF, blood, nose, throat, urine
- CSF may be normal; or have elevated white blood cells, neutrophils, and lymphs, only slightly elevated protein, and normal glucose; PCR shows HSV
- Electroencephalogram (EEG) abnormalities

Management

Invasive Treatment

- Possibly intracranial pressure monitoring

Nonpharmacologic Treatment

- Basic life support and resuscitation
- Airborne, contact, and droplet infection control precautions until organism identified
- Decrease environmental stimuli, specifically noise and lighting
- Position for comfort with head of bed slightly raised

Pharmacologic Treatment

- Acyclovir for herpes simplex virus
- Antiepileptics for seizures
- Antipyretics for fever
- Pain management
- Intravenous fluids to maintain fluid and electrolyte status

Patient and Family Education

- Disease process and treatment plan
- Isolation precautions
- Potential long-term complications

Outcomes and Follow-up

- The child will experience effective pain management.
- The child will receive prompt treatment for fever and seizures.
- The child will show signs of adequate hydration without fluid overload.
- The child will not develop cerebral edema, status epilepticus, cardiorespiratory failure, or syndrome of inappropriate antidiuretic hormone secretion (SIADH).
- The child will recover without neurologic, functional, or cognitive impairment.
- The family will verbalize an understanding of the disease and treatment plan.

BRAIN TUMORS

Description

Brain tumors are solid tumors originating from glial cells, nerve cells, epithelial cells, blood vessels, pineal gland, or hypophysis. Major childhood brain tumors, in order of prevalence, include astrocytoma, medulloblastoma, cerebellar astrocytoma, brainstem glioma, and ependymoma.

Etiology

The cause of brain tumors is unknown.

Incidence and Demographics

Brain cancer is the third most common cancer that occurs in children, and more than 70% of affected children will survive longer than 5 years.

TABLE 16-2.
INCIDENCE OF BRAIN TUMORS IN CHILDREN PER 100,000 BY AGE

< 1 YEAR	1-4 YEARS	5-9 YEARS	10-14 YEARS	15-19 YEARS
3.47	4.1	3.3	2.69	2.17

Risk Factors

- Past exposure to radiation
- Genetic disorders such as Li-Fraumeni syndrome, neurofibromatosis

Prevention and Screening

- No prevention or screening indicated

Assessment

History

- Headache that is worse in the morning
- Vomiting that is worse in the morning and not related to eating
- Frequent episodes of nausea and vomiting
- Irritability, fatigue
- Seizures
- Unusual sleepiness
- Change in activity level, behavior, personality

- Vision, hearing, or speech problems

Physical Exam

- Neuromuscular changes
  - Clumsiness, loss of balance
  - Weakness, poor fine motor control
  - Hypo- or hyperactive reflexes
  - Spasticity or paralysis
  - Positive Babinski sign
- Vital signs
  - Decreased pulse and respiratory rates
  - Increased blood pressure
  - Decreased pulse pressure
  - Hypo- or hyperthermia
  - Increased head size in infants and toddlers
- Cranial nerve neuropathy
  - Head tilt
  - Visual disturbances
- Other signs
  - Tense, bulging fontanel
  - Nuchal rigidity
  - Papilledema
  - Delayed attainment or loss of developmental milestones

Diagnostic Studies

- CT scan, PET scan
- MRI with gadolinium
- Angiogram
- Serum tumor marker test
- Biopsy during surgery
- Lumbar puncture, bone scan, bone marrow aspiration, chest radiography for staging

Management

Invasive Treatment

- Surgical resection of as much of tumor as possible

- Lasers to destroy tumor tissue
- Possible shunt placement for hydrocephalus
- Possible stem cell transplant

Nonpharmacologic Treatment

- Radiation therapy to shrink tumor
- Cooling blanket for hyperthermia after brain surgery
- Postoperative position determined by surgery
  - Nonoperative side
  - Infratentorial procedure: flat and side-lying
  - Supratentorial procedure: head elevated above heart level
- Postoperative saline eye drops if swelling prevents eye closure
- Quiet, dimly lit environment
- Ice bag to forehead for discomfort and swelling
- Available resources such as support groups, counseling, cancer camps

Pharmacologic Treatment

- Chemotherapy depending on specific type of tumor; oral, intravenous, intrathecal
- Corticosteroids or diuretics for brain edema
- Antiepileptics for seizures
- Pain management

Patient and Family Education

- Disease process and treatment plan
- Postoperative care
- Side effects of radiation and chemotherapy
- Care of residual problems
- Medication administration
- Safety measures such as helmet with active sports

Outcomes and Follow-up

- The child will return to his or her usual activities and school as soon as possible.
- The child will wear a helmet for active play or sports until the skull is healed.
- The child will adhere to activity restrictions.
- The child will experience minimal residual problems such as growth retardation, cranial nerve palsies, or cognitive, sensory, or motor impairment.

- The child and family will verbalize an understanding of the disease process and treatment plan.
- The child and family will access available resources.
- The family will utilize nonpharmacologic management strategies.

TRAUMATIC BRAIN INJURY

Description

Traumatic head injury (TBI) is trauma from impact and inertia forces that cause a broad spectrum of injury; the results range from full recovery to severe functional disability.

Etiology

The causes of head injury in children are numerous and include motor vehicle, pedestrian, and bicycle accidents; falls, near drowning, sports injuries, attempted suicide, and physical abuse. Head injury is the result of two forces, impact and inertia. Impact occurs when the head hits a surface or is struck by a moving object. Impact forces can cause scalp injury, skull fracture, contusion, or epidural hematoma. Inertia forces occur when the brain moves within the skull, tearing nerves and blood vessels. Concussion, diffuse injury, and subdural hematomas are the result of inertia forces.

Incidence and Demographics

Approximately 475,000 traumatic brain injuries occur annually in children between the ages of birth and 14 years. TBI is the leading cause of death in children older than 1 year of age.

Risk Factors

- Children from birth to age 5 years
- Adolescents
- Conduct disorder
- Attention-deficit hyperactivity disorder
- Prematurity
- Young parents
- Unstable family dynamics

Prevention and Screening

- Many head injuries are preventable, and screening involves evaluation after an injury.
  - Effective restraint of children in motor vehicles with car seats, booster seats, air bags, and position in the rear seat

- Driver education, night curfews, graduated licensing for adolescents
- Reduced speed limits and physical separation of pedestrians and traffic in areas frequented by children
- Bicycle and motorcycle helmets
- Protective equipment for sports and recreation activities
- Playground and water safety

Assessment

History

- Injury history
- Loss of consciousness
- Lethargy, confusion, irritability
- Severe headache
- Repeated vomiting
- Respiratory difficulty
- Seizures

Physical Exam

- Speech, vision, hearing, movement impairment
- Pupil changes
- Bulging fontanel
- Retinal hemorrhage
- Laceration or large bump on head
- CSF or blood in nasal or ear drainage

Diagnostic Studies

- CT scan
- MRI
- Radiographs

Management

Invasive Treatment

- Suture of lacerations or torn dura
- Surgical reduction of depressed skull fracture
- Possible craniectomy for brain swelling

- Hematoma evacuation
- Insertion of ventricular drains
- Intracranial pressure monitoring

Nonpharmacologic Treatment

- Basic life support and resuscitation
- Airway and oxygenation maintenance
- Spine stabilization
- Hyperventilation and elevating head of bed for increased intracranial pressure
- Decreased environmental stimuli initially
- Play and activity therapy
- Physical, occupational, and speech therapy
- Adaptive equipment such as crutches, walkers, wheelchairs
- Enteral feeding if unable to eat
- Treatment of vision or hearing impairment
- Special education for cognitive impairment

Pharmacologic Treatment

- Intravenous therapy to maintain fluid and electrolyte balance
- Total parenteral nutrition for those in coma state
- Antibiotics with lacerations or penetrating injury
- Medications such as mannitol, sedatives, or paralytics to treat increased intracranial pressure
- Barbiturate-induced coma and hypothermia
- Pain management
- Medications to treat spasticity and rigidity
    - Baclofen
    - Dantrolene (Dantrium)
    - Diazepam (Valium)
    - Botulinum toxin A (Botox)

Patient and Family Education

- Effects of injury and treatment plan
- Strategies to regain impaired function and promote normal development
- Strategies to prevent future injury
- Medication administration

- Skin care with mobility impairment
- Use of adaptive equipment
- Alternative feeding techniques
- Utilization of various professional disciplines
- Available resources such as support groups and counseling

Outcomes and Follow-up

- The child will maintain an open airway and adequate oxygenation.
- The child will not experience increased intracranial pressure.
- The child will maintain intact skin and a full range of motion.
- The child will receive adequate nutrition.
- The child will recover without long-term complications.
- The child will utilize adaptive equipment for impaired function.
- The family will verbalize an understanding of the injury, treatment plan, and residual disability.
- The family will demonstrate strategies to help the child regain function and promote normal development.
- The family will demonstrate the use of adaptive equipment, skin care, alternative feeding techniques, and medication administration.
- The family will utilize a variety of professional disciplines.
- The family will access available resources.

SPINAL CORD INJURIES

Description

Spinal cord injuries (SCIs) include compression, contusion, laceration, and transection of the spinal cord. Long-term function depends on the level of the injury. Complete SCI is defined as absence of motor and sensory function below the level of the lesion. With incomplete SCI, partial function remains.

Etiology

Causes of SCI in children include motor vehicle crashes, falls, birth injuries, lap belt injuries, sports injuries, and child abuse. Damage to the cord may also occur with nontraumatic causes such as tumors, cellular tissue damage, hemorrhage, inflammation, and edema. Injury results in temporary or permanent sensory or motor deficits, or both.

Incidence and Demographics

Incidence of SCI is 2 per 100,000 children each year. The prognosis for recovery in children is better than in adults because children have more rapid healing of bones and ligaments, as well as an increased potential for nerve regeneration.

Risk Factors

- Improper restraint in motor vehicles
- Serious head injury or trauma
- Age younger than 8 years

Prevention and Screening

- No screening indicated, but prevention is often possible
- Safe restraint in motor vehicles with car seats and booster seats
- Sports safety
- Age-appropriate supervision

Assessment

History

- History of trauma
- Local pain
- Muscle spasm
- Decreased range of neck motion
- Weakness

Physical Exam

- Flaccid muscle tone
- Numbness, tingling, burning sensation
- Loss of sensation
- Absence of deep tendon reflexes
- Weakness or paralysis
- Incontinence of bladder or bowel
- Loss of rectal tone
- Hypotension
- Bradycardia
- Temperature instability
- Autonomic dysreflexia

Diagnostic Studies

- MRI
- CT scan
- Radiography

Management

Invasive Treatment

- Decompression laminectomy
- Surgical intervention for paralytic scoliosis
- Tendon transfers to increase hand function
- Urinary diversion or bladder augmentation
- Insertion of functional electrical stimulation to increase motion and improve bowel and bladder function

Nonpharmacologic Treatment

- Cervical collar initially and spinal immobilization
- Ventilation support
- Possible lifelong ventilator support, phrenic nerve pacing, or both for high cervical injury
- Patient-triggered synchronous intermittent mandatory ventilation (SIMV-assist/ control mode) for midlevel injury
- Chest physical therapy
- Skin care and pressure ulcer prevention
- Pressure-relieving mattress
- DVT prophylaxis during first 12 months after injury
- Bowel and bladder management
- Prevention and management of autonomic dysreflexia
  - Elevate head
  - Loosen clothing
  - Empty bladder
  - Consistent bowel and bladder program
- Clean, intermittent catheterization for neurogenic bladder
- Bowel training program
- Promotion of normal development
- Physical and occupational therapy
- Mechanical or robotic orthoses

Pharmacologic Treatment

- Methylprednisolone (Solu-Medrol) to decrease inflammation
- Stool softeners or laxatives to promote regular bowel elimination
- Antihypertensive medication for autonomic dysreflexia
- Pamidronate (Aredia) for hypercalcemia
- Medication for chronic neuropathic pain
- Clonidine hydrochloride to improve ambulation with partial spinal cord injuries

Patient and Family Education

- Injury and treatment plan
- Bowel and bladder management strategies
- Skin care and prevention of pressure ulcers
- Prevention of latex allergy
- Use of adaptive equipment
- Signs of hypercalcemia
    - Behavior changes, malaise, lethargy
    - Nausea, vomiting, abdominal pain
    - Polyuria, polydipsia, dehydration
- Signs of autonomic dysreflexia
    - Headache
    - Profuse sweating, flushed skin
    - Blurred vision
    - Increased pulse rate
    - Anxiety
    - Nasal congestion
- Use of respiratory equipment, chest physical therapy
- DVT prevention
- Medication administration
- Implications for development of sexuality
- Available resources such as support groups and counseling

Outcomes and Follow-up

- The child will maintain open airway and effective respiration.
- The child will maintain or improve neurologic status.
- The child will maintain intact skin.
- The child will demonstrate adequate growth.
- The child will not develop latex allergy.
- The child will demonstrate effective bowel and bladder elimination.
- The child and family will utilize adaptive devices.
- The child will participate in a variety of environments, including home, school, childcare, neighborhood settings.
- The family will verbalize an understanding of the injury and treatment plan.
- The family will identify signs of autonomic dysreflexia and hypercalcemia.
- The family will demonstrate strategies to prevent autonomic dysreflexia and DVT.
- The family will utilize a variety of professional disciplines to determine therapy plan.
- The family will demonstrate medication administration.
- The family will discuss sexuality as the child matures.

LYME DISEASE

Description

Lyme disease is a tick-borne disorder caused by a spirochete *Borrelia burgdorferi* sensu stricto.

Etiology

The spirochete enters the skin through the bite of an infected deer tick and is disseminated through the blood and lymphatic systems. The incubation period is between 1 and 30 days, but late manifestations can occur months to years after the tick bite.

Incidence and Demographics

Lyme disease commonly occurs in the New England, Middle Atlantic, Upper Midwest, and Pacific Northwest states. The peak season is April through October. The average annual incidence is 66 per 100,000 children. The peak incidence of occurrence is in 5- to 9-year-old children and is more common in boys.

Risk Factors

- Exposure to ticks
- Inadequate protection

Prevention and Screening

- Prevention
    - Light-colored clothing
    - Long-sleeved shirt tucked into pants
    - Long pants tucked into socks
    - Avoid weedy, grassy areas and dense woods.
    - Cautious use of insect repellent
    - Tick prevention for pets
- Screening involves careful bare skin check for ticks after outside activity in suspect areas

Assessment

History

- History of tick bite or outside activity in suspect area

Physical Exam

- Early localized stage
    - Appears between 3 and 30 days after exposure
    - Erythema migrans (small painless, nonitchy red papule enlarging to form a ring with a red, raised border and a clear or necrotic center)
    - Chills, fever, headache, muscle aches, fatigue, malaise, lymphadenopathy
- Early disseminated stage
    - Appears 3–10 weeks after exposure
    - Multiple smaller, secondary erythema migrans
    - Systemic symptoms mentioned above
    - Joint pain and swelling
    - Dizziness, heart palpitation
    - Anorexia, stiff neck, lymphadenopathy, splenomegaly, conjunctivitis, sore throat, abdominal pain, cough
    - Carditis in about 1%
- Late stage
    - Intermittent, recurrent symptoms up to 12 months after exposure

- Arthritis of large joints
- Peripheral neuropathy

Diagnostic Studies

- Step 1: enzyme immunoassay
- Step 2: if step 1 is positive or indeterminant, immunoblot test (Western blot)
- Lumbar puncture will show Lyme disease–specific antibodies with CNS involvement

Management

Invasive Treatment

- No invasive management indicated

Nonpharmacologic Treatment

- Comfort measures

Pharmacologic Treatment

- Doxycycline (Vibramycin) for children 8 years and older
- Amoxicillin (Amoxil) for younger children
- Ceftriaxone (Rocephin) or penicillin for arthritis, carditis, CNS involvement

Patient and Family Education

- Disease process and treatment plan
- Medication administration
- Prevention of exposure to ticks
- Safe tick removal with fine-tipped tweezers

Outcomes and Follow-up

- The child will complete entire course of antibiotic therapy.
- The child will recover without arthritis, carditis, or CNS involvement.
- The child and family will identify strategies to prevent future exposure.
- The family will verbalize an understanding of the disease process and treatment plan.
- The family will demonstrate medication administration.

HYPOTHERMIA

Description

Cooling of body core below 35° C or 95° F.

Etiology

Body heat is lost via conduction, convection, or radiation. The body is unable to maintain heat production by exercise or metabolism.

Incidence and Demographics

Unusual with exception of trauma or accidental drowning

Risk Factors

- Prolonged exposure to cold environment
- Very young children with high ratio of body surface area to age
- Very thin children

Prevention and Screening

- Anticipation of cold conditions
- Knowledge of survival strategies
- Precautions against long exposure to severe cold
- No screening indicated

Assessment

History

- Presence of risk factors

Physical Exam

- Tachycardia progressing to bradycardia
- Rapid respiratory rate progressing to slow rate
- Vigorous shivering progressing to muscle rigidity
- Hypoactive bowel sounds
- Cold, pale extremities
- Decreased peripheral perfusion
- Impaired manual dexterity

- Impaired cognitive functioning
- Hypotension

Diagnostic Studies

- EKG shows cardiac arrhythmias
- Renal studies to evaluate function

Management

Invasive Treatment

- Possible peritoneal dialysis with warm fluid
- Possible hemodialysis
- Possible extracorporeal blood rewarming

Nonpharmacologic Treatment

- Remove wet clothing
- Warm, high-caloric liquids if conscious
- Warm, humidified oxygen
- Warm packs to groin, axilla, back of neck
- Basic life support to maintain ventilation

Pharmacologic Treatment

- Warm intravenous fluid to correct fluid and electrolyte imbalances

Patient and Family Education

- Strategies for cold survival
- Multiple clothing layers

Outcomes and Follow-up

- The child will maintain effective ventilation and perfusion.
- The child will exhibit adequate renal function.
- The child will exhibit adequate cognitive function.
- The child will have increasing body temperature.
- The child will have improved peripheral perfusion.
- The child and family will verbalize strategies for prevention.

HYPERTHERMIA

Description

Core body temperature exceeding set point, resulting from body creating more heat than it can eliminate. The set point is the body temperature regulated by a "thermostat" in the hypothalamus.

Etiology

Hyperthermia may be caused by internal or external conditions that raise the core body temperature.

Incidence and Demographics

Elevated temperatures related to infections are very common in children, but true hyperthermia is much less common.

Risk Factors

- Exposure to very hot environmental temperatures
- Aspirin ingestion
- Serotonin syndrome
- Seizures
- Hyperthyroidism

Prevention and Screening

Prevention of environmentally caused hyperthermia includes minimized sun exposure, avoidance of over-dressing. No screening is indicated.

Management

Invasive Treatment

No invasive treatment indicated.

Nonpharmacologic Treatment

- Cooling blanket or mattress
- Cool compresses
- Tepid tub bath
- Sponging one body part at a time with cool cloth

Pharmacologic Treatment

Antipyretics are not effective in hyperthermia.

Patient and Family Education

- Temperature measurement
- Nonpharmacologic treatment
- Prevention strategies

Outcomes and Follow-up

- The child with have decreasing body temperature.
- The child will not exhibit shivering during cooling process.
- The family will verbalize understanding of prevention strategies.
- The family will demonstrate temperature measurement.
- The family will verbalize understanding of nonpharmacologic treatment.

REFERENCES

American Cancer Society. (2012). *Brain and spinal cord tumors in children.* Retrieved from http://www.cancer.org/acs/groups/cid/documents/webcontent/003089-pdf.pdf

Appelboom, G., Zoller, S. D., Piazza, M. A., Szpalski, C., Bruce, B. A., McDowell, M. M., et al. (2011). Traumatic brain injury in pediatric patients. *Neurosurgical Focus, 31*(5). Retrieved from http://www.medscape.com/viewarticle/753232?src=mp&spon=9

Caviness, A. C. (2012). Spinal cord injury without radiographic abnormality (SCIWORA) in children. *UpToDate.* Retrieved from http://www.uptodate.com/contents/spinal-cord-injury-without-radiographic-abnormality-sciwora-in-children?source=see_link&anchor=H26107927#H26107927

Clore, E. T. (2010). Seizure precautions for pediatric bedside nurses. *Pediatric Nursing, 36*(4), 191–194.

Darras, B. T. (2011). Treatment of Duchenne and Becker muscular dystrophy. *UpToDate.* Retrieved from http://www.uptodate.com/contents/management-and-prognosis-of-cerebral-palsy?source=search_result&search=cerebral+palsy&selectedTitle=4%7E150

Fishman, M. A. (2010). Hydrocephalus. *UpToDate.* Retrieved from http://www.uptodate.com/contents/hydrocephalus?source=search_result&search=hydrocephalus&selectedTitle=1%7E150

Hardarson, H. S. (2012). Acute viral encephalitis in children and adolescents: Clinical manifestations and diagnosis. *UpToDate.* Retrieved from http://www.uptodate.com/contents/acute-viral-encephalitis-in-children-and-adolescents-clinical-manifestations-and-diagnosis?source=search_result&search=encephalitis+children&selectedTitle=2%7E150

Hardarson, H. S. (2012). Acute viral encephalitis in children and adolescents: Treatment and prevention. *UpToDate.* Retrieved from http://www.uptodate.com/contents/acute-viral-encephalitis-in-children-and-adolescents-treatment-and-prevention?source=search_result&search=encephalitis+children&selectedTitle=3%7E150

Hochberg, L., & Stone, J. (2012). Prenatal screening and diagnosis of neural tube defects. *UpToDate.* Retrieved from http://www.uptodate.com/contents/prenatal-screening-and-diagnosis-of-neural-tube-defects?source=see_link

Hockenberry, M. J., & Wilson, D. (2011). *Wong's nursing care of infants and children* (9th ed.). St. Louis, MO: Elsevier Mosby.

Kaplan, S. L. (2012). Clinical features and diagnosis of acute bacterial meningitis in children older than one month of age. *UpToDate.* Retrieved from http://www.uptodate.com/contents/clinical-features-and-diagnosis-of-acute-bacterial-meningitis-in-children-older-than-one-month-of-age?source=search_result&search=bacterial+meningitis+in+child&selectedTitle=1%7E150

McLone, D. G., & Bowman, R. M. (2011). Overview of the management of myelomeningocele (spina bifida). *UpToDate.* Retrieved from http://www.uptodate.com/contents/overview-of-the-management-of-myelomeningocele-spina-bifida?source=search_result&search=neural+tube+defects&selectedTitle=7%7E150

Miller, G. (2010). Epidemiology and etiology of cerebral palsy. *UpToDate.* Retrieved from http://www.uptodate.com/contents/epidemiology-and-etiology-of-cerebral-palsy?source=search_result&search=cerebral+palsy&selectedTitle=3%7E150

Miller, G. (2012). Clinical features of cerebral palsy. *UpToDate.* Retrieved from http://www.uptodate.com/contents/clinical-features-of-cerebral-palsy?source=search_result&search=cerebral+palsy&selectedTitle=1%7E150

Miller, G. (2012). Management and prognosis of cerebral palsy. *UpToDate*. Retrieved from http://www.uptodate.com/contents/management-and-prognosis-of-cerebral-palsy?source=search_result&search=cerebral+palsy&selectedTitle=4%7E150

National Cancer Institute. (2012). *General information about childhood brain and spinal cord tumors.* Retrieved from http://www.cancer.gov/cancertopics/pdq/treatment/childbrain/healthprofessional

Paul, S. P. (2011). Treatment and management of head injuries in children. *Emergency Nurse, 18*(10), 22–26.

Pickering, L. K., Baker, C. J., Kimberlin, D. W., & Long, S. S., (Eds.). (2009). *Red book: 2009 report of the Committee on Infectious Diseases* (28th ed.). Elk Grove Village, IL: American Academy of Pediatrics.

Russ, S. A., Larson, K., & Halfon, N. (2012). A national profile of childhood epilepsy and seizure disorder. *Pediatrics, 129*(2), 256–264.

Schachter, S. C. (2012). Risks associated with epilepsy and pregnancy. *UpToDate*. Retrieved from http://www.uptodate.com/contents/risks-associated-with-epilepsy-and-pregnancy?source=see_link&anchor=H4#H4

Wilfong, A. (2011). Treatment of seizures and epileptic syndromes in children. *UpToDate*. Retrieved from http://www.uptodate.com/contents/treatment-of-seizures-and-epileptic-syndromes-in-children?source=search_result&search=epilepsy+children&selectedTitle=5%7E150

CHAPTER 17

MUSCULOSKELETAL DISORDERS

Clara J. Richardson, MSN, RN-BC

DEVELOPMENTAL DYSPLASIAS OF THE HIP AND CONGENITAL DISLOCATED HIP

Description

Developmental dysplasia of the hip (DDH), previously referred to as congenital dislocated hip (CDH), is the abnormal anatomical relationship between the femoral head and the acetabulum. The degree of dysplasia may be described as preluxation, subluxation, or dislocation. In preluxation, also called acetabular dysplasia, the acetabulum is shallow and the head of the femur remains in place. In hip subluxation, the femoral head still makes contact with a part of the acetabulum, but is not in its normal position. The head of the femur makes no contact with the acetabulum in the dislocated hip.

Etiology

The etiology is multifactorial. Laxity of the surrounding ligaments may have a genetic component, predisposing the hip to movement. By the 11th week of gestation, the hip joint structures are fully formed but continue to grow, with the head of the femur growing faster than the acetabulum so mechanical forces can cause movement. Deeping of the acetabulum continues after birth.

Incidence and Demographics

Approximately 40% of newborns have initial mild hip instability. The incidence of persistent dysplasia is 3–5 per 1,000 infants.

Risk Factors

- Female gender
- First-born status
- Positive family history
- Breech position in utero
- Multiple fetuses
- Oligohydramnios, a decrease in amount of amniotic fluid
- Use of swaddling and cradle boards
- The majority of children with DDH have no identifiable risk factors.

Prevention and Screening

- There is no identified prevention for DDH.
- Screening of newborns is only done by experienced providers to prevent damage and to allow normal development of joint to continue. Those with identified risk factors should be evaluated at 2 weeks of age and regularly by primary provider.

Assessment

History

- History of risk factors

Physical Exam

- Positive Ortolani test: the examiner gently abducts the hip while applying forward pressure on the trochanter and then backward pressure from the thumbs, noting a palpable "clunk" as the femur head slips back into the acetabulum
- Positive Barlow test: hips are adducted and downward pressure is applied with a palpable "clunk" noted
- Positive Galeazzi sign: unequal knee height when infant is in supine position with knees flexed and hips adducted
- Asymmetry of gluteal thigh skin folds
- Limited hip abduction by 3 months of age
- Delayed walking
- Limping or walking on toes
- Waddling gait

Diagnostic Studies

- Ultrasound
- CT scan

Management

Invasive Treatment

- Closed or open reduction followed by spica cast for infants age 6–18 months
- Open reduction followed by spica cast for children age 18 months or older

Nonpharmacologic Treatment

- Abduction splint: Pavlik harness for infants younger than 6 months

Pharmacologic Treatment

- Pain management after surgical procedures

Patient and Family Education

- Nature of disorder and treatment plan
- Care of infant in Pavlik harness
  - Importance of keeping harness on, but also instructions on reapplication in case harness is removed
  - Undershirts under harness to protect skin and clothes over harness to keep it clean
  - Check for skin irritation 2–3 times each day
  - Avoid lotion, powder, and cream under harness
  - Positioning for feeding and car travel
  - Promoting normal development
- Care of infant in hip spica cast
  - Keep cast clean and dry with moisture barrier
  - Frequent diaper changes
  - Padding edges of cast to prevent skin irritation
  - Positioning for feeding and car travel
  - Promoting normal development
- Available resources for adaptable strollers and car seats

Outcomes and Follow-up

- The child will attain normal hip function.

- The child will not experience complications of treatment such as skin breakdown, femoral nerve palsy, femoral head damage or avascular necrosis, or early onset osteoarthritis of the hip.
- The family will verbalize an understanding of the care and maintenance of the Pavlik harness or hip spica cast.
- The family will provide safe transportation for child with harness or cast.
- The family will comply with scheduled follow-up visits.

CONGENITAL CLUBFOOT

Description

Clubfoot, talipes equinovarus, is a congenital deformity of the foot with four main features. The forefoot is inverted and adducted, the heel turns inward (varus), the ankle turns downward (equines), and the leg is rotated internally.

Etiology

The exact etiology of clubfoot is unknown, but is considered to be multifactorial. Foot development occurs during gestational weeks 9 and 10.

Incidence and Demographics

The incidence of clubfoot is 1–2 per 1,000 live births and presents bilaterally in about 50%.

Risk Factors

- Male gender
- Positive family history

Assessment

History

- History of risk factors

Physical Exam

- Smaller foot with soft heel pad
- Concave medial border
- Convex lateral border
- Deep transverse plantar crease
- Internally rotated heel
- Tight Achilles tendon with limited dorsiflexion

Diagnostic Studies

- Prenatal ultrasound
- Radiographs to identify severity
- Periodic radiographs or ultrasounds to monitor effectiveness of treatment

Management

Invasive Treatment

- At 6–12 months of age, after failure of nonsurgical methods
- Release of tight tendons with pin fixation
- Followed by casting for 2–3 months and corrective bracing

Nonpharmacologic Treatment

- Ponseti method for 8–12 weeks
  - Gentle manipulation and stretching of foot
  - Serial cast application every few days for 2 weeks, then at 1–2 week intervals
  - After casting for 8–12 weeks, corrective brace consisting of shoes with connecting bar that holds affected foot in hyperabducted position (Denis Browne splint)
  - Brace may be worn full-time for several months and then part-time for several years
- French physical therapy method
  - Daily physical therapy to stretch and stimulate muscles
  - Continuous passive motion machine for 16–18 hours per day
  - Splinting and taping until 2–3 years of age

Pharmacologic Treatment

- Pain management after surgical procedures

Patient and Family Education

- Nature of defect and treatment protocol
- Positioning, bathing, skin care, clothing
- Neurovascular, skin, pain assessment
- Care of cast, splint, or corrective brace

Outcomes and Follow-up

- The child will have a foot that is functional, mobile, and pain-free.
- The child will walk on the whole sole of the foot with the heel touching the floor.
- The family will verbalize an understanding of the defect and treatment plan.

- The family will demonstrate positioning, bathing, skin care, and clothing adaptations.
- The family will demonstrate care of appliance or cast.
- The family will identify and report neurovascular, skin, or comfort changes.

FRACTURES AND DISLOCATIONS

Description

There are four common types of bone fractures in children. Children's bones may bend up to 45 degrees without breaking, but the bone straightens slowly and has some degree of deformity; this is called a bend fracture. A buckle, or torus, fracture consists of a raised projection. A greenstick fracture is an incomplete fracture. Complete fractures divide the bone into segments. Children may have a fracture or injury of the growth plate, the physis. Growth plate injuries may result in shortened limb length or bone deformities. Fractures are accompanied by muscle contraction, soft tissue contusion, and bleeding. A dislocation involves abnormal position of bone ends in joint sockets.

Etiology

A bone fractures when it is subjected to more force than it can absorb. Fractures in children may occur during play, competitive sports, motor vehicle accidents, or physical maltreatment. Dislocations occur when direct or twisting trauma to ligaments forces bone ends and joint sockets into abnormal positions.

Incidence and Demographics

Approximately 27% of girls and 42% of boys will have a fracture during childhood. Children most commonly sustain fractures of the wrist, elbow, and clavicle. Fractures of the femur, pelvis, and tibia are the most common lower-extremity fractures in children. Growth plate injury accounts for about 25% of skeletal injuries in children.

The most common dislocations in children include phalanges, shoulders, elbows, hips, and knees.

Risk Factors

- Participation in high-risk activities such as contact sports, skateboarding
- Overweight and obesity
- Poor nutrition, particularly protein, vitamin D, and calcium deficiencies
- Excess intake of carbonated soft drinks
- Tobacco and alcohol use
- First fracture at young age

- Chronic conditions such as Duchenne muscular dystrophy, cystic fibrosis, cerebral palsy, sickle cell disease
- Disorders involving impaired motor skills, poor balance, postural instability
- Medical treatment such as immunosuppressive therapy, chemotherapy, corticosteroids, radiotherapy
- Family history
- Prenatal history of maternal smoking, poor nutrition, prematurity, very low birth weight

Prevention and Screening

- Protective gear for sports
- Safe, supervised playgrounds
- Motor vehicle safety measures
- Regular weightbearing exercise
- Accident prevention education
- Balanced diet, healthy body weight

Assessment

History

- History of risk factors
- Circumstances of injury: mechanism of injury, severity of trauma, description appropriate to injury, previous fractures or dislocations
- Possible physical abuse should be suspected in children with multiple fractures in various stages of healing, femur fractures in nonwalking children, midshaft ulna fractures, skull fractures, rib fractures, and scapula fractures

Physical Exam

- Observable deformity such as breaks in skin, swelling, bruising
- Pain, specifically point of maximum tenderness
- Decreased joint mobility
- Neurovascular status: including warmth, color, pulse, capillary refill, sensation
- Dislocations are characterized by pain, swelling, and joint immobility

Diagnostic Studies

- Radiographs, ultrasounds, CT scans
- Full radiographic skeletal survey or bone scan if physical maltreatment is suspected
- Growth plate injuries are graded I–V using the Salter-Harris system

Management

Invasive Treatment

- Open reduction
- Internal or external fixation

Nonpharmacologic Treatment

- Traction
- Procedural sedation, closed reduction and casting
- Splints, slings
- Elevation of extremities
- Dislocations are treated with mild sedation or local anesthesia, manual reduction, possibly immobilization followed by active range of motion

Pharmacologic Treatment

- Pain management
- Antispasmodics for muscle spasms

Patient and Family Education

- Cast care
- Pain management
- Signs of neurovascular compromise
- Safe ambulation with crutches, walkers, wheelchair
- Motor vehicle safely, specifically use of restraints
- Modifications of activities of daily living such as toileting or bathing
- Injury-prevention strategies for play, sports, and motor vehicles
- Strategies to promote balanced nutrition, weight control, and exercise

Outcomes and Follow-up

- The child's bone will heal without complications such as circulatory impairment, nerve injury, compartment syndrome, bone deformity or growth abnormalities, osteomyelitis, kidney stones, or pulmonary embolism.
- The child will not experience complications related to the cast such as cellulitis, abscess, or necrotizing fasciitis.
- The child and family will verbalize an understanding of cast care, pain management, signs of complications, safe ambulation, and activities of daily living.
- The child and family will verbalize an understanding of the injury prevention strategies.

- The child and family will verbalize an understanding of healthy nutrition, weight management, and exercise.
- The family will report signs of complications promptly.

LEGG-CALVÉ-PERTHES DISEASE

Description

Legg-Calvé-Perthes disease (LCPD) is a hip disorder involving avascular necrosis of the femoral head.

Etiology

The course of the disease follows four stages. The initial cause is unknown, but the disease leads to a temporary decrease in blood supply to the proximal femoral epiphysis, resulting in necrosis and flattening of the femoral head. The second stage is the fragmentation stage, with revascularization of the proximal femoral epiphysis and new bone formation. In the reossification, or healing stage, new bone is formed over an average of 4 years' time. The final stage involves either gradual remodeling of the femoral head or residual deformity.

Incidence and Demographics

LCPD occurs in children between the ages of 3 and 12 years, with a peak incidence at 5–7 years. It is four times more common in males and 10 times more common in Whites than in Blacks.

Risk Factors

- Family history
- Bone age and height lag behind peers

Prevention and Screening

- No prevention indicated
- Prompt evaluation of hip pain or limp in children

Assessment

History

- Vague history of mild trauma causing hip pain that resolved
- Pain of groin, thigh, or knee worsened by activity and relieved by rest
- Slow onset of a painful limp
- Joint stiffness

Physical Exam

- Limited internal rotation of hip
- Limited abduction of hip
- Pain with motion
- Limp with walking
- Muscle atrophy of thigh or buttocks
- Uneven limb lengths

Diagnostic Studies

- Radiographs to establish diagnosis and follow disease progression
- Bone scan
- MRI
- Arthrography, invasive imaging done under general anesthesia, to determine the best position of femoral head for healing

Management

Invasive Treatment

- Femoral osteotomy with pinning to hold femoral head in place
- Pelvic osteotomy with pinning to provide better coverage of the femoral head
- A combination of these is indicated in severe cases
- Surgical reconstruction and containment allows return to usual activities in 3 to 4 months

Nonpharmacologic Treatment

- Initial rest and no weight bearing
- Abduction traction to stretch surrounding muscles
- Progressively restoring mobility through physical therapy and aqua therapy
- Abduction bracing to maintain containment while allowing ambulation and motion of knee and ankle, but preventing weight bearing on affected hip
- Abduction casting for the same purpose as bracing
- Conservative treatment may last for 2 to 4 years, but bracing allows near-normal activity

Pharmacologic Treatment

- Pain management

Patient and Family Education

- Stages of the disease process
- Treatment protocol
- Medication schedule
- Pain management
- Physical therapy plan
- Application and care of containment appliance
- Activity restrictions

Outcomes and Follow-up

- The child will report comfort with adequate pain management.
- The child's femoral head will be securely contained in the acetabulum until healing is complete.
- The child will have a pain-free hip with full mobility.
- The child will not experience complications such as collapse of femoral head, subluxation of capital epiphysis, or degenerative arthritis.
- The child and family will verbalize an understanding of the disease process and treatment protocol.
- The child and family will demonstrate application and care of the containment device.
- The child and family will follow medication schedule, physical therapy, and activity restrictions.

OSTEOMYELITIS

Description

Osteomyelitis is a bacterial infection of the bone.

Etiology

Initial bacteremia may be caused by infection in another part of the body, puncture wound, open trauma, or surgical contamination. The bacteria deposited in the metaphysis cause cellulitis in the bone marrow. Exudate is then forced into the cortex of the bone. Infection may result in bone destruction, abscess formation, and accumulation of dead bone (sequestra).

Osteomyelitis in neonates is most often due to group B streptococcus and *Escherichia coli*. The most frequent causative organism in infants and children is *Staphylococcus aureus*. Other causes include group A streptococcus, *Streptococcus pneumoniae*, and community-associated methicillin-resistant *S. aureus* (MRSA).

Incidence and Demographics

Estimates of incidence vary depending on location, but the incidence overall is greater in those younger than 20 years of age. Approximately 25% of affected children are younger than age 2 years, and more than 50% are younger than age 5 years. Boys are affected twice as often as girls. More than 80% of cases occur in tubular bones, especially long bones such as the femur, tibia, or fibula.

Risk Factors

- Existing infection
- Open fractures
- Orthopedic hardware
- Puncture wound
- Indwelling vascular catheters
- Immunosuppression
- Infarcted areas of bone caused by sickle cell disease

Prevention and Screening

- Prompt effective treatment of bacterial infections
- Evaluation of unexplained bone pain accompanied by fever

Assessment

History

- History of risk factors
- History of surgery
- Bone pain with fever

Physical Exam

- Soft tissue redness, warmth, swelling, tenderness
- Limited joint range of motion
- Pathological fracture resulting from infection

Diagnostic Studies

- Elevated white blood cell count, platelet count, erythrocyte sedimentation rate (ESR), and C-reactive protein
- Positive bacterial cultures of blood, joint fluid, aspirated subperiosteal pus
- Bone biopsy if culture result is inconsistent
- MRI to identify extent of infection

- CT to show bone changes, soft tissue swelling, or abscess
- Radiographs show bone changes after 2–3 weeks.

Management

Invasive Treatment

- Surgical debridement of infection
- Draining of abscess
- Remove sequestra with chronic infection

Nonpharmacologic Treatment

- Position for comfort with support of affected extremity
- Avoid weight bearing until healing well underway
- Physical therapy to restore function
- Increased-calorie diet to compensate for decreased appetite
- Assess extremity for circulation, sensation, pain

Pharmacologic Treatment

- IV antibiotics until C-reactive protein returns to normal value, then oral antibiotics
- Nafcillin (Unipen), clindamycin (Cleocin), cefazolin (Ancef) for *S. aureus*
- Vancomycin (Vancocin) for methicillin-resistant *S. aureus*
- Cefotaxime (Claforan), oxacillin, or gentamycin (Garamycin) for neonates
- Pain and fever management

Patient and Family Education

- Nature of disease and treatment protocol
- Mobility restrictions
- Medication administration

Outcomes and Follow-up

- The child will exhibit signs of response to treatment such as fever relief, reduced local signs of infection, and return of lab values to normal limits.
- The child will report comfort with adequate pain management.
- The child will have a fully functional extremity with minimal bone damage.
- The child and family will verbalize an understanding of, and adhere to, the treatment protocol.
- The child and family will demonstrate correct use of mobility devices such as crutches or wheelchair.

JUVENILE IDIOPATHIC ARTHRITIS

Description

Juvenile idiopathic arthritis (JIA) is a chronic inflammatory disease of the joints with onset before 16 years of age that persists for at least 6 weeks.

Etiology

JIA is an autoimmune disease characterized by inflammation of the synovium, the lining of the joints, causing the synovium to produce excess fluid. The effusion leads to joint erosion and destruction, and fibrosis of the articular cartilage.

Incidence and Demographics

The incidence of JIA is 1 per 1,000 children, and it occurs more commonly in girls. Of the three major types, the prevalence is 40% polyarticular, 50% pauciarticular, and 10% systemic.

Risk Factors

- Family history of rheumatologic condition such as arthritis, psoriasis, or inflammatory bowel disease

Prevention and Screening

- No prevention or screening indicated

Assessment

History

- Morning stiffness
- Fatigue or irritability
- Fever
- Weight loss

Physical Exam

- Joint warmth, swelling, tenderness, loss of mobility
- Abnormal gait
- Pauciarticular (oligoarticular) JIA
  - Fewer than five affected joints
  - Knees and wrists most often affected
  - Can cause uveitis (inflammation of the iris, ciliary body, and choroid)

    - Uveitis may result in cataracts, glaucoma, loss of vision
    - Signs of uveitis include red eyes, diminished vision, unequal pupils, eye pain, and headaches
- Polyarticular JIA
    - Five or more affected joints
    - Usually symmetrical presentation
    - Hands and feet most often affected
- Systemic JIA
    - Symptoms occur before age 1 year
    - Daily high-spiking fevers
    - Intermittent rash
    - Variable joint involvement
    - Hepatosplenomegaly
    - Enlarged lymph nodes

Diagnostic Studies

- No diagnostic lab test for JIA
- Elevated white blood cells during flare-up of symptoms
- Elevated antinuclear antibodies (ANA) are indicative
- Elevated ANA indicates higher risk for uveitis
- Rheumatoid factor (RF) positive in some children
- Erythrocyte sedimentation rate (ESR) may be elevated
- Radiographs or MRI to show condition of joints
- Regular medication monitoring: CBC, liver enzymes, serum creatinine, annual tuberculin screening, antibody testing for hepatitis B and C

Management

Invasive Treatment

- No invasive management indicated for children

Nonpharmacologic Treatment

- Physical therapy to maintain muscle tone, improve mobility, prevent joint damage
- Occupational therapy to improve performance of activities of daily living
- Splinting during rest to relieve pain and prevent flexion deformity
- Heat or ice, massage
- Relaxation techniques, guided imagery, distraction to cope with discomfort

Pharmacologic Treatment

- Nonsteroidal antiinflammatory drugs (NSAIDs) to decrease inflammation, relieve pain, minimize joint damage: ibuprofen (Motrin), naproxen (Naprosyn)
- Disease-modifying antirheumatic drugs (DMARDs) to prevent bone and joint destruction by suppressing the immune system attack on joints: methotrexate, sulfasalazine (Azulfidine)
- TNF-α inhibitor to block binding of tumor necrosis factor with cell surface receptors, to reduce proinflammatory activity: etanercept (Enbrel), adalimumab (Humira)
- Glucocorticoid joint injections to decrease inflammation: triamcinolone hexacetonide (Aristospan)
- Immune modulator to decrease inflammation: abatacept (Orencia)
- Monoclonal antibody to decrease inflammation: rituximab (Rituxan)
- Immunological agent to decrease inflammation: Anakinra (Kineret)

Patient and Family Education

- Nature of disease process and treatment plan
- Splint therapy
- Nonpharmacologic management
- Medication administration
- Available support groups, counseling

Outcomes and Follow-up

- The child will have maximum mobility.
- The child will report comfort with effective pain management.
- The child will complete activities of daily living independently.
- The child will participate in age-appropriate physical activity.
- The child will experience minimal symptom flare-ups.
- The child will maintain growth within normal limits.
- The child will be screened regularly by an ophthalmologist.
- The child will receive regular medication-monitoring lab tests.
- The child and family will verbalize an understanding of the disease and treatment plan.
- The child and family will demonstrate splint therapy and strategies for nonpharmacologic management.
- The child and family will demonstrate effective medication administration.
- The child and family will report medication side effects promptly.
- The child and family will access available resources.

IDIOPATHIC SCOLIOSIS

Description

Idiopathic scoliosis (IS) is lateral spinal curvature of more than 10°. The disorder has three categories based on age of initial presentation. Infantile idiopathic scoliosis presents in children under the age of 3 years, the juvenile form between 3 and 10 years, and the adolescent form between 11 and 17 years.

Etiology

Wedging of one or more intervertebral discs along the spine is the most common deformity in IS. The cause of this wedging is not known. One possible explanation for the progression of IS is a cyclic relationship involving asymmetrical load, asymmetrical growth, and degree of wedging. Untreated scoliosis can lead to deformity of the thorax with pulmonary hypertension, pulmonary restrictive disease, and cor pulmonale.

Incidence and Demographics

Infantile scoliosis accounts for 0.5% of all IS, is usually detected by 6 months of age, is more common in boys, and usually resolves spontaneously without treatment by age 3 years. Juvenile scoliosis accounts for 10%–15% of cases, progresses rapidly, and usually requires surgical treatment.

Risk Factors

- Family history

Prevention and Screening

There is no prevention. Screening for girls at age 10 and 12 years, for boys at age 13 or 14 years, by physical exam, is recommended. Some states require school screening.

Assessment

History

- Progression of physical signs

Physical Exam

- Uneven shoulders, scapula, or waistline
- Visible or palpable spinal curve
- Scoliometer measurement of curve
- Asymmetrical rib prominence when bending at waist
- Tilt of pelvis
- Uneven gait, limp

Diagnostic Studies

- Radiography to evaluate degree of curve and skeletal maturity
- MRI scan

Management

Invasive Treatment

- Surgical correction for curves greater than 40°
- Spinal fusion
- Internal instrumentation with screws, rods to hold fusion in place
- Intravertebral stapling to prevent progression

Nonpharmacologic Treatment

- Treatment is not necessary if curve is less than 20° and nonprogressive
- External spinal orthotics (braces) for curves greater than 20°
- Cast stabilization if brace ineffective
- Halo traction for severe curves prior to other interventions
- Postoperative care
  - Pressure-relieving mattress
  - Long roll to turn, depending on specific surgery
  - Foley catheter or chest tube, depending on site of repair
  - Progressive ambulation and physical therapy

Pharmacologic Treatment

- Postoperative pain management
- Postoperative stool softeners to prevent constipation

Patient and Family Education

- Nature of defect and treatment plan
- Treatment options
- Postoperative care
- Care of external spinal orthotic or cast
- Pain management
- Progressive ambulation
- Signs of complications related to surgery, orthotic, cast, traction

Outcomes and Follow-up

- ▶ The child will have maximum mobility.
- ▶ The child's skin will remain intact.
- ▶ The child will participate in the exercise plan.
- ▶ The child will report effective postoperative pain management.
- ▶ The child will not experience constipation secondary to pain medication.
- ▶ The child will follow the plan for progressive ambulation.
- ▶ The child will plan strategies to cope with altered appearance because of an external device.
- ▶ The child and family will verbalize an understanding of the defect, treatment options, and plan of care.
- ▶ The child and family will demonstrate application and care of external orthotic.
- ▶ The child and family will comply with the treatment schedule for the external orthotic.
- ▶ The child and family will return to the clinic for regular orthotic modifications.

SLIPPED CAPITAL FEMORAL EPIPHYSIS

Description

Slipped capital femoral epiphysis (SCFE) is an acquired disorder of the hip in which the femoral capital epiphysis is displaced posteriorly and inferiorly. The condition occurs in preadolescent and adolescent children.

Etiology

The etiology is unknown, but seems to be related to an interaction between mechanical forces, such as obesity or injury, and endocrine alterations related to rapid growth and hormonal changes.

Incidence and Demographics

The incidence of SCFE is 2–10 per 100,000 children, and boys are affected in 60% of cases. The presentation is usually unilateral, but bilateral is in about 23%. The mean age at diagnosis is 13.5 years for boys and 12 years for girls. It is more common in Blacks, Native Americans, and Pacific Islanders.

Risk Factors

- ▶ Obesity
- ▶ Period of rapid growth
- ▶ Hypothyroidism
- ▶ Hyperparathyroidism

- Panhypopituitarism
- Growth hormone administration
- Renal osteodystrophy
- Previous radiation therapy

Prevention and Screening

- Screening is not indicated.
- Avoiding childhood obesity would decrease the risk of occurrence.

Assessment

History

- Groin, hip, thigh, or knee pain
- Exacerbation of pain after trauma such as a fall or sports injury

Physical Exam

- Limp or gait abnormalities
- Limited hip internal rotation
- Inability to bear weight with unstable SCFE
- Ability to bear weight with stable SCFE
- External rotation and abduction of hip with flexion
- Mild atrophy of thigh and gluteal muscles with chronic involvement

Diagnostic Studies

- Radiographs to show degree of slippage
- MRI to show bone edema around the growth plate if radiograph appears normal

Management

Invasive Treatment

- Stabilization with surgical placement of screw
- Radiographic guidance allows for small incision with minimal blood loss

Nonpharmacologic Treatment

- Crutches or wheelchair
- Partial or no weight bearing for 6–8 weeks following surgery
- Monitor incision for redness, swelling, or drainage
- Sports restrictions for 3–6 months

Pharmacologic Treatment

- Pain management

Patient and Family Education

- Nature of disease and treatment plan
- No weight bearing on affected leg to prevent further slippage
- Wound care and assessment
- Safe ambulation with crutches or wheelchair
- Importance of follow-up visits
- Strategies for weight control

Outcomes and Follow-up

- The child will adhere to mobility restrictions.
- The child's incision site will heal without infection.
- The child will demonstrate safe use of crutches or wheelchair.
- The child will not experience complications such as avascular necrosis of the femoral head, acute cartilage necrosis (chondrolysis), or early onset of degenerative arthritis.
- The child will receive monitoring for slippage of uninvolved hip.
- The child and family will verbalize an understanding of the disease process and treatment plan.
- The child and family will take steps to improve the child's diet and increase physical activity.
- The child and family will adhere to follow-up visit schedule.

BONE TUMORS

Description

Osteogenic sarcoma, also known as osteosarcoma, arises from the bone-forming cells. This cancer most commonly occurs in the distal femur and upper end of the humerus. Metastasis may involve other bones and the lung.

Ewing sarcoma is another primary bone tumor occurring in the bone (osseous) or in the soft tissue (extraosseous). Common sites include the extremity long bones, pelvis, chest wall, and spine. Metastasis is to lung, bone, and bone marrow.

Etiology

The cause is unknown.

Incidence and Demographics

Sarcomas account for 15% of all pediatric cancers and the 5-year survival rate for children with all types of sarcomas is 60%–70%. Osteosarcoma is slightly more common in males and in Black children. There is a significant peak during the adolescent growth spurt. Ewing sarcoma is slightly more common in boys and six times more common in White children.

TABLE 17-1. SARCOMA INCIDENCE PER 100,000 BY AGE

	1-4 YEARS	5-9 YEARS	10-14 YEARS	15-19 YEARS
Osteosarcoma	n/a	0.3	0.72	0.77
Ewing sarcoma	0.1	0.21	0.44	0.47

Risk Factors

- Osteosarcoma
  - Prior radiation or chemotherapy
  - Hereditary retinoblastoma
  - Li-Fraumeni, Rothmund-Thomson, and Werner syndromes
- Ewing sarcoma
  - Past history of hernia
  - Farming as parental occupation

Prevention and Screening

- No prevention or screening indicated

Assessment

History

- Osteosarcoma
  - Localized, dull, aching pain
  - Large, tender soft tissue mass
  - Pathologic fracture
- Ewing sarcoma
  - Intermittent, localized pain
  - Malaise
  - Low-grade fever

Physical Exam

- Limited mobility
- Fracture

Diagnostic Studies

- Radiographs
- MRI
- CT scan
- Bone scan
- Bone marrow biopsy
- Osteosarcoma: elevated alkaline phosphatase, LDH, erythrocyte sedimentation rate
- Ewing sarcoma: elevated white blood cell count, erythrocyte sedimentation rate, LDH

Management

Invasive Treatment

- Surgical resection
- Amputation
- Limb salvage surgery

Nonpharmacologic Treatment

- Radiation
- Prosthesis
- Physical therapy

Pharmacologic Treatment

- Osteosarcoma
    - Methotrexate
    - Doxorubicin (Adriamycin)
    - Cisplatin (Platinol)
    - Ifosfamide (Ifex)
- Ewing sarcoma
    - Vincristine (Oncovin)
    - Doxorubicin (Adriamycin)
    - Cyclophosphamide (Cytoxan)
    - Ifosfamide (Ifex)
    - Etoposide (VP-16, VePesid)
    - Dactinomycin (Actinomycin D)

Patient and Family Education

- Nature of disease and treatment options
- Preparation for diagnostic procedures
- Side effects of radiation and chemotherapy
- Signs of infection, anemia, low platelet count
- Infection prevention
- Strategies for coping with low platelet count, stomatitis, nausea and vomiting, constipation, decreased appetite, fatigue, alopecia
- Environmental mobility barriers
- Prosthesis camouflage if desired
- Available support groups, counseling, cancer camps

Outcomes and Follow-up

- The child will attain cancer-free status.
- The child will receive prompt treatment for complications of chemotherapy and radiation.
- The child will not experience infection.
- The child will have balanced nutritional intake.
- The child will report effective pain management.
- The child will plan strategies to deal with mobility and altered appearance.
- The child and family will verbalize an understanding of the disease, diagnostic procedures, and treatment options.
- The child and family will utilize strategies to cope with the effects of chemotherapy and radiation.
- The child and family will demonstrate care of prosthesis.
- The child and family will access available resources.

REFERENCES

Beukelman, T., Patkar, N. M., Saag, K. G., Tolleson-Rinehart, S., Cron, R. Q., DeWitt, E. M., et al. (2011). 2011 American College of Rheumatology recommendations for the treatment of juvenile idiopathic arthritis: Initiation and safety monitoring of therapeutic agents for the treatment of arthritis and systemic features. *Arthritis Care & Research, 63*(4), 465–482.

Boutis, K. (2010). Common pediatric fractures treated with minimal intervention. *Pediatric Emergency Care, 26*(2), 152–159.

Centers for Disease Control and Prevention. (2007). *United States cancer statistics.* Retrieved from http://apps.nccd.cdc.gov/uscs/childhoodcancerdetailedbyICCC.aspx

Clark, M. C. (2011). Overview of the causes of limp in children. *UpToDate.* Retrieved from http://www.uptodate.com/contents/overview-of-the-causes-of-limp-in-children?source=search_result&search=legg+calve+perthes+disease+children&selectedTitle=2%7E21

DeLaney, T. F., Hornicek, F. J., Lessnick, S. L., & Mankin, H. J. (2012). Epidemiology, pathology, and molecular genetics of the Ewing sarcoma family of tumors. *UpToDate.* Retrieved from http://www.uptodate.com/contents/epidemiology-pathology-and-molecular-genetics-of-the-ewing-sarcoma-family-of-tumors?source=search_result&search=risk+factors+for+Ewing+sarcoma&selectedTitle=1%7E57

Delasobera, B. E., Place, R., Howell, J., & Davis, J. E. (2011). Serious infectious complications related to extremity cast/splint placement in children. *Journal of Emergency Medicine, 41*(1). Retrieved from http://www.medscape.com/viewarticle/746890?src=mp&spon=9

Dimeglio, A., & Canavese, F. (2012). The French functional physical therapy method for the treatment of congenital clubfoot. *Journal of Pediatric Orthopaedics B, 21*(1), 30–39.

Heare, T., Hensley, M. A., & Dell'Orfano, S. (2009). Bone tumors: Osteosarcoma and Ewing's sarcoma. *Current Opinion in Pediatrics, 21,* 365–372.

Hockenberry, M. J., & Wilson, D. (2011). *Wong's nursing care of infants and children* (9th ed.). St. Louis, MO: Elsevier Mosby.

Jude, C. M., & Modarresi, S. (2012). Radiologic evaluation of the hip in infants, children, and adolescents. *UpToDate.* Retrieved from http://www.uptodate.com/contents/radiologic-evaluation-of-the-hip-in-infants-children-and-adolescents?source=search_result&search=legg+calve+perthes+disease+children&selectedTitle=3%7E21

Krogstad, P. (2012). Epidemiology, pathogenesis, and microbiology of hematogenous osteomyelitis in children. *UpToDate.* Retrieved from http://www.uptodate.com/contents/epidemiology-pathogenesis-and-microbiology-of-hematogenous-osteomyelitis-in-children?source=search_result&search=osteomyelitis+children&selectedTitle=4%7E150

Krogstad, P. (2012). Treatment of hematogenous osteomyelitis in children. *UpToDate.* Retrieved from http://www.uptodate.com/contents/treatment-of-hematogenous-osteomyelitis-in-children?source=search_result&search=osteomyelitis+children&selectedTitle=2%7E150

Larson, N. (2011). Early onset scoliosis: What the primary care provider needs to know and implications for practice. *Journal of the American Academy of Nurse Practitioners, 23*(8), 392–403.

Ludwig, J. A. (2008). Ewing sarcoma: Historical perspectives, current state-of-the-art, and opportunities for targeted therapy in the future. *Current Opinion in Oncology, 20,* 412–418.

Phillips, W. (2012). Epidemiology and pathogenesis of developmental dysplasia of the hip. *UpToDate.* Retrieved from http://www.uptodate.com/contents/epidemiology-and-pathogenesis-of-developmental-dysplasia-of-the-hip?source=see_link&anchor=H4#H3

Phillips, W. (2012). Treatment and outcome of developmental dysplasia of the hip. *UpToDate.* Retrieved from http://www.uptodate.com/contents/treatment-and-outcome-of-developmental-dysplasia-of-the-hip?source=search_result&search=developmental+dysplasia+of+hips+in+newborn&selectedTitle=2%7E150

Purcell, D., Varthi, A., & Lee, M. C. (2011). Slipped capital femoral epiphysis: Current concepts review. *Current Orthopaedic Practice, 22*(1), 81–89.

Stanley, L. C., & Ward-Smith, P. (2011). The diagnosis and management of juvenile idiopathic arthritis. *Journal of Pediatric Healthcare. 25*(3), 191–194.

Thompson, P. A., & Chintagumpala, M. (2012). Targeted therapy in bone and soft tissue sarcoma in children and adolescents. *Current Oncology Reports, 14,* 197–205.

Wang, L. L., Chintagumpala, M., & Gebhart, M. C. (2012). Osteosarcoma: Epidemiology, pathogenesis, clinical presentation, diagnosis, and histology. *UpToDate.* Retrieved from http://www.uptodate.com/contents/osteosarcoma-epidemiology-pathogenesis-clinical-presentation-diagnosis-and-histology?source=search_result&search=osteosarcoma+children&selectedTitle=1%7E80

Wick, J. M., Konze, J., Alexander, K., & Sweeney, C. (2009). Infantile and juvenile scoliosis: The crooked path to diagnosis and treatment. *AORN, 90*(3), 347–376.

Wu, G. S., & Pollock, A. N. (2011). Slipped capital femoral epiphysis. *Pediatric Emergency Care, 27*(11), 1095–1096.

CHAPTER 18

INTEGUMENTARY DISORDERS

Clara J. Richardson, MSN, RN-BC

ATOPIC DERMATITIS (ECZEMA)

Description

Atopic dermatitis, or eczema, is a chronic inflammatory skin disorder that usually begins in infancy and is associated with allergy.

Etiology

The cause is unknown, but seems to be related to structural abnormalities of the epidermis causing dry and sensitive skin combined with an immune reaction to a trigger such as soap, laundry detergent, skin infection, food, or inhaled allergens. For some children, exacerbation triggers include perspiration, dust, hard water, weeds, and stress.

Incidence and Demographics

Eczema affects up to 20% of children and the peak incidence is 18 months of age. About 95% of children with eczema have food allergy, asthma, or allergic rhinitis. Food allergy is the trigger for about 35% of children, with the most common allergens being milk and eggs. Less common triggers are soy, wheat, and peanuts.

Risk Factors

- Family history of eczema, asthma, food allergy, or allergic rhinitis

Prevention and Screening

- No prevention or screening indicated

Assessment

History

- Dry skin
- Sleep interruption
- Asthma or allergic rhinitis

Physical Exam

- Skin redness, dryness
- Itching
- Irritability
- Vesicles or papules with weeping, crusting
- Lichenification, thickened skin areas

Diagnostic studies

- No diagnostic studies indicated

Management

Invasive Treatment

- No invasive management indicated

Nonpharmacologic Treatment

- Twice daily lubrication with emollient such as Eucerin, Aquaphor, Cetaphil
- Avoid applying emollient immediately before or after topical medications
- Tepid bath with colloidal bath product or mild pH-neutral skin cleaner that is free of fragrance and dye
- Avoid triggers
- Cool wet compresses
- Hypoallergenic diet for identified food allergies
- Keep fingernails and toenails short
- Gloves or socks to prevent scratching

- Soft, cotton clothing and bedding
- Avoid overheating
- Mild laundry detergent without fabric softener

Pharmacologic Treatment

- Topical steroid (hydrocortisone) for acute exacerbation
- Topical calcineurin inhibitors for children age 2 years or older
  - Tacrolimus (Protopic)
  - Pimecrolimus (Elidel)
- Antihistamine for itching may improve sleep
  - Diphenhydramine (Benadryl)
  - Hydroxyzine (Atarax)
- Antibiotics or antifungals for secondary infection

Patient and Family Education

- Nature of condition and treatment plan
- Daily skin care
- Nonpharmacologic management
- Care during exacerbations
- Medication administration
- Signs of bacterial infection: worsening of lesions, fever, malaise

Outcomes and Follow-up

- The child will maintain intact skin.
- The child will show evidence of healing skin.
- The child will demonstrate relief from itching.
- The child will not develop a secondary bacterial infection.
- The family will verbalize an understanding of the diagnosis and treatment plan.
- The family will identify triggers that cause exacerbation.
- The family will demonstrate effective daily skin care and care during exacerbations.
- The family will demonstrate medication administration.
- The family will recognize and report signs of bacterial infection.

IMPETIGO

Description

Impetigo is a highly contagious bacterial infection of the skin.

Etiology

Staphylococcus aureus is the most common cause, with fewer cases from *Streptococcus pyogenes*. The organism affects the superficial epidermis layer of the skin and may be a primary or secondary infection. Impetigo may be spread by direct contact or indirectly by contact with clothing, toys, or towels.

Incidence and Demographics

Impetigo may occur at any age, but is most prevalent in children 2–5 years of age. The nonbullous form of impetigo accounts for approximately 70% of cases. The bullous form can occur at any age, but is most prevalent in newborns. The most common sites for the nonbullous form are face and limbs; for the bullous form, the most common sites are neck folds, nose, groin, and axillae.

Risk Factors

- Skin trauma
- High humidity
- Poor hygiene

Prevention and Screening

- Prevention consists of avoiding exposure
- No screening indicated

Assessment

History

- Insect bites
- Varicella
- Itchy, painful lesions

Physical Exam

- Nonbullous form: small vesicles or pustules that rupture, with honey-colored crusty exudate
- Bullous form: blisters that rupture easily, leaving erythematous lesions

- Occasionally, fever and lymphadenopathy

Diagnostic Studies

- Possibly culture of fluid from lesion

Management

Invasive Treatment

- No invasive management indicated

Nonpharmacologic Treatment

- Meticulous handwashing
- Daily bath, clothing change
- Wash clothing, bedding in hot water
- Avoid sharing towels, clothes
- Wash toys and avoid sharing with unaffected children

Pharmacologic Treatment

- Topical antibiotics for limited lesions
  - Mupirocin (Bactroban)
  - Fusidic acid
- Oral antibiotics for extensive disease
  - Amoxicillin/clavulanate (Augmentin)
  - Dicloxacillin (Dynapen)
  - Cephalexin (Keflex)
- Dilute sodium hypochlorite (bleach) baths two or three times per week

Patient and Family Education

- Diagnosis and treatment plan
- Medication administration
- Strategies to prevent spread of infection

Outcomes and Follow-up

- The child will regain clear, intact skin.
- The child will experience relief of itching.
- The child will not spread the infection to others.
- The family will verbalize an understanding of the diagnosis and treatment plan.

- The family will demonstrate medication administration.
- The family will identify strategies to prevent the spread of infection.

CELLULITIS

Description
Cellulitis is an acute bacterial infection of the skin and subcutaneous tissue.

Etiology
Common causative organisms are group A beta-hemolytic streptococci and *Staphylococcus aureus*, including methicillin-resistant *S. aureus* (MRSA). Areas most affected are face, lower extremities, periorbital, and perianal.

Incidence and Demographics
Each year, cellulitis is responsible for 1 in every 500 pediatric emergency department visits and 14 million outpatient visits.

Risk Factors
- Trauma or surgery
- Insect bite
- Abrasions
- Penetrating wound
- Preexisting skin infection

Prevention and Screening
- No prevention or screening indicated

Assessment

History
- Fever and chills
- Malaise
- History of risk factors

Physical Exam
- Erythema

- Edema
- Pain
- Possible drainage
- Hot and tender to touch
- Red streaking to surrounding skin

Diagnostic Studies

- Blood cultures or needle aspiration to identify causative organism
- CT scan to rule out abscess, a complication

Management

Invasive Treatment

- No invasive management for simple cellulitis
- Incision and drainage may be necessary for abscess

Nonpharmacologic Treatment

- Elevate affected extremity
- Warm moist compress
- Dressing to cover open areas
- Contact infection control precautions

Pharmacologic Treatment

- Oral amoxicillin, cephalexin (Keflex) or clindamycin (Cleocin)
- IV cefotaxime (Claforan), ceftriaxone (Rocephin), or vancomycin
- Pain management

Patient and Family Education

- Disease process and treatment plan
- Strategies to prevent spread of infection
- Nonpharmacologic management
- Medication administration

Outcomes and Follow-up

- The child's skin integrity is maintained with a decrease in symptoms.
- The child will experience effective pain management.
- The child will not experience abscess formation.

- The family will verbalize an understanding of the disease process and treatment plan.
- The family will identify strategies to prevent the spread of infection.
- The family will utilize nonpharmacologic management.
- The family will demonstrate effective pain management.

COMMUNICABLE DISEASES

Description

Communicable diseases with skin manifestations are illnesses caused by infectious agents.

Etiology

Exanthema subitum (Roseola)

- Human herpesvirus type 6 (HHV-6) transmitted through respiratory secretions
- Incubation period 5–15 days
- Complications: febrile seizures and rare cases of encephalitis

Erythema infectiosum (Fifth disease)

- Human parvovirus B19 (PV-B19) transmitted through respiratory droplets, blood products
- Incubation period 4–14 days
- Complication: aplastic crisis

Rubeola (Measles)

- Highly contagious virus transmitted through respiratory droplets
- Incubation period 10–12 days
- Time from exposure to rash appearance: 14 days
- Complications: otitis media, pneumonia, diarrhea; rarely, pneumonia, deafness, encephalitis, death

Rubella (German measles, 3-day measles)

- Virus transmitted through respiratory droplets, mother to fetus
- Incubation period 14–21 days
- Communicable 7 days before through 5 days after rash appearance
- Complications: rare cases of arthritis, encephalitis, or purpura
- Congenital deafness, eye abnormalities, congenital heart disease, cognitive impairment, fetal death

Varicella (Chickenpox)

- Varicella-zoster virus transmitted by respiratory droplets, contact with lesions, or from mother to fetus
- Incubation period up to 2–3 weeks
- Communicable 1 day before and up to 6 days after appearance of lesions
- Complications: secondary bacterial infection and, rarely, varicella encephalitis or varicella pneumonia

Incidence and Demographics

Exanthema subitum (Roseola)

- Most common in children younger than 3 years of age
- Occurrence peaks between 6 months and 15 months of age and in spring and autumn

Erythema infectiosum (Fifth disease)

- Most common in school-age children
- Peak occurrence in late winter or early spring

Rubeola (Measles)

- 0.02 per 100,000 people
- 55 cases in 2006

Rubella (German measles)

- No longer endemic in the United States
- 11 cases in 2006

Varicella (Chickenpox)

- 28.65 per 100,000 people
- Most cases occur in winter and early spring

Risk Factors

- Exposure to causative agent
- Immunocompromised state

Prevention and Screening

- Exanthema subitum (roseola): no prevention or screening
- Erythema infectiosum (fifth disease): no prevention or screening
- Rubeola (measles)
    - Measles, mumps, and rubella vaccine (MMR)

- First dose at 12–15 months of age and second at 4–6 years
- Rubella (German measles): see measles above
- Varicella (chickenpox)
  - Varicella vaccine
  - First dose at 12–15 months of age and second at 4–6 years
  - Postexposure varicella zoster immune globulin (VZIG) or intravenous immune globulin (IVIG) for susceptible individuals

Assessment

History

- Exanthema subitum (roseola): fever for about 3–4 days, decreased temperature, rash appearance, cold symptoms
- Erythema infectiosum (fifth disease): very mild with headache, low-grade fever, sore throat, malaise, nausea
- Rubeola (measles): fever, anorexia, cough, abdominal pain, cold symptoms
- Rubella (German measles): cough, sore throat, headache, low-grade fever, cold symptoms
- Varicella (chickenpox): low-grade fever, malaise, anorexia

Physical Exam

- Exanthema subitum (roseola)
  - Faint red, maculopapular, nonitching rash mainly on trunk that fades on pressure and lasts for 1–2 days
  - Inflamed throat
  - Cervical and postauricular lymphadenopathy
- Erythema infectiosum (fifth disease)
  - First stage: bright red, nonitching rash over cheeks ("slapped face" appearance) lasting 2–4 days
  - Second stage: red, maculopapular, nonitching rash on extremities appearing about 1 day after first stage and lasting about a week
  - Third stage: second stage rash fades into lacy pattern, appearing off and on for up to 3 weeks
- Rubeola (measles)
  - Progressive rash with discrete, red, maculopapular spots
  - Koplik spots: small, red, raised spots with whitish-bluish centers found on buccal mucosa
  - Conjunctivitis
  - Photophobia

- Generalized lymphadenopathy
- Rubella (German measles)
  - Progressive, pinkish-red, discrete, maculopapular rash
  - Fever
  - Conjunctivitis
  - Lymphadenopathy
- Varicella (chickenpox)
  - Itchy, red, papular rash becomes vesicular and then breaks, forming crusts by day 7
  - Rash may spread to mouth, conjunctivae, genital area
  - Irritability
  - Lymphadenopathy

Diagnostic Studies

- Diagnosis based on symptoms

Management

Invasive Treatment

- No invasive management indicated

Nonpharmacologic Treatment

- Rest
- Extra fluids
- Low lighting for measles
- Warm soaks to eyes for measles
- Mittens at night to prevent scratching with chickenpox
- Isolate from susceptible individuals
- Droplet infection control precautions
- Airborne infection control precautions for rubeola (measles)
- Airborne and contact infection control precautions for varicella (chickenpox)

Pharmacologic Treatment

- Acetaminophen (Tylenol) or ibuprofen (Motrin) for fever or discomfort
- Antihistamine (Benadryl) for itching
- Antiviral agent, acyclovir (Zovirax)

Patient and Family Education

- Disease process
- Prevention of transmission
- Comfort measures
- Fever control
- Medication administration

Outcomes and Follow-up

- The child will experience relief from fever, discomfort, and itching.
- The child will not experience complications.
- The child will maintain skin integrity.
- The family will verbalize an understanding of the disease.
- The family will utilize strategies to prevent the spread of infection.
- The family will demonstrate comfort measures and medication administration.

FUNGAL INFECTIONS

Description

Fungal infections are superficial skin infections caused by dermatophytes, a group of fungi. The three most common fungal infections affecting children are tinea capitis (ringworm of the scalp), tinea corporis (ringworm of the skin), and candidiasis (moniliasis), which grows in warm, moist areas of the body.

Etiology

- Tinea capitis is caused by *Trichophyton tonsurans, Trichophyton mentagrophytes, Microsporum audouinii,* and *Microsporum canis.* The fungus penetrates the hair cuticle and moves into the hair shaft. The infection is visible in 12–14 days, when the hair grows, becomes brittle, and breaks in 3–4 weeks. It can be transmitted by direct contact or indirectly by clothing, bedding, toys, combs, phones, and household pets.
- Tinea corporis is caused by *Trichophyton rubrum, Trichophyton mentagrophytes, M. canis, and Epidermophyton.* Fungi live on the skin and subsist by metabolizing skin keratin. Tinea corporis is transmitted by skin-to-skin contact or acquired from household pets.
- Candidiasis is caused by *Candida albicans*, a yeastlike fungus that invades mucus membranes. It is transmitted by person-to-person contact or acquired from contaminated articles. It can also be passed from mother to baby during delivery.

Incidence and Demographics

- Tinea capitis is more prevalent in Blacks and in children between the ages of 3 and 9 years.
- Tinea corporis occurs at all ages and often in association with tinea capitis.
- Candidiasis occurs at all ages and is the most common invasive fungal infection.

Risk Factors

- Tendency toward other allergic reactions (tinea capitis and corporis)
- Altered immune status, antibiotic therapy, very low birth weight (candidiasis)

Prevention and Screening

- Screening of others in household, classroom, or daycare
- Treatment of asymptomatic family members with medication and shampoo
- Avoid sharing hair brushes, towels, clothing
- Mouth care and diaper care

Assessment

History

- Exposure

Physical Exam

- Tinea capitis
    - Hair loss and breaking
    - Erythema of the scalp
    - Scaling and itching
    - Oval patches
    - Cervical lymphadenopathy
    - Black dots on scalp due to broken hairs
    - Pustules
    - Spongy, raised, draining lesions called kerion indicate secondary infection
    - Scarring if kerion not treated
- Tinea corporis
    - Round or oval patch
    - Erythema
    - Scaly vesicular or pustular border
    - Possible fine, itchy, papulovesicular rash

- Candidiasis may manifest as oral lesions (thrush) or as diaper dermatitis
  - Erythema
  - White exudates
  - Peeling and bleeding
  - Itching
  - Pain

Diagnostic Studies

- Microscopic visualization
- Wood's ultraviolet lamp
- Culture or PCR

Management

Invasive Treatment

- No invasive management indicated

Nonpharmacologic Treatment

- Tinea capitis
  - 1%–2.5% selenium sulfide shampoos to decrease scaling and itching
  - Cleaning environment
  - Personal hygiene
  - Consider treatment for all household members
- Tinea corporis
  - Cleaning environment
  - Personal hygiene
- Candidiasis
  - Mouth care
  - Strategies to prevent diaper dermatitis

Pharmacologic Treatment

- Tinea capitis: oral antifungals
  - Griseofulvin (Fulvicin)
  - Terbinafine (Lamisil)
  - Fluconazole (Diflucan)
  - Prednisolone (Orapred) for kerions
- Tinea corporis: topical antifungals

    - Miconazole (Mycostatin)
    - Clotrimazole (Lotrimin)
    - Terbinafine (Lamisil)
    - Oral griseofulvin (Fulvicin) if unresponsive to topical
- Candidiasis: topical antifungals
    - Nystatin (Mycostatin)
    - Miconazole (Monistat)
    - Clotrimazole (Lotrimin)
    - Fluconazole (Diflucan)

Patient and Family Education

- Disease process and treatment plan
- Strategies to prevention spread of infection
- Nonpharmacologic management
- Medication administration

Outcomes and Follow-up

- The child will recover with intact, lesion-free skin.
- The family will verbalize an understanding of the disease and treatment plan.
- The family will demonstrate medication administration.
- The family will identify strategies to prevent the spread of infection.
- The family will demonstrate nonpharmacologic management.

PARASITIC INFESTATIONS

Description

Two common parasitic skin infestations in children are scabies and head lice.

Etiology

Scabies is caused by a mite called *Sarcoptes scabiei* that burrows under the skin, leaving a trail of eggs and feces. The incubation period is 4–6 weeks after first exposure, but only 1–4 days on subsequent exposure. Symptoms are the result of a hypersensitivity reaction to the mites. Usual sites of infestation in children are finger webs, wrists, axillae, elbows, and buttocks.

Pediculus humanus capitis is caused by parasitic insects, head lice. The female lays eggs with a glue-like substance at the base of the hair shaft. The eggs hatch in 8–10 days and the nymphes feed on blood. Symptoms are caused by a reaction to lice saliva injected into the scalp during feeding. Usual sites are behind the ears and near the neck.

Incidence and Demographics

Head lice occur most often in preschool and school-age children and their families. Blacks rarely get head lice.

Risk Factors

- Scabies
    - Prolonged personal skin-to-skin contact
    - Crowded living conditions
    - Immunocompromised state
- Head lice
    - Head-to-head contact
    - Less commonly, from shared head-contact items such as hats and hairbrushes

Prevention and Screening

- Scabies
    - Treat household contacts
    - Wash contaminated bedding and clothing in hot water and dryer
- Head lice
    - Treat household contacts
    - Wash contaminated bedding and clothing in hot water and dry in dryer
    - Store items that cannot be washed in sealed plastic bag for 2 weeks
    - Soak combs and brushes for 1 hour in alcohol or wash in hot water
    - Recheck every few days for 2–3 weeks after infestation
    - Avoid sharing of hair gear

Assessment

History

- History of symptoms or exposure

Physical Exam

- Scabies

- Pruritus, especially intense at night
- Burrow looks like a short, wavy, grayish or white line
- Papules are small and red, changing to vesicles and pustules
- Scratching leads to excoriation and secondary infection
- Crusted appearance indicates hyperinfestation

- Head lice
  - Pruritus
  - Sensation of something moving
  - Secondary lesions from scratching

Diagnostic Studies

- Scabies
  - Microscopic examination of skin scrapings
- Head lice
  - Presence of nits or live lice on inspection

Management

Invasive Treatment

- No invasive management indicated

Nonpharmacologic Treatment

- Scabies
  - Cool baths to relieve itching
  - Avoid scratching, which can lead to secondary bacterial infection
  - Wash contaminated bedding and clothing in hot water and dry in dryer
  - Use contact infection control precautions for first 24 hours after treatment
- Head lice
  - Wash clothing and bedding used within the last 2 days
  - Avoid rewashing hair for at least 1 day after treatment
  - Remove nits with nit comb
  - Use contact infection control precautions for first 4 hours after treatment

Pharmacologic Treatment

- Scabies
  - Permethrin 5% (Elimite) topical solution in single overnight application; bathe after 8–14 hours

- Oral antihistamine or topical corticosteroid for itching that may last several weeks after treatment
- Treat all members of household at the same time

- Head lice
  - Pyrethrins (A-200, Pronto, Rid)
  - Permethrin (Nix)
  - Benzyl alcohol 5%
  - Malathion (Ovide): flammable; avoid hair dryer
  - Spinosad (Natroba): one treatment kills lice and prevents nits from hatching
  - Wash hair over sink, not in shower or bath

Patient and Family Education

- Diagnosis and treatment plan
- Medication administration
- Nonpharmacologic management
- Strategies to prevent spread

Outcomes and Follow-up

- The child will be parasite-free after treatment.
- The child will maintain intact skin with no secondary infection.
- The family will verbalize an understanding of the diagnosis and treatment plan.
- The family will demonstrate medication administration.
- The family will utilize nonpharmacologic management strategies.
- The family will identify strategies to prevent the spread of infestation.

ACNE VULGARIS

Description

Acne is an inflammatory skin condition characterized by obstruction of sebaceous follicles.

Etiology

Excessive sebum and desquamated epithelial cells clog pores, *Propionibacterium acnes* proliferates and causes an inflammatory reaction.

Incidence and Demographics

Almost all adolescents have acne to some degree, but 15%–20% develop moderate to severe acne. Acne begins earlier in girls, but affects more boys.

Risk Factors

- Family history
- Cosmetics containing lanolin, petrolatum, lauryl alcohol, butyl stearate, and oleic acid
- Polycystic ovary syndrome
- Hot, humid environments
- Some antiepileptic medications
- Some anticancer medications
- Anabolic steroid use
- Smoking worsens severe acne

Prevention and Screening

- Avoidance of risk factors may help prevent acne

Assessment

History

- Presence of acne
- Psychological impairment such as social inhibition, anxiety, embarrassment, depression, anger

Physical Exam

- Noninflammatory open comedones, called blackheads
- Noninflammatory closed comedones, called whiteheads
- Reddened papules, pustules, nodules, or cysts
- Scarring may appear as ice-pick marks or be more hypertrophic

Diagnostic Studies

- No diagnostic studies indicated

Management

Invasive Treatment

- Injection of intralesional steroid, triamcinolone acetonide into acne cysts
- Subcision, punch excision of scars

- Laser resurfacing, dermabrasion, chemical peels for scars

Nonpharmacologic Treatment

- Nonabrasive, nonalkaline skin cleanser
- Handwashing
- Avoid squeezing or picking, which increases scarring
- Keep hair shampooed and away from face

Pharmacologic Treatment

- Over-the-counter benzoyl peroxide
- Topical antibacterials
    - Erythromycin
    - Clindamycin (Cleocin)
    - Tetracycline
- Topical retinoids to loosen comedones, anti-inflammatory
    - Tretinoin (Retin-A)
    - Isotretinoin (Accutane)
    - Adapalene (Differin)
    - Tazarotene (Tazorac)
    - Retinoids affect fetus, requires pregnancy prevention
- Systemic antibiotics
    - Tetracycline
    - Doxycycline (Vibramycin)
- Hormonal treatment with oral contraceptive pill to decrease sebum

Patient and Family Education

- Disease process
- Treatment options
- Skin care
- Available resources such as support groups, counseling, discount offers on expensive medications

Outcomes and Follow-up

- The child will have a decrease in lesions and heal without scarring.
- The child will demonstrate effective skin care.
- The child will access available resources.

- The child will report relief of psychological stressors.
- The child and family will discuss treatment options and agree on plan of care.

BURNS

Description

A burn is tissue injury from contact with heat, extreme cold, chemicals, electricity, or radiation.

Etiology

Thermal injuries result from scalds, hot objects, and flame. Children sustain electrical burns from inserting conductive objects into outlets or chewing on electrical cords. Chemicals may be spilled on skin, splashed in eyes, or ingested. Burn injuries from radiation or extreme cold are rare in children. The body's response to a burn is local and systemic according to the severity of the injury.

- Local response
  - Vasodilation causes increased hydrostatic pressure in the vessels, which, coupled with increased capillary permeability, moves fluid into the interstitial spaces, causing edema
  - Fluid lost from the burn wound
  - Fluid shifts, decreased cardiac output, and edema lead to capillary stasis with tissue ischemia
- Systemic response
  - Significant decrease in cardiac output and fluid loss, can result in burn shock.
  - Fluid shift to interstitial spaces can compress the vessels, causing compartment syndrome.
  - Reduced renal blood flow can cause acute renal failure.
  - Ischemia of the gastrointestinal tract can cause necrosis.
  - Gastric acid production is decreased for up to 3 days, but then accelerates rapidly and can lead to ulceration.
  - Increased cortisol and catecholamines initiate hypermetabolism that may cause rapid protein breakdown, lipid catabolism, and muscle wasting.
  - Anemia and metabolic acidosis occur.
  - Production of growth hormone diminishes and growth is delayed.

Incidence and Demographics

An average of 496 children ages 14 years or younger die each year due to burn injury, and 107,170 sustain nonfatal bury injuries. Scald burns from hot liquids or steam are most common. Burn injuries are more common in males and in children younger than 5 years. Deaths from burns are 2–3 times higher in Native Americans and Blacks than in Whites.

Risk Factors

- Young children are more likely to sustain burn injury
- Use of heating devices such as kerosene heaters and wood-burning stoves
- Inadequate supervision by adults
- Lack of home safety precautions

Prevention and Screening

There is no screening, but there are many ways to prevent burns in children.

- Kitchen safety
    - Use stove guards; keep pot handles and hot liquids out of reach
    - Avoid tablecloths and drinking hot liquids with child on lap
    - Keep child out of kitchen during food preparation
- Bath safety
    - Lower temperature of water heaters to 120° F
    - Constant supervision of young children
- Home safety
    - Keep matches, lighters, candles, flammables out of reach
    - Keep electrical cords out of reach; use outlet covers
    - Working smoke detectors, emergency escape plan
    - Flame-retardant sleepwear
- Outside safety
    - No fireworks for children
    - Keep children away from grills, fire pits
    - Sun protection

Assessment

History

- Details of burn injury

Physical Exam

- Extent of injury: total body surface area (TBSA) burned
- Depth of injury

TABLE 18–1.
CLASSIFICATION OF BURNS

1ST DEGREE	Superficial	Red, pain, epidermis only
2ND DEGREE	Partial thickness	Blisters, pain, swelling of epidermis and dermis
3RD DEGREE	Full thickness	White, brown, charred, blisters, little or no pain
4TH DEGREE	Full thickness	Involves skin, muscle, and bone

- Severity of injury
  - Minor: < 10% TBSA, partial thickness, outpatient or short-term admission
  - Moderate: 10%–20% TBSA, partial thickness, hospital with expertise in burn care
  - Major: > 20% TBSA, all full thickness, specialized burn center
- Inhalation injury
  - Facial or neck edema
  - Singed nasal hairs
  - Hoarseness
  - Difficulty breathing
  - Stridor, wheezing, rales
  - Restricted chest movement due to encircling burn

Diagnostic Studies

- Arterial blood gases reflect metabolic acidosis
- Chest radiography shows effect on airways
- Complete blood count shows elevated hematocrit, blood urea nitrogen, and creatinine
- Type and cross-match for blood replacement
- Coagulation studies
- Chemistry panel shows altered concentrations of potassium, sodium, chloride, bicarbonate
- Urinalysis shows hematuria, myoglobinuria with electrical burns
- Electrocardiogram (ECG)

Management

Invasive Treatment

- Escharotomy (incision of burned tissue) to relieve compartment syndrome
- Excision and debridement
- Skin grafts provide permanent coverage
- Cultured epithelium grown from the child's skin
- Reconstructive plastic surgery

Nonpharmacologic Treatment

- Basic life support and resuscitation
- Intubation and artificial ventilation for > 20% TBSA or inhalation injury
- 100% humidified oxygen to relieve carbon monoxide poisoning
- Nasogastric tube for decompression
- Early high-protein, high-carbohydrate enteral feeding
- Increase environmental temperature to 31.5° C (88.7° F)
- Foley catheter to monitor urine output
- Cool compresses only for < 10% TBSA burned
- Hydrotherapy
- Flush chemical burns with water for 20 minutes
- Temporary skin substitutes to promote healing
  - Allograft (homograft) cadaver skin lasts about 14 days
  - Porcine xenograft lasts 2–3 days
  - Synthetic skin coverings for partial thickness burns such as Xeroform petroleum dressing, Biobrane silicone mesh, DuoDerm hydrocolloid dressing, OpSite or Tegaderm transparent adhesive film
  - Artificial skin (Integra) for partial or full thickness burns
- Protective isolation infection control precautions
- Pressure-sensitive mattress, joint splints at night
- Physical therapy and range of motion
- Pressure garments to reduce scarring
- Scar massage and moisturizers such as Eucerin, Nivea, or cocoa butter

Pharmacologic Treatment

- Fluid resuscitation to maintain urine output of 1–2 mL/kg/hr and specific gravity
- Intravenous albumin after 18–24 hrs to maintain serum level
- Topical antimicrobials
  - Silver sulfadiazine (Silvadene)
  - Mafenide (Sulfamylon)
  - Bacitracin for small areas of minor burn
- Histamine-2 (H2) receptor antagonist therapy, antacids, or both to prevent stress ulcer
- Opthalmic ointment for eye abrasions
- Tetanus immunoprophylaxis
- Pain management with morphine, fentanyl, midazolam (Versed)
- Anesthetic agents for procedures such as nitrous oxide, propofol, or ketamine

Patient and Family Education

- Extent and implications of burn injury
- Treatment plan
- Preparation for procedures
- Medication administration
- Feeding techniques
- Promotion of age-appropriate activity
- Promotion of coping with altered appearance
- Prevention of future injury
- Available resources such as support groups, counseling, burn camps

Outcomes and Follow-up

- The child will maintain open airway and effective circulation.
- The child will maintain body temperature between 98.6° F and 100.5° F (37° C and 38° C).
- The child will maintain fluid and electrolyte balance.
- The child will show evidence of wound healing.
- The child will receive adequate nutrition.
- The child will attain optimal mobility.
- The child will experience effective pain management.
- The child will not experience complications such as pneumonia, respiratory failure, wound infection, or septicemia.
- The family will verbalize an understanding of the burn injury and treatment plan.

- The family will demonstrate effective pain management, including use of medications and nonpharmacological interventions to help child cope with pain.
- The family will monitor skin grafts for signs of infection and bleeding.
- The family will utilize prevention strategies to prevent future injury.

REFERENCES

Baddour, L. M. (2011). Cellulitis and erysipelas. *UpToDate*. Retrieved from http://www.uptodate.com/contents/cellulitis-and-erysipelas?source=see_link

Baddour, L. M. (2012). Impetigo. *UpToDate*. Retrieved from http://www.uptodate.com/contents/impetigo?source=search_result&search=impetigo&selectedTitle=1%7E71

Bangert, S., Levy, M., & Hebert, A. A. (2012). Bacterial resistance and impetigo treatment trends: A review. *Pediatric Dermatology, 29*(1), 1–6.

Centers for Disease Control and Prevention. (2012). *Measles (rubeola)*. Retrieved from http://www.cdc.gov/measles/index.html

Dempster, J., Jani, B., & Daly, T. (2011). Managing eczema in children – a treatment update. *The Journal of Family Practice, 60*(11), 660–668.

Hockenberry, M. J., & Wilson, D. (2011). *Wong's nursing care of infants and children* (9th ed.). St. Louis, MO: Elsevier Mosby.

Nicol, N. H. (2011). Efficacy and safety considerations in topical treatments for atopic dermatitis. *Pediatric Nursing, 37*(6), 295–301.

Pickering, L. K., Baker, C. J., Kimberlin, D. W., & Long, S. S. (Eds.). (2009). *Red book: 2009 report of the Committee on Infectious Diseases* (28th ed.). Elk Grove Village, IL: American Academy of Pediatrics.

Safe Kids Worldwide (SKW). (2011). *Burn and scalds safety in the USA*. Washington (DC): SKW. Retrieved from http://www.safekids.org/assets/docs/ourwork/research/2011-burns-and-scalds.doc

Williams, H. C., Dellavalle, R. P., & Garner, S. (2012). Acne vulgaris. *Lancet, 379,* 361–372.

CHAPTER 19

MENTAL HEALTH ISSUES IN THE CHILD: ACUTE AND CHRONIC

Mary Jo Gilmer, PhD, MBA, RN-BC, FAAN, and
Paula Chiplis, PhD, RN, CPNP

Numerous mental health issues begin in childhood. With early identification of problems, treatment modalities can be used to prevent or reduce symptoms that may interfere with activities of daily living. Autism, eating disorders, substance abuse, and depression are some of the challenges facing many families as their children develop.

AUTISM

Description

Autism is a group of developmental disabilities defined by significant impairments in social interaction and communication skills, usually evident before age 3 years.

Etiology

Many theories are under study, but no definitive cause has been identified. It is typically viewed as a behavioral disorder resulting from abnormal brain function.

Incidence and Demographics

- ~1 in 500 children, with males affected four times as often as females

Risk Factors

More common among siblings than in general population. Puberty has been identified as a crucial stage for showing either improvement or deterioration.

Prevention and Screening

- No known prevention for autism

Diagnosing autism spectrum disorders (ASD) can be difficult, because there is no medical test, like a blood test, to diagnose the disorders. Providers may conduct a developmental screening and a comprehensive diagnostic evaluation that includes hearing and vision screening, genetic testing, and neurological testing to make a diagnosis.

Assessment

- Physical exam
- Denver Developmental Screening Test (DDST)
    - May include evaluation of the following signs and symptoms:
        - Impaired in three domains: communication, social interaction, and repetitive behaviors
        - Withdraws from reality
        - Appears indifferent or aversive to affection or physical contact
        - May develop seizure disorders or schizophrenia
- Interference with intellect may result in appearance of being cognitively impaired
- Lack of meaningful relationships
- Apathy
- Looseness of associations
- Unpredictable, uncontrolled behavior
- May refuse to eat

Management

- Prioritize nursing diagnoses and problem list as above
- Psychotherapy focused on developmental level of child
- Medications: stimulants, neuroleptics, lithium
    - Use of reminders and incentives to enhance compliance

Patient and Family Education

- Provide consistent routine in familiar environment
- Set consistent limits
- Prevent self-destructive behavior
- Encourage verbalization
- Physical contact on a regular basis
- Referrals to community resources

Outcomes and Follow-up

- Meta-analyses show that early intensive behavioral interventions have a positive effect on intellectual and adaptive functioning.
- Ongoing follow-up of verbal IQ, language (receptive and expressive), and socialization is important.

FAILURE TO THRIVE (FTT)

Description

Growth failure is defined as weight or height falling below the 5th percentile for a child's age, or a weight loss curve that crosses > 2 percentile lines on the National Center for Health Statistics growth chart.

Etiology

The cause is often classified as organic (resulting from a physiological condition, such as congenital health defects, neurologic lesions, malabsorption syndrome, chronic infections, gastroesophageal reflux, endocrine dysfunction, or cystic fibrosis). Nonorganic FTT is related to psychosocial factors such as poverty, health beliefs, lack of emotional and sensory stimulation, or family stress (parental depression, substance abuse, acute grief).

Incidence and Demographics

Approximately 5% of infants and children are below the 5th percentile for height or weight and may be diagnosed as FTT. Nonorganic causes are more common than organic FTT.

Risk Factors

- An infant or child with physical, or psychosocial conditions, or both, as described above
- Psychosocial problems in the family, including food insecurity and poverty

Prevention and Screening

- Parental education about infant and childhood development may minimize risk of development of FTT.
- Routine well-child check-ups are useful for screening.

Assessment

- Physical and developmental exams may include evaluation of the following signs and symptoms:
    - Failure to meet developmental milestones
    - Withdrawn
    - Eating disorders
    - Avoidance of eye-to-eye contact
    - Stiff or unyielding body posture

Management

- Prioritize nursing diagnoses and problem list as above
- Treat physical cause of FTT through surgery or medications
- Assist families with relational issues

Patient and Family Education

- Focus on supervision and feeding advice rather than repeated measurements that imply poor parenting
- May involve a multidisciplinary healthcare team, behavior modification, and hospitalization
- Consistent caregiver, provision of optimum nutrients, positive feeding environment
- Provide emotional support to parent
- Confidence-building with parent

Outcomes and Follow-up

- Evidence suggests improvement in outcomes for infants with severe growth and development delays.
- Follow-up should include ongoing assessments and educational interventions.
- Care should be taken to avoid instilling unnecessary anxiety in parents.

DEVELOPMENTAL DISABILITY

Description

Developmental disability is a mental or physical disability that is evident before the age of 22 years and likely to continue indefinitely.

Etiology

- Learning disability, which is frequently found in association with medical conditions such as lead poisoning, fragile X syndrome, fetal alcohol syndrome
- Impaired motor skills with no definitive cause but may be a response to a chronic illness

Incidence and Demographics

- Developmental disabilities occur in 1 in 6 children in the United States.
- The number of children with select developmental disabilities (autism, attention-deficit hyperactivity disorder, and other developmental delays) has increased, requiring more health and education services.

Risk Factors

- Perinatal brain injury or infection
- Growth or nutrition problems
- Chromosomal abnormalities
- Extreme prematurity
- Poor maternal diet and absent or minimal health care
- Abuse

Prevention

- Health promotion
- Education of parents regarding normal growth and development

Screening

- Denver II, both parent observation and direct observation; the Developmental Screening Tool has long been the standard for developmental screening
    - Ages and Stages Questionnaire (ASQ), a parental report of child development, is easy to implement, takes little provider time, and has relatively high specificity and sensitivity for identifying children with developmental delays

Assessment

Includes evaluation of the following signs and symptoms:

- Difficulty with fluidity and flexibility of thinking
- Dislike of ambiguity (black-and-white thinkers)
- Tendency to concentrate on one aspect of a situation while neglecting others
- Difficulty prioritizing and breaking down tasks into manageable projects
- Tendency to have highly focused areas of expertise and interests
- Tendency for poor generalization skill
- Communication and social problems
    - Idiosyncratic speech
    - Inability to perceive social cues
    - Difficulty utilizing or understanding nonverbal communication
    - Frequent miscommunications and misunderstandings
    - Tendency toward one-sided conversations
    - Tendency to ask many questions, especially when uncomfortable
    - Tendency to return to familiar, rote questions or subjects of personal interest when anxious
    - Intrusive behavior
    - Poor understanding of the impact of behavior on others
    - Difficulty making and keeping friends

Management

- Early intervention and special education classes
- Prioritize nursing diagnoses and problem list
    - Be specific when making suggestions for change.
    - Practice different ways of handling tough situations the patient is likely to encounter.
    - Work on building coping skills rather than insight.
    - Slow down speech.
    - Use visuals whenever possible to reinforce your verbal messages.
    - Draw pictures.
    - Write down suggestions for change in brief, outline form.
    - Present information one item at a time.
    - Ask for feedback after each item to ensure clear comprehension.

Patient and Family Education

- Include a variety of support and education services for children, families, and caregivers
  - Down Syndrome Association
  - Autism Society
  - United Cerebral Palsy

Outcomes and Follow-up

- Best outcomes with early intervention
- Follow-up needed for ongoing evaluations to mitigate sequelae

ENURESIS

Description

Enuresis is involuntary or intentional micturition in inappropriate places, including clothing.

Etiology

Contributing factors include a slower rate of physical development, positive family history, and lengthy duration of sleep in infancy. Enuresis is primarily an alteration of neuromuscular bladder functioning, generally benign and self-limiting.

Incidence and Demographics

- Types:
  - Primary (enuresis in a child who has never been dry)
  - Secondary (enuresis in a child who was previously dry)
  - Nocturnal (nighttime enuresis: bedwetting)
    - More common in boys
    - Resolves spontaneously at 6 to 8 years of age in 15% of cases
  - Diurnal (daytime: wetting clothes)

Risk Factors

May have comorbidity with sickle cell disease, diabetes, urinary tract infection, developmental disorders, learning problems, or behavioral difficulties

Prevention and Screening

- Exact mechanism of enuresis is poorly understood and multifactorial, making prevention and screening difficult, but simple measures include:
    - Evaluation of cormorbidities such as diabetes, urinarty tract infection
    - Decreased fluid intake in evening

Assessment

Includes evaluation of the following signs and symptoms:

- Urgency
- Acute discomfort
- Restlessness
- Urinary frequency

Management

- Conditioning therapy: training the child to awaken with a stimulus initiated when the child voids (most effective)
- Retention control training: child drinks lots of fluid and retains as long as possible to stretch the bladder
- Waking schedule: parents wake the child during the night at intervals to void
- Medications: tricyclic antidepressants, antidiuretics, and antispasmodics (least effective)

Patient and Family Education

- Education about the condition
- Encourage and support child and parents
- Teach parents side effects of medications

Outcomes and Follow-up

- Comorbidity of behavioral problems is 2–4 times higher in children with enuresis in all epidemiologic studies.
- Emotional impact of enuresis on a child and family can be considerable. Children with enuresis are commonly punished and are at significant risk of emotional and physical abuse.
- Numerous studies report feelings of embarrassment and anxiety in children with enuresis; loss of self-esteem, and effects on self-perception, interpersonal relationships, quality of life, and school performance. These outcomes necessitate folllow-up child and family therapy.

ATTENTION DEFICIT DISORDER (ADD) AND ATTENTION-DEFICIT HYPERACTIVITY DISORDER (ADHD)

Description

These disorders are degrees of inattention, impulsivity, and hyperactivity beyond normal disturbances occurring at this stage of childhood development

Etiology

The causes are multifactorial including physiologic, genetic, and environmental factors

Incidence and Demographics

- 6% of school-age children
- Affects boys 3 times as often as girls

Risk Factors

- Higher risk in children with family members with ADD or ADHD
- May be associated with substance abuse, learning disabilities, conduct disorders, depression, and antisocial personality disorders

Prevention and Screening

- Though there is no proven way to prevent ADHD, early identification and treatment may prevent many of the problems associated with ADHD.

Assessment

Includes evaluation of the following signs and symptoms:

- Excessive impulsivity
- Inappropriately attentive
- Short attention span
- Hyperactivity may or may not be present.
- Difficulty with organization

Management

- Therapy, counseling
- Medications: methylphenidate (Ritalin), amphetamine and dextroamphetamine (adderall), pemoline (Cylert), dextroamphetamine (Dexedrine)

Patient and Family Education

- Help plan activities to balance energy expenditure and quiet time
- Set realistic, attainable goals
- Structure situations for limited stimulation
- Consistent discipline
- Plan activities to ensure some success

Outcomes and Follow-up

- Children with ADHD exhibit impaired academic functioning and perform more poorly on cognitive tasks than children developing typically.
- Children with ADHD are more often characterized as having low self-esteem and poor social functioning.
- Careful monitoring of medication and counseling are important components of follow-up.

OVERWEIGHT AND OBESITY

Description

The excessive accumulation of body fat relative to lean body mass is the most common nutritional concern of childhood. Children who are overweight or obese are at risk of remaining overweight or obese in adulthood. This is a major and growing health problem in the United States.

Etiology

Obesity is caused by caloric intake that exceeds needs, usually coupled with decreased activity.

Incidence and Demographics

Approximately 17% (or 12.5 million) of children and adolescents age 2–19 years are obese. Since 1980, the prevalence of obesity among children and adolescents has almost tripled. There are significant racial and ethnic disparities in the prevalence of obesity among American children and adolescents. In 2007–2008, Hispanic boys age 2 to 19 years were significantly more likely to be obese than non-Hispanic White boys, and non-Hispanic Black girls were significantly more likely to be obese than non-Hispanic White girls.

Risk Factors

- 5% of obese children have an underlying medical condition (e.g., hypothyroidism, adrenal hypercorticoidism, hyperinsulinism, central nervous system damage).

Other risk factors include:

- Diet: regularly eating high-calorie foods, such as fast foods, baked goods, and vending machine snacks
- Lack of exercise: inactive leisure activities, such as watching television or playing video games
- Family history: genetic or environmental predisposition
- Psychological factors: overeating may be a coping strategy
- Socioeconomic factors: frozen foods and inexpensive food fillers often contain a lot of salt and fats

Assessment

- Children with body mass index above the 95th percentile are obese.
- Children at 85th to 94th percentile are overweight.

Management

- Best management is prevention through education, because diet modification is difficult to maintain
- Increase physical activity
- Behavior modification
- Medications: appetite suppressants may be habit-forming and are not recommended
- Surgery: gastric bypass surgery is not recommended

Patient and Family Education

- Assess motivation
- Encourage personal responsibility
- Nutrition counseling (foods low in fat, smaller portions)

Outcomes and Follow-up

- Outcomes depend on treatment modalities; family therapy and other sources of support for eating and activity change are important.
- Follow-up of ongoing family therapy is needed to reduce the socioeconomic and psychosocial burdens of obesity in adult life.
- Evaluation of potential lifelong consequences of the following discorders is also needed:
    - High blood pressure, high cholesterol, type 2 diabetes, sleep apnea, joint problems, musculoskeletal disorders, fatty liver disease, gallstones, and gastroesophageal reflux disease.

ANOREXIA NERVOSA AND BULIMIA

Description

- Anorexia: Eating disorder characterized by refusal to maintain body weight within a normal range. Anorexic individuals feel hungry, but deny it.
- Bulimia: Eating disorder characterized by repeated binge-eating followed by purging through induced vomiting, laxatives, or excessive exercise.

Etiology

- Relentless pursuit of being thin
- Strongly dependent on parents
- Searching for sense of control
- Abnormalities of hypothalamic-pituitary and end-organ function

Incidence and Demographics

- Mainly occurs in White, middle–upper class females
- High achievers
- 0.5%–1% of young females

Risk Factors

- Gender (female)
- Age (teens through early 20s)
- Family history of eating disorders
- Emotional disorders such as depression, anxiety, or obsessive–compulsive disorders
- Dieting with subsequent positive reinforcement
- Transitions like going away to college or a relationship breakup
- Involvement in sports, work, and artistic activities

Prevention and Screening

- Be attentive and intervene when physical, emotional, social, and familial issues arise.
- Deemphasize appearance and obsession with one's body.
- Foster the development of self-esteem and self-respect.
- Maintain ongoing well-child check-ups.

Assessment

- Nutritional assessment
- Health interview

- Evaluate for the following symptoms:
  - Self-imposed starvation
  - Frequent strenuous exercise
  - Social isolation
  - Secondary amenorrhea
  - Bradycardia
  - Decreased blood pressure
  - Hypothermia
  - Dental caries (particularly with bulimia)

Management

- Psychotherapy
- Family therapy
- Malnutrition reversal

Patient and Family Education

- Strengthen self-esteem
- Family support

Outcomes and Follow-up

- Improved outcome in younger patients
- Around 25% of previous inpatients may require another admission
- Recovery uncommon for at least 3 years; requires long-term follow-up
- Recovery rates usually increase with longer follow-up
- Poor prognosis with chronic anorexia nervosa

SUBSTANCE ABUSE

(See also Chapter 7, Life Situations and Adaptive and Maladaptive Responses)

Description

Overindulgence in and dependence on a drug or other chemical, leading to effects that are detrimental to the individual's physical and mental health or the welfare of others

Etiology

Most substance abuse begins with experimentation. The substance is then used occasionally, and gradually becomes an integral part of a lifestyle.

Incidence and Demographics

- 4% of adolescents report daily use of alcohol.
- 1%–2% of adolescents report regular use of "hard drugs."

Risk Factors

- Parental substance abuse
- Child abuse or neglect
- Single-parent families
- Stressful life events
- Inadequate coping mechanisms

Prevention and Screening

- Provide factual information about risks of substance abuse
- Teach children how to refuse drugs and alcohol
- CRAFFT is a mnemonic acronym of first letters of key words to screen adolescents for substance abuse

C: Have you ever ridden in a CAR driven by someone (including yourself) who was "high" or had been using alcohol or drugs?
R: Do you ever use alcohol or drugs to RELAX, feel better about yourself, or fit in?
A: Do you ever use alcohol/drugs while you are by yourself, ALONE?
F: Do you ever FORGET things you did while using alcohol or drugs?
F: Do your family or FRIENDS ever tell you that you should cut down on your drinking or drug use?
T: Have you gotten into TROUBLE while you were using alcohol or drugs?

Assessment

Varies with substance abused

- Interviews
- Drug Use Inventory
- Alcohol Use Inventory
- Toxicology
- Physical assessment for the following symptoms:

- Nausea, vomiting
- Slurred speech
- Poor coordination
- Hypertension
- Weight loss
- Flashbacks
- Hallucinations
- Gastritis
- Respiratory depression
- Coma
- Death
- Irreversible damage to central nervous system

Management

- Rehabilitation
- Foster healthy interdependent relationships

Patient and Family Education

- Foster feelings of self-worth
- Sensitivity to developmental transitions

Outcomes and Follow-up

- Outcomes improve when the entire family is treated
- Systematic follow-up of children after treatment should be implemented to determine instances of drug-free behavior or possible need for additional treatment

DEPRESSION

Description

Depression is a psychiatric disorder that generally includes a state of unhappiness or hopelessness and manifests in many different ways in childhood, depending on developmental stage and language and cognitive development.

- Acute: usually temporary after an event such as death of a parent or close friend
- Chronic: related to illness or disability

Incidence and Demographics

- Approximately 3% to 5% of all children

Risk Factors

- Chronic illness such as diabetes
- Female gender
- Puberty
- Parental depression
- Neglect or abuse
- Socioeconomic deprivations
- Loss of loved one or loss of romantic relationship
- Anxiety disorder
- ADHD
- Smoking

Prevention and Screening

- None

Assessment

- Child Depression Inventory
- Beck Depression Inventory
- Center for Epidemiological Studies-Depression Scale for Children
- Reynolds Child Depression Scale
- Careful history and evaluation of child
- Evaluate for:
  - Persistent feelings of hopelessness
  - Dejection
  - Poor concentration
  - Lack of energy
  - Inability to sleep
  - Suicidal tendencies

Management

- Counseling
- Psychotherapy

- Family therapy
- Cognitive therapy
- Education about coping skills
- Environmental therapy
- Medications (tricycle antidepressants, selective serotonin reuptake inhibitors [SSRIs]). SSRIs may, however, increase the risk for suicidal thinking and behavior.

Patient and Family Education

- Family education regarding meds (take 2–4 weeks to reach therapeutic effect; monitor for side effects)

Outcomes and Follow-up

- Systematic depression treatment improves clinical outcomes and reduces healthcare costs.
- Long-term treatment promotes stability of remission.

SUICIDE

Description

Suicide is deliberate self-injury with intent to die.

- Suicide ideation: preoccupation with thoughts of committing suicide
- Suicide intent: injury intended to result in death but unsuccessful

Incidence and Demographics

- Whites age 15–24: 18.5% males, 3.3% females
- Blacks age 15–24: 15% males, 2.2% females
- Hispanics age 15–24: 13.4% males, 2.8% females

Risk Factors

- Depression
- Alcohol or drug use
- Impulsivity
- Feelings of guilt
- Body image problems
- Gender identity questions
- Difficult family situation

- Lack of effective social support

Prevention and Screening

- School curricula focused on the problem
- Inservice training for teachers and staff to help identify students at risk of suicide and provision of strategies to take when students have been identified
- Schoolwide suicide screening that involves class- or schoolwide self-report screening to identify potentially suicidal adolescents.

Assessment

- Ask adolescent screening questions
  - Do you consider yourself a happy person?
  - Have you ever been so upset you wanted to be dead?
  - Have you ever thought about hurting yourself?
  - Have you ever had a plan to hurt yourself?
  - Have you ever attempted to kill yourself?

Management

- Ensure safety
- Preventive care
  - Counseling
  - Psychotherapy
  - Family therapy
- Confidentiality may not be possible to honor for safety's sake
- Show of caring and understanding
- Express commitment

Patient and Family Education

Warning signs include:

- Suicidal threats in the form of direct and indirect statements
- Suicide notes and plans
- Prior suicidal behavior
- Making final arrangements (e.g., giving away prized possessions)
- Preoccupation with death
- Changes in behavior, appearance, thoughts, feelings, or a combination of these

Outcomes and Follow-up

- Follow up with family, if needed, to enhance:
    - Family support, cohesion, and good communication
    - Peer support and close social networks
    - School and community connectedness
    - Adaptive coping and problem-solving skills, including conflict resolution
    - Self-esteem, sense of purpose

LOSS AND GRIEF, DEATH AND DYING

(See also Chapter 7, Life Situations and Adaptive and Maladaptive Responses)

Description

The concept "grief" is derived from a Latin word *gravere,* meaning to burden or to cause distress. Lindemann's (1944) seminal work noted that grieving persons display heightened irritability and anger, and may withdraw socially, despite efforts of others to support them. However, definitions continue to be vague and ambiguous. Bowlby's attachment theory (1969) refers to the state and quality of an individual's connections with others. A threat of loss typically results in anxiety and the actual loss usually leads to sorrow. Since grief has not been shown to progress in a rigid manner, it is described as a dynamic process with a broad range of feelings and reactions. Individuals may experience a variety of physical sensations, thoughts, behaviors, and feelings after a loss.

Etiology

To help a child dealing with death, nurses must be aware of the child's understanding and previous experience with death. The concept of death develops through stages according to a child's cognitive abilities. Death as irreversible, inevitable, and universal is not understood by many children until preadolescence, although the concept is certainly influenced by parental attitudes and explanations as well as personal experiences.

Incidence and Demographics

While about 50,000 children in the United States die each year, children are also faced with grief associated with deaths of parents, friends, grandparents, or even pets.

Risk Factors for Complicated Grief

- Inadequate support system or friendships
- Feelings of guilt
- Inability to talk about feelings

- History of depression or anxiety
- Violent or sudden death

Prevention and Screening

- None

Assessment

- Reactions may be physical, psychological, cognitive, or combinations of these
  - Frequent illness, overeating or underrating, insomnia
  - Antisocial behavior, depression, compulsions
  - Forgetfulness, difficulty concentrating
  - May be ongoing
- Influencing factors
  - Amount of social support
  - Prior positive coping skills
  - Open family communication style
  - Spiritual and religious beliefs
  - Anticipatory grief

Management

Going through grief is hard work and a process that takes time. In severe cases, cognitive–behavioral methods for treating symptoms and stress relief, along with interpersonal techniques to encourage reengagement with the world, may be helpful.

- Be in touch with your own feelings
- Be compassionate and unafraid to show your caring and concern
- Encourage expression of feeling
- Provide support and active listening; use silence and presence
- Recognize that a child's serious illness affects the entire family
- Encourage family's participation in child's care, including siblings and extended family members as desired
- Provide private area for parents and family members near child's bedside.
- Assist parents in identifying and utilizing support systems
- Encourage family members directly involved in the patient's care to take care of themselves and to seek medical care if they fail to adequately care for themselves
- Facilitate addressing of parents' spiritual needs and rituals as desired

- Facilitate memory-making between child and family as desired (e.g., videotaping, scrapbooking)
- Identify and document patient, family, and caregiver needs related to anticipatory grieving (National Hospice and Palliative Care Organization, 2006).

Patient and Family Education

- Provide anticipatory guidance about disease progression and dying process as parent(s) desire.
- Seek opportunities to provide honest information, without being evasive, and do so in a sensitive manner.

Outcomes and Follow-up

- Assess for indications of complicated grief.
- Remember that there is no time limit for the grieving process.
- Follow up with families, so they do not feel abandoned.

CHILD ABUSE AND NEGLECT

(See also Chapter 7, Life Situations and Adaptive and Maladaptive Responses)

Description

One of the most significant social concerns affecting infants and children, child abuse may be classified as intentional physical abuse or neglect, emotional abuse or neglect, or sexual abuse.

Etiology

A precise cause of abuse is unknown, but its etiology is influenced by parental characteristics, the child's characteristics, and environmental characteristics. It is the interaction among several factors that increases the risk for abuse.

Incidence and Demographics

- In the United States, approximately 800,000 to 1,000,000 children per year
    - Approximately 68% neglect
    - 20% physical abuse
    - 12% sexual abuse

Risk Factors

- Parents who were abused

- Socially isolated families
- Children of teen mothers
- Parents with low self-esteem
- Parents who use drugs
- Parents with poor understanding of typical childhood development
- Child's temperament
- Child's position in family
- Premature infants
- Children of a difficult pregnancy

Prevention and Screening

- Strengthen families through education about normal growth and development.
- Role model positive parenting.
- Provide community parent support groups.
- Provide access to hotline resources.

Assessment

- Physical
  - Bruises on face, back, buttocks, torso
  - Welts in patterns descriptive of objects used
  - Burns on soles of feet, palms of hands
  - Fractures such as spiral or dislocation, or multiple fractures in various stages of healing
- Sexual
  - Bruises, bleeding, lacerations of external genitalia
  - Penile discharge
  - Recurrent urinary tract infections
  - Sexually transmitted infections
  - Inappropriate acting out of sexual behavior
- Neglect
  - Most common form of maltreatment
  - Failure of adult legally responsible for child's welfare to provide basic needs and adequate level of care
  - Physical neglect is deprivation of good, clothing, shelter, education, health care
  - Emotional neglect is absence of attention, affection, and nurturing

Management

- Prevention is best strategy
- Protect child from further injury
- Mandatory reporting of even suspected child abuse
- Support child
- Support parents
- Treat child's injuries or neglect

Patient and Family Education

- Typical child development
- Health promotion
- Conflict resolution
- Coping strategies

Outcomes and Follow-up

- With support and education, parents may demonstrate an understanding of the normal expectations for their child and refrain from further abuse or neglect.
- Follow-up should include:
    - Observing child for additional physical or emotional neglect or abuse
    - Interviewing parents regarding their knowledge of child's physical and developmental needs
    - Investigating community programs aimed at preventing child maltreatment

REFERENCES

Ball, J. W., Bindler, R. C., & Cowen, K. J. (2010). *Child health nursing: Partnering with children & families* (2nd ed.). East Rutherford, NJ: Pearson.

Bowden, V. R., & Greenberg, C. S. (2009). *Children and their families: The continuum of care: Text and study guide package* (2nd ed.). Philadelphia: Lippincott Williams & Wilkins.

Bowlby, J. (1969/82). *Attachment and loss. Volume 1: Attachment.* New York: Basic Books.

Centers for Disease Control and Prevention. (2009). *Overweight and obesity: NHANES surveys (1976–1980 and 2003–2006).* Retrieved from http://www.cdc.gov/obesity/childhood/prevalence.html

Fischbach, F. T., & Dunning, M. B. (2009). *A manual of laboratory and diagnostic tests* (8th ed.). Philadelphia: Lippincott Williams & Wilkins.

Hagan, J. F., Shaw, J. S., & Duncan, P. M. (Eds.). (2007). *Bright futures: Guidelines for health supervision of infants, children, and adolescents* (3rd ed.). Elk Grove Village, IL: American Academy of Pediatrics.

Hockenberry, M. J., & Wilson, D. (2011). *Wong's nursing care of infants and children* (9th ed.). St. Louis, MO: Elsevier/Mosby.

Joint Commission, The. (2010). *Meeting the Joint Commission's 2011 national patient safety goals.* Oakbrook Terrace, IL: Joint Commission Resources.

Lindemann, E. (1944). Symptomatology and management of acute grief. *American Journal of Psychiatry, 101*(3), 141–149.

National Hospice and Palliative Care Association. (2006). *Grief and healing.* Retrieved from http://www.nhpco.org/i4a/links/?pageid=3287&showTitle=1#Grief and Healing

Ogden, C. L., Carroll, M., National Center for Health Statistics (U.S.), & Division of Nutrition Examination. (2010). *Prevalence of obesity among children and adolescents: United States, trends 1963–1965 through 2007–2008.* Retrieved from http://www.cdc.gov/nchs/data/hestat/obesity_child_07_08/obesity_child_07_08.htm

Pillitteri, A. (2009). *Maternal & child health nursing: Care of the childbearing & childrearing family* (6th ed.). Philadelphia: Lippincott Williams & Wilkins.

Polit, D. F., & Beck, C. T. (2009). *Essentials of nursing research: Appraising evidence for nursing practice* (7th ed.). Philadelphia: Lippincott Williams & Wilkins.

Stuart, G. W. (2009). *Principles and practice of psychiatric nursing* (9th ed.). St. Louis, MO: Mosby/Elsevier.

Tschudy, M. M., Arcara, K. M., Johns Hopkins Hospital, & Children's Medical and Surgical Center. (2012). *The Harriet Lane handbook: A manual for pediatric house officers* (19th ed.). Philadelphia: Elsevier Mosby.

U.S. Department of Health and Human Services, Administration for Children and Families, Administration on Children, Youth and Families, & Children's Bureau. (2010). *Child maltreatment 2009.* Retrieved from http://www.acf.hhs.gov/programs/cb/pubs/cm09/cm09.pdf

CHAPTER 20

HEALTH MAINTENANCE, PROMOTION, AND WELLNESS

Mary Jo Gilmer, PhD, MBA, RN-BC, FAAN

Health maintenance, promotion, and wellness include physical, cognitive, emotional, and social dimensions.

- *Health maintenance* refers to activities that prevent disease or injury, thus preserving health.
- *Health promotion* refers to activities that promote well-being or health according to an individual's potential. Thus, individuals with disabilities can be healthy if they adapt to their condition.
- *Wellness* refers to a healthy balance of body, mind, and spirit, resulting in an overall feeling of wholeness or well-being.
- *Health supervision* refers to services that focus on growth and development, screening, health promotion at key developmental stages, and services that prevent diseases and injuries and treat diseases. Health supervision is the core of primary care pediatrics and general pediatrics.

TABLE 20-1.
AGE, WEIGHT, HEIGHT, AND DEVELOPMENTAL ISSUES

AGE GROUP	AGE	WEIGHT	HEAD CIRCUMFERENCE	PHYSICAL DEVELOPMENT ISSUES
Newborn	Birth–1 week	2.7–4 kg (6–9 lbs)	33–35 cm (13–14 in)	Transition to extra-uterine well-being
Infant	1 week–1 yr	Weekly gain 140–200 g (5–7 oz)	35–48 cm (14–19 in)	Developmental milestones
Toddler/ Preschooler	> 1–5 yrs	14.5 kg (32 lbs) @ 3 yrs 16.5 kg (36.5 lbs) @ 4 yrs	48–52 cm (19–20.5 in)	Gross and fine motor skills
School Age	> 5–12 yrs	18.5 kg (41 lbs) @ 5 yrs		Cognitive development
Adolescent	> 12–18 yrs	Wt gain 7–30 kg (15–65 lbs)		Sexual development, menarche

Immunizations

A rapid decline in the number of infectious diseases during the 20th century has been a dramatic benefit of the widespread use of immunizations. The recommended schedule begins during infancy. Visit http://www.cdc.gov/vaccines/recs/schedules/child-schedule.htm for the Centers for Disease Control and Prevention's recommendations for immunization schedules.

Preterm infants should receive full doses of vaccines at the appropriate chronologic age.

Hepatitis B

Preservative-free Hep B (Recombivax HB, no mercury) is now available.

- *Reaction:* Few side effects
- *Nursing Responsibilities:* Administer IM in vastus lateralis of newborns or in deltoid for older infants and children. First dose should be given within 12 hours of birth. Can be administered simultaneously at separate site with DTaP, MMR, and Hib. Should not be given to children allergic to baker's yeast.

Hepatitis A

- *Reaction:* Few side effects; no severe reactions; erythema at site
- *Nursing Responsibilities:* Dose 2 should be given at least 6 months after first dose.

Diphtheria

- *Reaction:* Fever within 24–48 hours; soreness, redness, and swelling at site; behavioral changes (e.g., fussy, fretful, anorexia, unusual crying)

- *Nursing Responsibilities:* Withhold for encephalopathy ≤ 7 days after previous DTaP. Advise of potential side effects and have parents call for neurological symptoms and temperature ≥ 40.5° C (104.9° F). Boosters given every 10 years after DTaP/DTP vaccine series.

Tetanus

- *Reaction:* Same as for diphtheria, plus urticaria and malaise; may have delayed onset, lump at site that lasts weeks or months but eventually disappears, or both
- *Nursing Responsibilities:* Boosters every 10 years after DTaP/DTP vaccine series

Pertussis

- *Reaction:* Same as for tetanus, plus loss of consciousness, convulsions, inconsolable crying episodes, generalized or focal neurologic signs, systemic allergic reaction. Acellular pertussis vaccine has fewer local and systemic side effects (such as redness at site, fever, and irritability) than the whole-cell pertussis vaccine.

Polio

- *Reaction:* Inactivated poliovirus vaccine (IPV) is now recommended because of the rare risk of vaccine-associated paralysis. This change increased cost and the number of injections necessary.
- *Nursing Responsibilities:* Four doses are needed and only IPV is used in the United States. Contraindicated if anaphylactive response to neomycin or streptomycin.

Measles

- *Reaction:* To the live, attenuated vaccine: anorexia, malaise, rash, and fever 7–10 days after administration
- *Nursing Responsibilities:* Advise parents of side effects and use of acetaminophen for fever

Mumps

- *Reaction:* To the live, attenuated vaccine: brief, mild fever
- *Nursing Responsibilities:* Should ***not*** be administered to infants < 12 months because maternal antibodies can interfere with immune response. Recommended for all individuals born after 1957 who are at risk for the disease.

Rubella

- *Reaction:* To the live, attenuated vaccine: fever, lymphadenopathy, mild rash lasting 1–2 days, arthritis, arthralgia, and paresthesia of hands and fingers 2 weeks after vaccination
- *Nursing Responsibilities:* Advise of side effects, especially of time delay of joint pain, assuring parents that symptoms will disappear. May cross placental barrier and the immunization should not be given to pregnant women. Contraindicated with known immunodeficiency. Recommend acetaminophen if needed for fever or discomfort.

Haemophilus influenzae Type B (Hib)

- *Reaction:* Mild pain and redness, low-grade fever
- *Nursing Responsibilities:* Advise parents of side effects and use of acetaminophen for fever

Varicella (Chickenpox, VZV)

- *Reaction:* To live attenuated vaccine: local soreness or swelling, fever, rash
- *Nursing Responsibilities:* Advise of side effects. Recommend acetaminophen if needed. Should not be given to infants prior to 12 months of age. Has been shown to be effective for at least 11 years. Contraindicated with HIV, known immunodeficiency, pregnancy.

Pneumonococcal

- *Reaction:* Local tenderness, fever, anorexia
- *Nursing Responsibilities:* Now recommended for children at 2, 4, 6 and 12–15 months of age

Influenza

- *Reaction:* Soreness, fever, aches
- *Nursing Responsibilities:* Recommended annually for children ≥ 6 months of age. Administer in early fall before flu season begins and repeat annually. Do not administer to any flu vaccine to children with hypersensitivity to eggs. FluMist may be given nasally in 2 doses 4 weeks apart instead of injection to children 2 years and older. Children in contact with immunocompromised individuals should get the injection rather than FluMist.

Meningococcal

- *Reaction:* MCV4: Pain at site, fever, headache, fatigue, chills, anorexia, vomiting, diarrhea, rash. MPSV4: Pain at site, redness, fever, urticaria, wheezing, rash.
- *Nursing Responsibilities:* Explain benefits, especially in adolescents and young children. Recommended for children with sickle cell anemia, but contraindicated in persons allergic to diphtheria toxoid or latex.

Human Papilloma Virus (HPV)

- *Reaction:* Local irritation, fever
- *Nursing Responsibilities:* Recommended for children (not before age 9) and adolescents to prevent HPV-related cancer. Three doses needed: HPV2 or HPV4 for females, HPV4 for males. Contraindicated with pregnancy or hypersensitivity to yeast.

Inactivated vaccines may result in limited side effects such as local tenderness, erythema, fever, drowsiness, and irritability. These responses usually occur within a few hours or days. Live vaccines such as MMR may result in unfavorable reactions 30 to 60 days after administration.

Administration

Immunizations may be given intramuscularly (IM) or subcutaneously (sub-Q; MMR, varicella, and meningococcal). The needle length should be selected to suit the amount of a child's sub-Q tissue. Needle gauge should be as small as possible to deliver the medication; 25- to 30-gauge needles are least painful, but larger diameter may be necessary for viscous medications. Ensuring the correct dose of a medication given is a shared responsibility of the practitioner and the nurse. Children may unexpectedly react with severity to some drugs, and care should be taken to monitor children carefully.

ANTICIPATORY GUIDANCE AND PATIENT SAFETY (HOME, HOSPITAL, AND COMMUNITY)

Falls

Although falls are more common after an infant has learned to roll over (~4 months), they can occur at any age. Caregivers should be encouraged to get in the habit of raising side rails all the way and never leaving a child on a changing table unattended, even when restrained. Infant seats, high chairs, swings, and walkers also present challenges to preventing falls. Never leave an unattended infant on a raised surface; the safest place may be the floor. To prevent falls once an infant is mobile, gates should be used at the tops and bottoms of any stairs. Furniture should be kept away from windows.

Poisoning

Because of their curiosity and impulsivity, young children are particularly vulnerable to poisoning. The most frequent cause is improper storage in the home. Toddlers are very quick and can swallow a whole bottle of aspirin in seconds. Parents should be advised to call a Poison Control Center before initiating an intervention. General first aid for various types of poisoning is described below.

- ***Caustics and Corrosives*** (Drano, lye)
  - Do not induce vomiting, because a substance that burns on the way down can burn on the way back up. The child needs emergent care with a lavage tube to suction out the poison.
- ***Hydrocarbons*** (gasoline, cleaning solutions)
  - Treat like caustics or corrosives and do not induce vomiting. These substances are usually excreted through the lungs and may cause respiratory depression.
- ***Medications***
  - Syrup of ipecac is no longer recommended because it may result in prolonged vomiting. In its place, activated charcoal, which is an odorless, tasteless, fine black powder that adsorbs many compounds, may be mixed with soda for a child to drink.

- *Metals*
  - There is no normal excretory mechanism to rid the body of metal ingestion, so chelation therapy is typically used to bind with the metal for rapid and safe excretion.

INJURY PREVENTION

Vehicular Safety

Motor vehicle accidents remain the leading cause of accidental death in children under 9 years of age. Car seats for infants and young children are mandatory in all states. The safest location for an infant is in the rear seat, facing backwards. Children under age 12 years should ride in the rear seat in vehicles with airbags.

Toy Safety

Although toys are integral to a child's play, they can be hazardous and it is the nurse's responsibility to ensure toy safety in a hospital setting. If a child is receiving oxygen therapy, electrical or friction toys are contraindicated; sparks may cause the oxygen to ignite. Toys with small parts should be avoided in children younger than 3 years of age. Latex balloons are also not appropriate because a young child may choke on a piece of latex if the balloon breaks.

ADOLESCENT ISSUES

Sexuality

Anticipatory guidance can help prevent unfortunate choices teens may make that negatively affect their futures. Many children report never having been informed about puberty development and sexuality issues. Education should consist of information about normal anatomy and physiology, using correct terminology that adolescents can understand. They also need to know about biological processes and the mechanics of conception, so they can make informed decisions about intimate relationships and their future.

Smoking and Drug Use

The prevalence of smoking has decreased in recent years, but it continues to be the most common cause of preventable death. While the dangers of smoking prevail at any age, it is particularly important to prevent smoking at a young age because of its addictive nature. Although experimentation with illegal drugs is widespread, most teens do not become high-risk users. Nurses can play an important role in administering educational programs to prevent smoking and drug use as part of holistic anticipatory guidance toward a healthy lifestyle.

Community-Based Screening and Resources

- ***Newborn universal screening for metabolic disorders and hemoglobinopathy:*** At birth or 1 week. Screening for conditions varies by state and results must be documented.
- ***Hearing:*** At birth or in the first month; a normal result must be documented by the 2-month visit or further evaluation is needed. Congenital hearing loss should be identified before 3 months of age. Hearing should be evaluated at the 4-year, 5-year, 8-year, and 10-year visits.
- ***Vision:*** Screening should be done at an early age and at regular intervals (AAP, 2003). Infants and children should be assessed for visual acuity, peripheral vision, color vision, and ocular alignment.
  - *Visual acuity*
    - In infants, check for light perception and test of ability to follow an object.
    - Fixed pupils, strabismus, nystagmus, or setting sun sign all indicate visual loss or other serious concerns.
    - A common test for visual acuity in children is the Snellen chart, with lines of letters of decreasing size.
    - If a child is unable to read letters, a tumbling E test can be used and a child is asked to point the direction the E is facing.
    - Typically by the time an infant is 3 to 4 months, she or he has the ability to view one visual field with both eyes simultaneously.
  - *Peripheral vision:* It is useful with older children to check their ability to fix their eyesight on a space directly in front of them, and then move an object such as a pencil, asking the child to indicate when she or he can no longer see it.
  - *Color vision:*
    - Tests for color vision use a series of pictures composed of spots of one color in the background and an object in the foreground composed of spots of a color often confused with the background.
    - Almost 10% of White males are assessed as having poor color vision.
  - *Ocular alignment*
    - Typically, by the time infants are 3 to 4 months old, they can see a visual field with both eyes simultaneously.
    - However, with strabismus (cross-eye), one eye deviates.
    - The weak eye may become lazy over time.
    - The corneal light reflex test is used to determine alignment by indicating whether a light falls symmetrically within each pupil when the light is shined directly into the child's eyes.
    - Another test is the cover test, in which a child is asked to look at an object and then one eye is covered and movements of the uncovered eye are observed.

- ***Anemia:*** At 4 months, test hemoglobin and hematocrit for preterm, low birth weight, and those fed non–iron-fortified formula. At 12-month, 2-year, 3-year, and all other visits, ask risk assessment questions asking about limited access or avoidance of high-iron-rich foods, for example, vegan diet.
- ***Oral health:*** At 6 months, question feeding practices (e.g., bottle in bed) and examine teeth. At 12 months, refer to dentist with visits every 6 months.
- ***Lead:*** At 12 months and 2 years, test those in high-prevalence areas or with Medicaid insurance. Ask environmental risk questions at 6 months, 9 months, 12 months, 18 months, 2 years, 3 years, 4 years, 5 years, and 6 years: Does the child live in a building built before 1950, or built before 1978 and recently renovated? Test refugee children 6 months to 16 years old upon entering the United States and repeat for those 6 months to 6 years of age 3 to 6 months after permanent placement.
- ***Tuberculosis:*** A tuberculin skin test (TST) is a screening test used to determine if a child has been infected with the tubercle bacillus. Universal screening is no longer recommended by AAP; screening is done only when a child is at high risk for contracting the disease.
- ***Autism:*** Screen at 18-month and 2-year visits with an autism-specific screening tool.
- ***Blood pressure:*** Annually beginning at 3-year visit. Prior to 3 years old, monitor according to risk conditions such as prematurity, very low birth weight, renal disease, congenital heart disease, or other neonatal complications.
- ***Body mass index (BMI) and weight for length:*** Assess weight, length, and weight for length every visit from birth until the 18-month visit. Beginning at 2-year visit, BMI for age percentile according to standing height.
- ***Dyslipidemia***
  - *Fasting lipoprotein profile* (total cholesterol, LDL, HDL, and triglycerides): Once in late adolescence.
  - *Dyslipidemia risk assessment:* At 2-year, 4-year, 6-year, 8-year, and 10-year visits and then annually according to risk for coronary artery disease given family history, BMI, or health behaviors.
  - *Fasting lipid profile:* For all persons with a BMI ≥85th percentile, even if no other risk factors are present.
- ***Sexually transmitted infections (STI)***
  - For sexually active youth, annual screen for chlamydia and gonorrhea
  - Selective HIV screen for sexually active youth with positive response to risk assessment (injection drug users, men who have sex with men, women who have unprotected sex with multiple partners, persons who exchange sex for money or drugs, persons treated for sexually transmitted infection, people who are bisexual, partners of those with HIV)
- ***Pregnancy:*** Sexually active females who report late menses or amenorrhea
- ***Cervical dysplasia:*** Females 3 years after onset of sexual activity or at age 21

- ***Alcohol or drug use:*** Risk assessment at every adolescent visit (Have you ever had an alcoholic drink? Have you ever used marijuana or another drug to get high?). A positive response should trigger the use of a screening tool, such as CRAFFT, designed for use with teens in primary care settings.
- ***Developmental and behavioral assessment:*** At every visit
- ***Scoliosis:*** Girls twice at 5th and 7th grade and boys once at 8th or 9th grade
- ***Denver Developmental Screening Tool (DDST II):*** This is a revised developmental screening tool with 125 items used to determine relative areas of advancement or delay in development.

Barriers to Care

- ***Access:*** May be a concern related to socioeconomic conditions, physical constraints, mental status, transportation, finances, lack of insurance, or many other barriers to care.
- ***Availability:*** Individuals living in rural areas may have limited availability of services, but limited access to the services that do exist may be related to social standing, economic status, and poor health.
- ***Culture:*** Barriers to care may be related to lack of family support, transportation difficulties, or family mistrust of Western medicine.
- ***Health literacy:*** Ability of parents and adolescents to obtain, process, and understand health information and services needed to make appropriate health decisions for themselves

REFERENCES

American Academy of Pediatrics, & Pickering, L. K. (Eds.). (2009). *Red book: 2009 report of the Committee on Infectious Diseases* (28th ed.). Elk Grove Village, IL: American Academy of Pediatrics.

Ball, J. W., Bindler, R. C., & Cowen, K. J. (2010). *Child health nursing: Partnering with children & families* (2nd ed.). East Rutherford, NJ: Pearson.

Bowden, V. R., & Greenberg, C. S. (2009). *Children and their families: The continuum of care, 2nd ed: Text and study guide package.* Philadelphia: Lippincott Williams & Wilkins.

Centers for Disease Control and Prevention. (2011). *Vaccines & immunizations: Recommendations and guidelines: 2012 child & adolescent immunization schedules.* Retrieved from http://www.cdc.gov/vaccines/recs/schedules/downloads/child/7-18yrs-schedule-pr.pdf

Fischbach, F. T., & Dunning, M. B. (2009). *A manual of laboratory and diagnostic tests* (8th ed.). Philadelphia: Lippincott Williams & Wilkins.

Hagan, J. F., Shaw, J. S., & Duncan, P. M. (Eds.). (2007). *Bright futures: Guidelines for health supervision of infants, children, and adolescents* (3rd ed.). Elk Grove Village, IL: American Academy of Pediatrics.

Hockenberry, M. J., & Wilson, D. (2011). *Wong's nursing care of infants and children* (9th ed.). St. Louis, MO: Elsevier/Mosby.

Joint Commission, The. (2010). *Meeting the Joint Commission's 2011 national patient safety goals.* Oakbrook Terrace, IL: Joint Commission Resources.

National Association of Pediatric Nurse Practitioners, Society of Pediatric Nurses, & American Nurses Association. (2008). *Pediatric nursing: Scope and standards of practice.* Silver Spring, MD: American Nurses Association.

Pillitteri, A. (2009). *Maternal & child health nursing: Care of the childbearing & childrearing family* (6th ed.). Philadelphia: Lippincott Williams & Wilkins.

Tschudy, M. M., Arcara, K. M., Johns Hopkins Hospital, & Children's Medical and Surgical Center. (2012). *The Harriet Lane handbook: A manual for pediatric house officers* (19th ed.). Philadelphia: Elsevier Mosby.

Wilson, B. A., Shannon, M. T., Shields, K., & Geoff, W. (2011). *Pearson nurse's drug guide 2012.* New York: Pearson.

Internet Resources

- ***Advisory Committee on Immunization Practices (ACIP within CDC)*** www.cdc.gov/vaccines: Provides education for public and healthcare providers, school requirements, vaccine laws.
- ***American Academy of Pediatrics (AAP)*** www.aap.org: Organization of physicians committed to physical, mental, and social health for all infants, children, adolescents, and young adults.
- ***Medicaid*** www.medicaid.gov: A state-administered health insurance program of joint federal and state responsibility, available to low-income individuals and families who fit into an eligibility group. Payments are sent directly to healthcare providers.

CHAPTER 21

MANAGEMENT AND LEADERSHIP

Mary Jo Gilmer, PhD, MBA, RN-BC, FAAN

Pediatric nurses may be in management roles or be managed by other nurses. Each pediatric nurse has an opportunity to be a leader—at the individual unit or hospital, or at the community or national level, advocating for children and their families, pediatric health care and policy, and pediatric nursing.

PRINCIPLES OF MANAGEMENT

- Leadership styles
  - Autocratic
    - Power lies with leader
    - Leader makes decision and informs group
      - Group without options
  - Democratic
    - Group comes to decision
    - Leader facilitates group member involvement and decision-making
  - Laissez-faire
    - Leader does not direct group
    - Group may not be functional without leader
    - Work may not be accomplished

- Reactionary
  - Leader is not change-directed
  - Leader deals with situations after problems occur
- Transformational
  - Leader empowers members to create change by creating a shared vision
  - Driving forces are organizational goals

- Principles of effective leadership
  - Model expected behavior.
  - Inspire a vision for improvement.
  - Challenge the process at all levels.
    - Encourage thinking outside the box.
    - Don't accept current thinking or processes as the only way.
  - Enable others.
  - Current change processes may confine those with great ideas.
  - Encourage those you manage.
    - Get to know their professional goals and personal drives.
- Change theories
  - Transtheoretical model
    - Precontemplation
      - Denial and blaming common
      - Feel change is not needed
    - Contemplation
      - Need for change recognized
      - Fear, anxiety, and ambivalence about actual change
    - Preparation
      - Planning for change
      - Exploration of options
        - Process of change
        - What change is actually necessary, needed, or wanted
    - Action
      - Actual change occurs; may affect several areas
        - Behavior and attitudes
        - Structure and personnel
        - Process and work flow

      - Endpoint and measures of success
    - Maintenance
      - Change is continued.
      - Change is not a linear process.
      - Individuals cycle up and down through the stages of change.
    - Terminal stage
      - Previous behavior no longer desirable
      - Persons see new behavior, process, and endpoint as normal
  - Organizational change
    - Barriers to change
      - Personnel
        - Seen as opposite of own interest
        - Assumptions and inaccuracies about effect of change
        - Do not value the proposed change
        - Change seen as unnecessary
        - Work stress does not leave energy for change
      - Systems
        - Stable systems are resistant to change
    - Forces promoting change
      - Personnel
        - Agree with need for change
        - Generation of, or agreement with, idea for the change
        - Change reduces workload
        - Idols and peers agree with change
      - Systems
        - Change decreases work
        - Pilot project of change with open evaluation of process and outcomes
        - Change implemented with enthusiasm by leadership team
- Conflict resolution
  - Goals
    - Resolution of dispute while meeting the needs of all parties
    - Satisfaction through compromise rather than concession
  - Methods of conflict resolution
    - Active listening

        - Reflecting, restating, summarizing
    - Mediation
        - Third-party involvement in negotiation, with goal of compromise that is agreeable to both parties
    - Arbitration
        - Third-party involvement as decision maker. Both parties may be legally bound by the decision of arbitrator.
    - Litigation
- Strategies for conflict resolution
    - Accomodation
        - Passive way of resolving conflict by providing false reassurance instead of dealing with the issues
    - Collaboration
        - Both parties work together to find a mutually satisfying solution
    - Competition
        - Use of power to force resolution
    - Smoothing
        - Compliments opponent, downplays differences, focuses on minor areas of agreement

- Supervision and delegation
    - Nurses may be in the situation of supervising or delegating tasks to licensed or unlicensed personnel.
    - Stay within the state's nurse practice act
        - Nurse responsible for knowing which nursing tasks may be delegated
    - Supervision and training of new nurses and new employees
        - Education on policies and procedures
        - Task-oriented with new nurses
        - Progression from direct supervision to resource for questions
        - Promotion of critical thinking skills
            - Case-based scenarios to promote critical thinking
            - Case studies and simulations

ORGANIZATIONAL STRUCTURE

- Mission statement
    - Written documentation of the purpose of the organization
        - Range from one sentence to multipage documents
        - Includes "Who, What, Why, and How" the purpose will be accomplished
    - Should be the driving force of the organization
        - Goals
        - Commitments
        - Values
- Institutional policy
    - Employee management
        - Illness and vacation
        - Hiring and firing
        - Counseling and disciplinary action
    - Patient care policies and procedure guidelines
        - Frequency of vital signs during administration of blood products
        - Care of a central line
        - Obtaining blood cultures
    - Standards of care
        - Family-centered care model
        - Asthma care model
        - Pathway for care of a child with community-acquired pneumonia
- Chain of command
    - Accessible document that delineates the chain of command within an organization
    - Appropriate pathway of escalation for problems or concerns
        - Escalation stops when satisfactory answer obtained
        - Sample issues
            - Nurse feels patient assignment is inappropriate or unsafe
            - Nurse feels harassed by another employee
            - Nurse feels disciplined unjustly
    - Example for a bedside nurse
        - Self-charge nurse to shift supervisor or head nurse to nursing department director to nursing division director to chief nursing officer
        - If still unsatisfied, nurse may escalate outside of workplace to state nurses' organization

PROFESSIONAL DEVELOPMENT

- Employer requirements
  - Yearly requirements
    - Health and safety
      - Fire safety
      - Tuberculosis skin testing
      - Equipment operations and functioning
      - Security of patient information
      - Disaster awareness
    - Ability to practice
    - Evaluations
      - Peers
      - Supervisors
      - Assessment for presence of complaints
- Self-development
  - Up-to-date licensure
  - Continuing education programs
    - Conferences
    - Self-study programs
    - Development and presentation of programs
  - Certifications
    - Basic life support
    - Specialty certifications
    - Pediatric Advanced Life Support (PALS)
  - Professional organizations
    - Membership
    - Involvement
      - Committee work
      - Task forces
      - Office holder

REFERENCES

Ball, J. W., Bindler, R. C., & Cowen, K. J. (2010). *Child health nursing: Partnering with children & families* (2nd ed.). East Rutherford, NJ: Pearson.

Hagan, J. F., Shaw, J. S., & Duncan, P. M. (Eds.). (2007). *Bright futures: Guidelines for health supervision of infants, children, and adolescents* (3rd ed.). Elk Grove Village, IL: American Academy of Pediatrics.

Joint Commission, The. (2010). *Meeting the Joint Commission's 2011 national patient safety goals*. Oakbrook Terrace, IL: Joint Commission Resources.

Marquis, B. L., & Huston, C. J. (2011). *Leadership roles and management functions in nursing: Theory and application* (7th ed.). Philadelphia: Lippincott Williams & Wilkins.

Pillitteri, A. (2009). *Maternal & child health nursing: Care of the childbearing & childrearing family* (6th ed.). Philadelphia: Lippincott Williams & Wilkins.

Polit, D. F., & Beck, C. T. (2009). *Essentials of nursing research: Appraising evidence for nursing practice* (7th ed.). Philadelphia: Lippincott Williams & Wilkins.

Stuart, G. W. (2009). *Principles and practice of psychiatric nursing* (9th ed.). St. Louis, MO: Mosby/Elsevier.

CHAPTER 22

RESEARCH

Mary Jo Gilmer, PhD, MBA, RN-BC, FAAN

STEPS OF THE RESEARCH PROCESS

- Identify a problem that can be studied.
- Review the literature.
- Define the theoretical framework.
- Ask the research question or formulate the hypothesis.
- Design the study.
    - Identify the population, sample, variables, and methods of measurement.
    - Build in appropriate controls to minimize bias.
- Get institutional review board (IRB) approval.
- Conduct the study.
- Collect data.
- Design the database and enter data.
- Analyze and interpret the data.
- Disseminate findings.

USE OF RESEARCH IN PRACTICE

- There is a delay of 17 years before new knowledge is used in practice (Clancy, 2003).
- Only 60% of American patients with chronic diseases receive recommended care (Schuster et al., 1998).

EVIDENCE-BASED PRACTICE

Evidence-based practice (EBP) is more than applied science. It is nursing practice that is based on research findings, the consensus of experts, available resources, and patient preference to optimize patient outcomes. It deemphasizes opinion, unsystematic clinical experience, intuition, and traditional practice. The randomized controlled trial (RCT) design is the most valid type of evidence.

- Why EBP now?
  - Growth of information
  - Delay in implementing new knowledge
  - Decline in knowledge of best care
  - Sophisticated consumer pressure
- Steps of EBP
  - Identify an EBP question.
  - Search for evidence.
  - Critically evaluate the evidence.
  - Develop recommendations for practice.
  - Integrate the evidence into practice.
  - Measure outcomes to evaluate the effectiveness or improved patient outcomes.

CLINICAL PRACTICE GUIDELINES

Clinical practice guidelines define standards of care and help in decision-making about specific diseases. They are based on clinical evidence and expert consensus.

- A *clinical pathway* is a method for managing a defined group of patients in a period of time. A clinical pathway explicitly states the goals and key elements of care based on evidence-based medicine (EBM) guidelines, best practice, and patient expectations.
- *Knowledge translation* is the use of research findings in clinical practice. It is a nonlinear process that involves not only research findings but also new knowledge that is created from the dynamic interaction of the people and groups who come together to solve health problems. Knowledge translation methods include clinical pathways, audit and feedback, academic detailing, reminders, and local opinion leaders. These initiatives are instituted at the level of a particular hospital or agency with respect to a certain condition.
- *Best practice in nursing* is today's popular phrase that refers to the use of interventions and techniques that are based on research and known to promote a higher quality of care. It is a generic phrase that isn't equivalent to EBP, which is a more rigorous concept. With the explosion of valuable practice-related research and reports, the astute nurse keeps abreast of current recommendations for the highest quality care of patients and families.

REFERENCES

Hagan, J. F., Shaw, J. S., & Duncan, P. M. (Eds.). (2007). *Bright futures: Guidelines for health supervision of infants, children, and adolescents* (3rd ed.). Elk Grove Village, IL: American Academy of Pediatrics.

Joint Commission, the. (2010). *Meeting the Joint Commission's 2011 national patient safety goals*. Oakbrook Terrace, IL: Joint Commission Resources.

Marquis, B. L., & Huston, C. J. (2011). *Leadership roles and management functions in nursing: Theory and application* (7th ed.). Philadelphia: Lippincott Williams & Wilkins.

National Association of Pediatric Nurse Practitioners, Society of Pediatric Nurses, & American Nurses Association. (2008). *Pediatric nursing: Scope and standards of practice*. Silver Spring, MD: American Nurses Association.

Pillitteri, A. (2009). *Maternal & child health nursing: Care of the childbearing & childrearing family* (6th ed.). Philadelphia: Lippincott Williams & Wilkins.

Polit, D. F., & Beck, C. T. (2009). *Essentials of nursing research: Appraising evidence for nursing practice* (7th ed.). Philadelphia: Lippincott Williams & Wilkins.

CHAPTER 23

LEGAL AND ETHICAL ISSUES

Mary Jo Gilmer, PhD, MBA, RN-BC, FAAN, and
Karen Corlett, MSN, RN-BC, CPNP-AC/PC, PNP-BC

Legal definitions vary by state law. This chapter is intended not to delineate laws, but as a reference for concepts related to legal questions and ethical dilemmas.

GUIDELINES FOR THE PRACTICE AND DELIVERY OF HEALTH CARE

- Federal requirements
  - Medicaid and Medicare requirements
    - Definitions of appropriate care, treatment, billing
  - Health Insurance Portability and Accountability Act (HIPAA)
    - Privacy of patient information
  - Emergency access to care without regard to race, gender, or ability to pay
- Regulatory requirements
  - Federal, state, or local guidelines or statutes, such as
    - The Joint Commission (formerly JCAHO)
      - Implements and evaluates practices for the improvement of patient safety
      - Provides accreditation to hospitals that meet criteria
        - Marker of safe practices
        - Accreditation necessary for Medicare reimbursement

        - Clinical Laboratory Improvement Amendments (CLIA)
            - Describe safe and appropriate laboratory policies
            - Provide certification for compliant clinical laboratories
        - Centers for Disease Control and Prevention
            - Requirements and regulations for reporting and tracking of contagious diseases
            - State health departments may have stricter or looser reporting criteria

- Professional nursing practice
    - Term "registered nurse" protected as to definition and use
    - Licensure
        - State-by-state regulation of the registered nurse
        - Grants permission to practice the profession of nursing within the state
        - Regulatory board charged with ensuring a minimum level of safety to the public
        - Many states part of a "compact" to improve portability of nurses from state to state without undergoing relicensing procedures
            - Each state in the compact accepts the nursing licensure of other states within the compact
    - Certification
        - National recognition of expertise within a particular specialty by a certifying body
            - Requirements for acquisition of certification
            - Requirements for maintenance of professional certification
        - Recognition of excellence, but not authority to practice
    - Nurse Practice Acts
        - State definition of the legal aspects of the practice of nursing within that state
        - It is the nurse's responsibility to read, understand, and stay within his or her state nurse practice act.
        - Violation of nurse practice acts can result in disciplinary action.
    - Standards of practice
        - National Association of Pediatric Nurse Practitioners (NAPNAP), Society of Pediatric Nurses (SPN), and American Nurses Association (ANA), *Pediatric Nursing: Scope and Standards of Practice* (2008)
        - Sixteen standards describing the process and responsibilities for both generalist and advanced practice nurses who care for pediatric patients and their families. The standards and scope include
            - Clinical components of the nursing process

  - Evaluation of nursing process and professional practice
  - Quality
  - Education and research
  - Leadership
  - Teamwork and communication
  - Advocacy
- Standards of Professional Performance for the Pediatric Nurse
  - Systematically evaluates the quality and effectiveness of pediatric nursing practice
  - Evaluates her or his own nursing practice in relation to professional practice standards and relevant statutes and regulations
  - Acquires and maintains current knowledge in pediatric nursing practice
  - Contributes to the professional development of peers, colleagues, and others
  - Makes decisions and takes actions on behalf of children and their families that are determined in an ethical manner
  - Collaborates with the child, family, and healthcare providers in providing patient care
  - Uses research findings in practice
  - Considers factors related to safety, effectiveness, and cost in planning and delivering care
- Other international, national, specialty organization, institutional, or practice-related guidelines for practice such as
  - American Nurses Association *Code of Ethics for Nurses with Interpretative Statements*: guidelines for ethical practice
  - CDC Guidelines for Immunization Practices
  - Society of Pediatric Nurses statement on Safe Staffing Practices
  - Institutional policies such as frequency of vital signs during administration of blood products
  - Unit policies such as placement of patients on cardio-respiratory monitoring devices

REIMBURSEMENT

- Most registered nurses do not bill directly for their services
- Anyone involved in billing is responsible for awareness of the billing process and mandatory reporting of unlawful practices
    - How the charge is generated
    - How the bill is prepared
    - Who is billed for the care
    - Where the money is distributed once received
    - HIPAA protection throughout the billing process
- Medicaid and Medicare as the gold standard for billing requirements
    - Documentation of care
        - Adequate for fee charged
    - Appropriate level of care billed for
        - Underbilling and overbilling both illegal
        - Cannot "unbundle" care
            - For example, cardiac surgeon must charge to repair Tetralogy of Fallot rather than billing for VSD closure and repair of pulmonary stenosis
        - Cannot "double dip"
            - If employed by department of nursing, cost of nursing care is typically rolled into the daily room charge; a nurse cannot also submit a separate bill for a dressing change
            - Those employed by another entity may be able to bill for procedures, care, or consultation

AUTHORITY FOR DECISION-MAKING

- Adults have authority for their own medical decision-making
    - Definition of "adult" varies by state and by situation
        - Reaching age definition of legal adult (18 years)
        - A minor who is legally married, has joined the military, lives on his or her own and is financially self-supporting, or has given birth may be considered an adult by legal definitions (emancipated)
    - Incapacitated adults (illness, injury, or incompetence)
        - Next of kin or delineated medical decision-maker to give authorization for health care
- Those not of legal age or emancipated must have consent of a parent or guardian to receive health care

- Physical custody of child does not imply legal custody
  - Many complex situations
    - Divorce
    - Remarriage
    - In-process adoptions
    - Incapacitated or injured parents or guardians
    - Children in protective custody
  - Consult legal counsel for assistance if any question
- Special situations where minor children *may* have ability to receive care without parental consent (state by state definitions for emancipation)
  - Pregnancy care or prevention
  - Testing and treatment for sexually transmitted infections
  - Treatment for drug or alcohol use or abuse
  - Suspected or substantiated abuse or neglect of a minor child
  - Emergent situation in which two physicians agree delay of care would adversely affect child

▶ Informed consent

- Responsibility of healthcare provider to inform parent or guardian, or patient, or both of the proposed treatment, risks, benefits, and alternatives in terms they can understand
  - Opportunity for questions and clarifications
  - Parent or guardian can refuse to give consent to some or all of proposed treatments
  - Nurses typically sign as witness to event
    - Role as advocate for patient and family understanding
    - Consult state law for definition of responsibility

▶ Assent of minor children

- Minor agrees to allow procedure
- Age-appropriate explanation of procedure
- May be requirement for assent in pediatric research studies

▶ Limitation of life-saving treatment

- Involve judicial system if medical team believes treatment is beneficial to child and parent or guardian denies it
  - Support for family and child if court intervenes to order treatment

▶ Limitation of care

- Mechanism for advance directive for those classified as legal adults
  - Facilitate discussion with patient, parent, or both for those with chronic illness and known risk of death
  - Age and developmentally appropriate approach to discussion
    - Involve child life for ongoing support and therapies
  - Limitation of resuscitation discussed with parent or guardian

ETHICAL DILEMMAS

- Patient care situation with no clear-cut correct answer
- Typically is difference of opinion on appropriate care
  - Difference can be between
    - Providers
    - Parents
    - Parents and providers
    - Hospital or agency and providers or parents
    - Insurance coverage and any of the above
- Principles of ethical decision-making
  - Respect for autonomy
    - The ability of persons to make their own decisions in a manner appropriate for themselves
    - Respect of each individual's own decision
  - Beneficence
    - Helping others is primary motivator
  - Nonmaleficence
    - Avoidance of harm is driving force
  - Justice
    - Allocation of resources
    - Respect of rights
    - Respect of morals
    - Respect of beliefs
- Ethical theories
  - Deontology
    - An ethical position that judges the morality of an action based on rules or principles

        - Rules and principles guide decision-making
        - Concepts of right and wrong
        - Consequences not the major decision-driver
    - Teleology
        - Outcome as most important event
        - Outcome justifies the means
    - Virtue
        - Intent is the most important concept
        - Outcome is trumped by the intent of the decision-maker
    - Care
        - The wishes or assumed wishes of the patient are of utmost concern.
    - Utilitarianism
        - The good of society is of utmost concern.
        - The benefit of the outcome is compared to the relative cost of the action.
            - Cost can be defined as monetary, pain, suffering, risk to others, energy expenditure, etc.

NURSING RESPONSIBILITIES

- Explore own ethical viewpoint
- Professional relationship with patient and family
    - ANA statement
- Support of patient and family during ethical discussions
- Escalating ethical dilemmas through appropriate channels
    - Hospital ethics committees
    - Legal counsel

REFERENCES

Ball, J. W., Bindler, R. C., & Cowen, K. J. (2010). *Child health nursing: Partnering with children & families* (2nd ed.). East Rutherford, NJ: Pearson.

Bowden, V. R., & Greenberg, C. S. (2009). *Children and their families: The continuum of care* (2nd ed).: Text and study guide package. Philadelphia: Lippincott Williams & Wilkins.

Hockenberry, M. J., & Wilson, D. (2011). *Wong's nursing care of infants and children* (9th ed.). St. Louis, MO: Elsevier/Mosby.

Joint Commission, The. (2010). *Meeting the Joint Commission's 2011 national patient safety goals.* Oakbrook Terrace, IL: Joint Commission Resources.

Jonsen, A. R., Siegler, M., & Winslade, W. J. (2010). *Clinical ethics: A practical approach to ethical decisions in clinical medicine* (7th ed.). New York: McGraw-Hill Medical.

Marquis, B. L., & Huston, C. J. (2011). *Leadership roles and management functions in nursing: Theory and application* (7th ed.). Philadelphia: Lippincott Williams & Wilkins.

National Association of Pediatric Nurse Practitioners, Society of Pediatric Nurses, & American Nurses Association. (2008). *Pediatric nursing: Scope and standards of practice.* Silver Spring, MD: American Nurses Association.

Polit, D. F., & Beck, C. T. (2009). *Essentials of nursing research: Appraising evidence for nursing practice* (7th ed.). Philadelphia: Lippincott Williams & Wilkins.

APPENDIX A

REVIEW QUESTIONS

1. A 7-year-old child was recently hospitalized with a respiratory infection and has special needs related to her autism. She lives with her mother, two sisters, and grandmother. Which of the following describes the family's composition?

   a. Blended family
   b. Nuclear family
   c. Same-gender family
   d. Extended family

2. When conducting an initial assessment of a 5-year-old child, which of the following would be the best approach for the nurse to take?

   a. Ask the child if she is allergic to anything
   b. Request the child's mother step out of the room
   c. Ask the child's mother what approach would work best
   d. Ask the child's grandmother to explain the child's behaviors

3. An infant weighed 2.90 kg at birth. Now, at her 6-month well-child checkup, she weighs 12.75 lbs. How would you describe her weight gain?

   a. Normal for age
   b. Small for age
   c. Large for age
   d. Excessive for age

4. Parents of a 4-month-old infant bring their blue and nonbreathing baby to the emergency room where she is diagnosed with sudden infant death syndrome. Which of the following is most appropriate to say to the parents?

   a. Do you know how to do CPR?
   b. Tell me more about how you found her.
   c. Why did you put the pillow in bed with her?
   d. What did you do after you put her in bed for the evening?

5. The father of a 2½-year-old toddler tells the nurse he is frustrated by the child's temper tantrums and that the child says "No" to every question. Although the father realizes this is common behavior among toddlers, he doesn't understand the etiology of the behavior. The nurse explains that toddlers act this way as a normal expression of their desire to:

   a. Increase their independence
   b. Gratify oral fixation
   c. Develop a sense of trust
   d. Assert how industrious they are

6. Parents of an 18-month old toddler are worried about their child's behaviors and propensity to have accidents and get hurt. Which of the following recommendations should the nurse make to this parent?

    a. Allow your child to learn by trial and error.

    b. Reward your child's good behaviors, and ignore the bad behaviors.

    c. Punish your child when he does something wrong.

    d. Consistently enforce well-defined limits, such as no playing on the stairs.

7. An infant with retinoblastoma will exhibit which of the following?

    a. Absent red reflex

    b. Eyes that gaze in one direction

    c. Inability to visually track an object

    d. Nystagmus

8. Which visual disorder is characterized by an abnormal growth of blood vessels, resulting in their death and formation of scar tissue?

    a. Amblyopia

    b. Cerebral visual impairment

    c. Optic nerve hypoplasia

    d. Retinopathy of prematurity

9. A mother calls the clinic because she suspects that her baby has otitis media. The baby has been pulling at her ear and crying all morning, but has recently relaxed and is not longer crying. The nurse offers which advice?

    a. "Call back if she starts crying again."

    b. "Don't worry. It sounds like she's fine now."

    c. "Give her Tylenol and call tomorrow if she's not better."

    d. "Her eardrum may have torn. Bring her in today."

10. A 2-year-old arrives at the emergency department with a sore throat, fever of 104° (40° C) F, extreme agitation, and profuse drooling. What should the nurse do first?

    a. Alert the ED physician

    b. Call the child life specialist to help calm the child

    c. Examine the child's throat using a tongue blade for clear visualization

    d. Start an intravenous line

11. Which study provides a definitive diagnosis of cystic fibrosis?

   a. Chest radiography
   b. Pulmonary function test
   c. Sputum culture
   d. Sweat chloride test

12. Research has identified which of the following as a protective factor against sudden infant death syndrome?

   a. Avoidance of pacifier at bedtime
   b. Breastfeeding
   c. Consistent use of video monitoring device
   d. Well-supported side-sleeping position

13. A group of parents whose children attend a local daycare center are receiving nutritional guidance from a pediatric nurse. The nurse should recommend which of the follow ways to encourage good nutritional habits for preschool children?

   a. Offer snacks 1 hour after a meal if the child does not like or eat what is being served.
   b. Allow children to eat only what they want.
   c. Insist children eat all of the food on their plates.
   d. Serve nutritious foods that all family members will eat.

14. Parents of a preschooler are worried that their child has difficulty going to sleep at night. Which of the following is a strategy that should be used to help in the situation?

   a. Allow the child to fall asleep in the parents' room.
   b. Have an established routine for winding down before bedtime.
   c. Have one parent lie down with the child until she or he falls asleep.
   d. Insist the child take a longer nap to make up for lost nighttime sleep.

15. Accidents are a major cause of health concerns in the preschooler. Which of the following comments made by the parent of a preschooler shows understanding of the need to be alert for potential injuries and accidents?

   a. "Now that my daughter doesn't put everything in her mouth, I no longer have to keep locks on all my cleaning supplies."
   b. "I have the phone number of the Poison Control Center programmed into my phone."
   c. "My daughter needs to wear a helmet when she rides her bike in the street, but not in the backyard."
   d. "After my daughter's sixth birthday, she can sit beside me in the front seat of the car."

16. Which of the following activities demonstrates Erikson's developmental task for the school-age child?

    a. The child is learning who can be trusted.
    b. The child depends on older siblings to tell him how to complete his homework.
    c. The child is focused on a chosen profession when her education is completed.
    d. The child likes to engage in tasks that can be carried through to completion.

17. Typical adolescents engage in risky behaviors related to the developmental stage when:

    a. They cannot think logically.
    b. They see themselves as invincible.
    c. They have no understanding of the rules.
    d. They cannot concentrate for long periods of time.

18. The mother of a 3-month-old infant asks a nurse at the well-child clinic when solid foods can be added to the baby's diet. Which of the following is the most appropriate response?

    a. It's OK to feed cereal to your baby now if he seems hungry after your breast milk.
    b. Babies should only have breast milk until they are 12 months old.
    c. As long as you space introduction of solid foods by at least 5 days, you may begin to give pureed vegetables and fruits now.
    d. You may feed your baby rice cereal at 4–6 months.

19. Which medication should a parent use when her asthmatic child starts to wheeze during a soccer game?

    a. Albuterol
    b. Budesonide (Pulmicort)
    c. Epinephrine
    d. Ipratropium bromide (Atrovent)

20. Nursing care of the child with nephrotic syndrome includes regular urine dipstick monitoring for:

    a. Blood
    b. Glucose
    c. Ketones
    d. Protein

21. Which diagnostic study would provide the most specific information about possible vesicoureteral reflux?

- **a.** Renal biopsy
- **b.** Serum creatinine
- **c.** Urine culture and sensitivity
- **d.** Voiding cystourethrogram

22. After the birth of a son with hypospadias, parents need to know that this condition:

- **a.** Can be prevented in the future by earlier prenatal care
- **b.** Is easily correctable with one simple surgical procedure
- **c.** May require a temporary urinary catheter after repair
- **d.** Requires prompt circumcision to prevent urinary tract infection

23. Which nursing intervention is the highest priority when caring for an infant awaiting surgery for Wilms tumor?

- **a.** Meticulous skin care for edema that characterizes this condition
- **b.** Posting a sign on the crib stating "no abdominal palpation"
- **c.** Scheduled administration of morphine for this painful tumor
- **d.** Strict adherence to protective infection prevention precautions

24. A 16-year-old girl complains of labial tingling, itching, and burning. Physical examination reveals redness, but no visible lesion. This presentation is most indicative of which sexually transmitted infection?

- **a.** Chlamydia
- **b.** Genital herpes
- **c.** Human papillomavirus
- **d.** Syphilis

25. A 5-year-old child has been involved in a motor vehicle accident and is now hospitalized in skeletal traction for a fractured femur. Which of the following activities would be developmentally appropriate to assist with the child's growth?

- **a.** Putting together a 100-piece jigsaw puzzle
- **b.** Watching TV
- **c.** Playing with puppets
- **d.** Stacking blocks to build towers

26. A nurse is asked to administer an oral medication to a child with a feeding tube. Proper administration includes

- **a.** Pushing very slowly on the plunger of the administration syringe to gently administer the medication through the tube
- **b.** Flushing the tubing with normal saline before and after administration of the medication
- **c.** Checking tube placement, and then administering medication by gravity flow, flushing adequately
- **d.** Dissolving tablet in a premeasured amount of fluid, measuring into a syringe, and giving slowly into the side of the mouth to prevent clogging of the feeding tube

27. When administering an IM injection to an 11-month-old infant, which is the most appropriate site?

- **a.** Dorsogluteal
- **b.** Deltoid
- **c.** Vastus lateralis
- **d.** Ventrogluteal

28. A 5-year-old child received thermal burns during a house fire. She is scheduled for a dressing change that will produce moderate pain. Which of the following interventions should the nurse perform?

- **a.** Administer pain medication prior to the procedure.
- **b.** Tell the child she can play video games during and for 1 hour after the dressing change if she remains still during the procedure.
- **c.** Tell the child pain medication is available if she needs it during the procedure.
- **d.** Inform the child that her mother can stay with her if she doesn't cry during the dressing change.

29. A school-age child is hospitalized with a life-limiting condition that has progressed to a terminal state. Which of the following interventions is most appropriate for the nurse caring for the child?

- **a.** Reassure the child everything will be OK.
- **b.** Tell the child that having the condition and being in the hospital is not a punishment for any thoughts or actions.
- **c.** Provide information about the child's condition, medications, and procedures.
- **d.** Perform all care for the child and let her rest.

30. A 6-year-old child fell at the playground at school and is being treated in the emergency room for a head contusion. Nursing history shows the child lives at home with her mother, who is a single parent. The discharge instructions include waking the child every hour during the night to assess her for further head injury. In which of the following situations should the nurse intervene to prevent discharge?

- **a.** The nurse smells alcohol on the mother's breath.
- **b.** The child states her head hurts and she just wants to go home.
- **c.** The mother verbalizes fear about taking the child home.
- **d.** The mother doesn't have insurance or resources for a follow-up visit.

31. Which of these lab results indicates type 1 diabetes?

- **a.** Glycated hemoglobin (A1C) of 6.0%
- **b.** Fasting glucose level of 130 mg/dL
- **c.** Random glucose level of 180 mg/dL
- **d.** Two-hour oral 75g glucose tolerance test of 160 mg/dL

32. The nurse notices a line of dark, thick, velvety skin along the back neck crease of an adolescent boy. This finding is often present with which condition?

- **a.** Diabetes insipidus
- **b.** Hyperthyroidism
- **c.** Type 1 diabetes
- **d.** Type 2 diabetes

33. The child with cystic fibrosis is at risk for developing which endocrine disorder?

- **a.** Central diabetes insipidus
- **b.** Growth hormone deficiency
- **c.** Type 1 diabetes
- **d.** Type 2 diabetes

34. In planning education for the family of a child treated with synthetic growth hormone, the nurse needs to include:

- **a.** Common side effects such as abdominal pain, diarrhea, nausea, and vomiting
- **b.** Injection technique for daily administration
- **c.** Monthly monitoring of growth measurements
- **d.** Return appointment schedule for monthly intravenous administration

35. A child presents at the endocrinology clinic with sore throat, high fever, and severe leukopenia. Which medication is responsible?

   a. Desmopressin acetate
   b. Levothyroxine
   c. Propylthiouracil
   d. Thyroid stimulating immunoglobulin

36. Lymph node biopsy reveals presence of Reed-Sternberg cells, abnormal B lymphocytes, in which disorder?

   a. Hemophilia
   b. Hodgkin's disease
   c. Idiopathic thrombocytopenia
   d. Sickle cell disease

37. A nurse is confronted with an ethical dilemma. Which of the following documents will probably be most beneficial in helping resolve the concern?

   a. ANA Code of Ethics
   b. Health Insurance Portability and Accountability Act (HIPAA)
   c. Patient Care Partnership
   d. The Joint Commission

38. A nurse from the Adult Medical Unit has been asked to work on the Pediatric Unit today. Which of the following patients should the pediatric charge nurse assign to the float nurse?

   a. A toddler admitted last night who has epiglottitis
   b. A preschooler who had surgical fixation yesterday of a fractured humerus
   c. A preschooler scheduled for excision of a Wilm's tumor tomorrow
   d. An infant returning from surgical repair of a cleft lip and palate

39. During a staff meeting, a nurse manager identifies a conflict between the staff members of different shifts about restocking supplies. When the manager says "Let's all try harder to be nicer to each other by stocking as we go," which resolution strategy is the manager using?

   a. Accommodation
   b. Collaboration
   c. Competition
   d. Smoothing

40. A 7-year-old with suspected peanut allergy experiences stridor and dyspnea after eating a cookie at a neighbor's home. His father should administer which medication?

- **a.** Albuterol
- **b.** Diphenhydramine (Benadryl)
- **c.** Epinephrine
- **d.** Prednisolone (Orapred)

41. The mother of a 10-year-old complains that her daughter "zones out frequently and just seems to be daydreaming." She denies any concurrent movement changes or loss of consciousness. This behavior may be indicative of which type of seizure?

- **a.** Absence seizures
- **b.** Complex partial seizures
- **c.** Myoclonic seizures
- **d.** Simple partial seizures

42. Which diagnostic study is performed periodically to monitor potential medication side effects in children with juvenile idiopathic arthritis (JIA)?

- **a.** Antinuclear antibodies
- **b.** Liver enzymes
- **c.** Rheumatoid factor
- **d.** White blood cells

43. A 14-year-old boy is being discharged from the hospital after treatment for slipped capital femoral epiphysis (SCFE). The nurse should include information about which of the following?

- **a.** Complete bed rest for 1 week
- **b.** Restricted weight bearing for 6 months
- **c.** Return to sports when incision is healed
- **d.** Sports restrictions for at least 3 months

APPENDIX B

ANSWERS TO THE REVIEW QUESTIONS

1. **Correct Answer: D.** An extended family includes one or both parents, one or more children, and other family members such as a grandparent. A blended family includes at least one stepparent, step-sibling, or half-sibling. A same-sex family includes two parents of the same gender, who may or may not have children. A nuclear family includes two parents and their children.

2. **Correct Answer: C.** Parents are generally the best resource for help in understanding their child's needs and behaviors.

3. **Correct Answer: A.** Infants typically double their birth weight at 6 months.

4. **Correct Answer: B.** This is an open-ended request to gain more information about the circumstances. The other options are all judgmental.

5. **Correct Answer: A.** Toddlers are in the developmental stage of autonomy versus shame and doubt. When they say "No," they are asserting their autonomy or independence. An infant is in Erikson's stage of trust versus mistrust and Piaget's stage of autonomy versus shame and doubt. Completing a project is part of the school-age child's developmental need for industry versus inferiority.

6. **Correct Answer: D.** While toddlers are curious and often try to extend their limits, those in authority need to be consistent in defining boundaries to limit injuries. Allowing them to learn by trial and error or ignoring their bad behavior may lead to catastrophes, and punishing them for something they don't understand is unduly harsh.

7. **Correct answer: A.** The red reflex in a child with retinoblastoma may be absent or have an abnormal appearance.

8. **Correct answer: D.** This process is characteristic of retinopathy of prematurity.

9. **Correct answer: D.** In otitis media, rupture of tympanic membrane provides release of fluid with relief of pressure and pain.

10. **Correct answer: A.** This presentation indicates epiglottitis, a medical emergency requiring rapid intervention with possible intubation or tracheostomy. Examining the throat or starting an IV could precipitate closure of the airway.

11. **Correct answer: D.** Diagnosis of cystic fibrosis is based on pilocarpine iontophoresis (sweat chloride test) showing chloride level at or above 60 mmol/L.

12. **Correct answer: B.** Research has shown breastfeeding to be a protective factor. Pacifier use and back-only sleeping position are also considered protective.

13. **Correct Answer: D.** Many preschoolers learn by example, and seeing other family members try new foods and eat healthy foods will foster good eating behaviors. Insisting children eat everything on their plates can lead to feelings of guilt and even overindulgence. Serving snacks as alternatives to healthy food at mealtime does not promote healthy habits.

14. **Correct Answer: B.** The child's falling asleep in the his or her own bed is preferred, and it is important for even young children to learn to console themselves without a hovering parent. An established routine is important for children's sense of security and well-being. Extending naps may not necessarily be a good replacement for inability to fall asleep at night.

15. **Correct Answer: B.** Even after the sensorimotor stage is over, preschoolers still may put things in their mouths, and parents need to know appropriate resources in response to poisoning. The safest place for children to sit is in the back seat, and bicycle helmets should be worn whenever a child is on a bicycle or tricycle.

16. **Correct Answer: D.** The school-age child is typically in Erikson's stage of industry versus inferiority. Completing tasks and being successful are important goals of this stage.

17. **Correct Answer: B.** Adolescents use formal operational thought with abstract reasoning and logical thought. Their attention span has increased over that of school-age children, but they tend to take risks as they stretch their limits and think bad things only happen to others.

18. **Correct Answer: D.** Solid foods are not recommended until the infant is at least 4 months, and rice cereal is the food of choice.

19. **Correct answer: A.** Albuterol is a quick-relief, short-acting beta 2–agonist used as first-line treatment. Epinephrine is used for status asthmaticus, and the other two are controller medications.

20. **Correct answer: D.** In nephrotic syndrome, the glomeruli are more permeable to protein. Checking urine protein is used to monitor effectiveness of treatment and possible relapse.

21. **Correct answer: D.** Voiding cystourethrogram (VCUG) will show the degree of urine reflux into the ureters and the presence of structural abnormalities.

22. **Correct answer: C.** A urinary catheter may be used after surgical repair. Hypospadias is not related to timing of prenatal care. Several surgeries may be required, and the foreskin may be used during the repair.

23. **Correct answer: B.** Abdominal palpation may rupture the tumor.

24. **Correct answer: B.** Outbreaks of genital herpes are usually preceded by tingling, itching, and burning followed by appearance of lesions.

25. **Correct answer: C.** Appropriate activities for a 5-year-old in traction are consistent with their magical thinking and developmental needs. A 100-piece jigsaw could be frustrating, and building a tower with blocks is more appropriate for a younger child. Watching TV is passive and unimaginative.

26. **Correct answer: C.** Placement of the feeding tube should be checked before administering medications, and normal saline is not used to flush the meds. They should be given by gravity flow and not forcefully with a plunger. If a feeding tube is in place, meds should not generally be given by mouth.

27. **Correct answer: C.** Until a child has been walking for a year, IM injections should be given in the vastus lateralis.

28. **Correct answer: A.** Medication should be given BEFORE a known painful procedure because less medication may be required to prevent the pain than if medication is held until the child is already experiencing pain. Telling a child it's OK to cry when something is painful allows for honest communication.

29. **Correct answer: C.** Honesty is important in interactions with children, especially at the end of life. Allowing them to live fully until they die is essential to their well-being.

30. **Correct answer: A.** In being an advocate for the child, the nurse needs to ensure the mother is capable of completing hourly monitoring of the child at home. A person who is chemically impaired may not be able to do the hourly assessments. After the fall and associated head contusions, head pain is an expected finding. Education about the hourly assessments and appropriate interventions following the assessments will hopefully help reduce the mother's fears. Lack of insurance should not contraindicate discharge.

31. **Correct answer: B.** A fasting glucose level greater than or equal to 126 mg/dL.

32. **Correct answer: D.** This skin feature, acanthosis nigricans, is often found in children with type 2 diabetes.

33. **Correct answer: C.** With cystic fibrosis, thick secretions may block the pancreatic ducts and lead to progressive fibrosis. As fibrosis continues, the number of islets of Langerhans decreases and eventually limits insulin production.

34. **Correct answer: B.** Synthetic growth hormone is administered by daily injection. Gastrointestinal side effects do not occur, and growth is monitored every 3–6 months.

35. **Correct answer: C.** This reaction requires discontinuing the antithyroid medication propylthiouracil.

36. **Correct answer: B.** Reed-Sternberg cells are present in Hodgkin's disease.

37. **Correct answer: A.** The ANA Code of Ethics was specifically developed to assist nurses with ethical dilemmas, using a set of principles. The other options all have some relationship to ethical nursing care, but not with the same specificity.

38. **Correct answer: B.** The child with a fracture has a condition that is less pediatric-specific than the other options. Care of this child requires the least in-depth understanding of developmental issues.

39. **Correct answer: D.** The definition of smoothing includes interactions where differences are downplayed, and the focus is on minor areas of agreement while accomplishing the task at hand. Accommodation is a very passive way of resolving conflict without dealing with the issue. Collaboration involves both parties working together to find a mutually satisfying solution. Competition involves the use of power to force resolution.

40. **Correct answer: C.** These symptoms indicate systemic allergic reaction, or anaphylaxis. Epinephrine is first-line therapy because of its immediate onset.

41. **Correct answer: A.** Absence seizures, characterized by very brief loss of consciousness with minimal change is muscle tone, are often mistaken for daydreaming.

42. **Correct answer: B.** Liver enzymes are checked to monitor for liver disease, a side effect of medications used for JIA. Elevated antinuclear antibodies and rheumatoid factor are indicative of JIA, and white blood cells are elevated during symptom flares.

43. **Correct answer: D.** Sports restrictions are necessary for 3–6 months, and are not determined by healing of incision. Bedrest is not necessary, but weight bearing is restricted for 6–8 weeks.

INDEX

INDEX

A

B

C

D

E

F

G

H

I

J

K

L

M

N

O

P

R

S

T

U

V

W

Z

ABOUT THE AUTHORS

Mary Jo Gilmer, PhD, MBA, RN-BC, FAAN, currently the Director of Pediatric Palliative Care Research Team at Vanderbilt University, is a graduate of Michigan State University's School of Nursing. She began her career in nursing at Children's Memorial Hospital in Chicago, Illinois while she completed her MSN at the University of Illinois. She worked as a Clinical Specialist in Pediatric Cardiovascular Surgery before receiving a Commonwealth Fund Executive Nurse Fellowship to pursue an MBA at Queens University. Dr. Gilmer earned her PhD in nursing at University of North Carolina -Chapel Hill.

Before coming to Vanderbilt, Dr. Gilmer was on the faculty at Queens University from 1983 to 1998. Throughout her career, she has received numerous awards for her research and teaching expertise: National Co-Alliance for Teaching Excellence Award; Great 100, North Carolina Foundation for Nursing Award; Sigma Theta Research Award; McColl Faculty Research Award; Julia Hereford Teaching Award; and Excellence in Teaching Award from Educational Resources, Inc. She has been a leader in several international healthcare projects, including initiatives in Belize, Uganda, China, Italy, and Ecuador.

Beginning in 2002, Dr. Gilmer's research and practice have focused on enhancing care of children with life-threatening conditions. Her work at Monroe Carell Jr. Children's Hospital at Vanderbilt involved establishing an interdisciplinary team to develop research initiatives, clinical services in palliative care, education and training, and support services in palliative care. Her current research is focused on parent–sibling bereavement after a child dies from cancer and parent–child communication about cancer.

Clara J. Richardson, MSN, RN-BC, is a graduate of DePaul University and Indiana University. Clara has been a pediatric nurse for her entire career. Currently based in Colorado, she is a Clinical Development Professional for Banner Health, responsible for providing pediatric clinical education for Banner's 11 Western Region hospitals. Prior to joining Banner, Clara spent 29 years teaching theory and clinical pediatric nursing at Purdue University.

Clara has been certified as a pediatric nurse by the American Nurses Credentialing Center since 1997. Additional certifications include American Heart Association Basic Life Support Instructor and Pediatric Advanced Life Support Instructor. She is a member of Sigma Theta Tau International, Society of Pediatric Nurses, Association for Nursing Professional Development, and Nurses Christian Fellowship. Clara has authored multiple journal articles and book chapters related to nursing education and child health care.

Review and Resource Manual

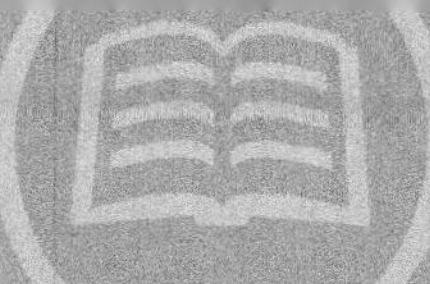

Pediatric Nursing

Addendum to the 3rd Edition

CONTINUING EDUCATION RESOURCE

NURSING CERTIFICATION REVIEW MANUAL

CLINICAL PRACTICE RESOURCE

Mary Jo Gilmer, PhD, MBA, RN-BC, FAAN

NURSING KNOWLEDGE CENTER

The American Nurses Credentialing Center (ANCC), a subsidiary of the American Nurses Association (ANA), provides individuals and organizations throughout the nursing profession with the resources they need to achieve practice excellence. ANCC's internationally renowned credentialing programs certify nurses in specialty practice areas; recognize healthcare organizations for promoting safe, positive work environments through the Magnet Recognition Program® and the Pathway to Excellence® Program; and accredit providers of continuing nursing education. In addition, the ANCC's Institute for Credentialing Innovation provides leading-edge information, education services, and products to support its core credentialing programs.

8515 Georgia Ave., Suite 400
Silver Spring, MD 20910

Contents

Introduction to the *Pediatric Nursing Review & Resource Manual Addendum*

Appropriate nursing management of children and their families continues to progress as understanding of specific needs and goals change. Evolution of their needs and advances in technology affect the practice of pediatric nurses. The Nursing Knowledge Center recognizes the importance of staying abreast of these changes. This addendum includes information from the revised test content outline to ensure the *Pediatric Nursing Review and Resource Manual* is up to date. This revision to the test content outline includes information about use of complementary therapies, patient safety and risk reduction, family-centered care, teaching strategies, and the professional role of the pediatric nurse.

This additional information will assist you with successful completion of the certification exam and may be used as a guideline for your practice. While this addendum highlights these content areas, it is not meant to be all-inclusive. For detailed information, we encourage you to explore the topics, using the pediatric reference list. We hope you will find this content useful as a study guide and a source of information for your practice.

If you have questions about this addendum or the review manual, please send an email to revmanuals@ana.org.

—Mary Jo Gilmer, PhD, MBA, RN-BC, FAAN

I. ASSESSMENT, DIAGNOSIS, PLANNING, AND OUTCOMES

A. COMPLEMENTARY AND ALTERNATIVE HEALTHCARE PRACTICES

Complementary and alternative healthcare practices (CAM) may be used as supplements to medical and nursing care. They are often referred to as complementary therapies when they are used as adjuncts to conventional care and as alternative therapies when they are used in place of conventional care. Recently, the use of CAM has increased in the general population.

Among pediatric populations, CAM interventions such as herbal supplements, acupuncture, coining, cupping, and dietary modifications are reportedly used by 2% to 20%–30% of children. Higher rates have been reported among children with specific medical conditions, such as pediatric cancer, rheumatoid arthritis, epilepsy, and cystic fibrosis, where 30%–70% of patients employ CAM therapies (Emerich, Braeunig, Clement, Ludtke, & Huber, 2014; Gilmour, Harrison, Cohen, & Vohra, 2011; Grossoehme, Cotton & McPhail, 2013; Italia, Wolfenstetter, & Teuner, 2014; Ladas, Lin, Antillion et al., 2014).

Herbal supplements

Herbal therapy may be consumed internally as pills, powders, tinctures, or syrups, and is often brewed into teas. Ointments and shampoos are sometimes applied to the skin, scalp, or mucous membranes. The parts of a plant used for medicinal purposes include flowers, stems, leaves, roots, seeds, and berries. Essential oils give plants their characteristic aromas and are generally classified as volatile oils composed of complex hydrocarbons extracted from plants. Aromatherapy involves inhalation of volatile oils focused on treatment of specific health concerns. Carminatives aid in expelling gas from the gastrointestinal tract. Fixed oils are nonvolatile oils, such as mineral oil or safflower oil, and may be used as carriers for the essential oils. Resins are semisolid substances found in plants and are generally applied topically.

Children respond to herbal supplements quite differently than adults (Perry, Hunt, & Ernst, 2011). The absorption, distribution, metabolism, and excretion of some substances differs significantly from adults. Children have proportionately larger livers than adults and may detoxify herbs more efficiently. However, their central nervous and immune systems are not as well developed as adults'; consequently, children may be more sensitive to adverse effects of herbs. Known cathartics such as senna and aloe and known diuretics such as herbal teas and juniper oil may result in significant dehydration and electrolyte disturbance when used in young children. Another concern is the susceptibility of some children to the adverse effects of herbs. Some plants may provoke allergic manifestations such as contact dermatitis, conjunctivitis, wheezing, photosensitization, or rhinitis.

Long-term consequences of use of herbal therapy include carcinogenicity, toxicity to a fetus, and concerns with lactation and breastfeeding infants. Chemicals in some plants are known carcinogens, but their effects on humans have not been thoroughly investigated. Research continues on possible toxic effects of herbs on the reproductive systems of children. Regulation of herbal products and dietary supplements is limited unless a products has been conclusively shown to be detrimental to health.

Interactions with families should include discussions about parental beliefs regarding CAM, and parents are often reticent to begin that conversation. Along with explanations of conventional therapies, nurses may explore and document parental CAM use. Nurses need to help parents understand that "natural" does not equate with "safe." Herbal therapy may have beneficial results, but may also result in unanticipated toxicity. The best interests of the child need to stay at the forefront of treatment, and clinicians may support parental decisions to use CAM when the risk of harm is low, and potential benefits are backed by scientific evidence (Woolf, 2003).

Acupuncture

An increasingly popular method of managing some symptoms, acupuncture is one of the CAM therapies frequently recommended by family physicians. The use of dry needles has been practiced in China for over 2000 years as a form of bioenergetic healing. Specific acupoints serve as targets in efforts to restore "qi" energy. With children, acupuncture is embraced as a potential treatment for pediatric pain, infant distress, allergies, constipation, enuresis, neurologic disabilities, laryngospasms, and vomiting. More work is needed to establish evidence to support its use as empirically valid for childhood conditions (Gold, Nicolaou, Katz, Benaron, & Yu, 2009). Interestingly, research suggests that children may tolerate use of these needles better than drug therapies, but some pediatric acupuncturists use noninvasive treatments such as low-level electrical stimulation or magnets without penetrating the skin (Golianu, Hey, & Brooks, 2014; Vinson, Yeh, Davis, & Logan, 2014).

Hot stones

Stone massage involves use of water-treated stones placed over specific body parts. Stones are typically basalt or polished and hardened lava stones. Heating takes place in an electric roaster with water. Stones used are generally hot, but cool stones may be used when inflammation exists.

Prior to placing the stones, the muscles may be pretreated. Stones are gradually placed along pressure points and can result in relief very quickly. The stone massage elicits "kundalini" energy, a Sanskrit word often described as the creative potential in man. Stone massage has been used by Native Americans and Europeans as long ago as 1500 B.C.

Some of the stated benefits derived from stone therapy include relaxation, release of toxins, pain reduction, improved circulation, and stress reduction. In addition, the therapy may result in a deep meditation that helps the body to re-energize. These responses have the potential to make this CAM useful in treatment of anxiety, stress, back pain, insomnia, depression, and arthritis. Although effects are not well documented, a recent study (Manikanda & Chandrasehara, 2014) that demonstrated participants in kundalini yoga showed better resting heart rate and blood pressures than the control group.

Cupping

Another CAM used primarily in Russian, Asian, and Mexican cultures is cupping, in which a heated cup is applied to the skin. This treatment has been mistakenly identified as abuse when it causes bruises. Knowledge of the values, beliefs, and practices of various cultures, coupled with a thorough history, may aid in a diagnosis and avoid unfounded accusations of abuse (Hannan, 2014).

Coining

While coining is a CAM used less frequently than other treatments, it is important for nurses to be aware of the practice. Sometimes called *cao gio*, this treatment involves application of ointment to the skin followed by rubbing the skin with a coin or a spoon until petechiae can be seen. This results in a symmetrical pattern of bruises typically on the child's back, shoulders, temples, or forehead. As with cupping, the resulting marks can be mistaken for abuse (Hannan, 2014).

Ketogenic diet

A ketogenic diet is a CAM treatment for children with seizures not responsive to medications. The diet consists of foods with high fat, low carbohydrate, and adequate proteins, and has been shown to be effective in about 50% of children with intractable epilepsy. The mechanism of action is that the diet forces the body to burn fats instead of carbohydrates for energy. When there are few carbohydrates in the diet, the liver converts fat into fatty acids and ketones. The ketones can replace glucose as an energy source. An elevated level of ketones in the blood results in a state of ketosis, which may lead to a reduction in seizures (Freeman, Kossoff, & Hartman, A., 2007).

B. SUPPORT SYSTEMS CONSISTENT WITH PATIENTS' AND GUARDIANS' PREFERENCES

Assessment of beliefs, values, and goals will enable nurses to provide supportive care to children while considering patients' and guardians' preferences and hopes. Families, friends, and experiences contribute to a patient's sense of identity and world views. Nurses working with vulnerable children need to be aware of their own values and beliefs in order to help empower children without imposing their own ideas.

Values

A value is often defined as something considered to be of high worth. It is a principle, a standard, or a quality held in high regard that guides the way people live their lives. Values often influence decisions and judgments and may affect the support nurses provide to children and their families (Wynia, Papadakis, Sullivan, & Hafferty, 2014).

Values are derived from many sources:

- Family
- Education
- Spirituality
- Peers
- Media
- Culture
- Significant life events

Values provide the framework for what individuals perceive as right and wrong. A key responsibility of a pediatric nurse is to refrain from influencing a child or family decision based on the nurse's values. Instead, every effort should be made to support a patient's values.

Beliefs

Beliefs generally are derived from real-life experiences and are an important part of one's identity. Beliefs may be religious, cultural, or moral and reflect the core of a person as he or she lives his or her life. Preexisting beliefs are often related to stereotypes of people's characteristics such as sexual orientation, age, health, and rights. These stereotypes may affect the ways in which nurses interact with patients and may lead to a denial of children's rights, respect, and dignity. For this reason, stereotyping must be avoided for optimal care of children and their families (Helman, 2014).

II. IMPLEMENTATION AND EVALUATION

A. PATIENT SAFETY AND RISK REDUCTION

Patient abduction and elopement

An "abduction" is an unapproved removal of any infant, child, or adolescent from an expected location within the facility. An "elopement" occurs when a child or adolescent intentionally leaves an expected location within the hospital or clinic without informing the healthcare team of intent or destination.

Infants and young children are particularly easy to abduct because of their preverbal development and portability. Adolescents are more likely to elope because of their own unique social and developmental stage.

Pediatric visitors and patients considered to be at a higher risk include

- All infants and young children due to preverbal developmental age and portability,
- Children who are the subject of custody disputes,
- Children who are under surveillance by child protective services,
- Children whose parents are unable to stay during hospitalization,
- Patients who are at risk for suicide, and
- Patients who are involved in the legal system.

Care needs to be taken to

- Secure and monitor all entrances to and exits from child-care areas,
- Allow elevators leaving the area to function only with use of card reader or ID badge, and
- Monitor high-risk patients carefully.

Transfers and transports

Moving ill children within and between healthcare facilities involves inherent risks. Each institution should have a formalized plan for transfers and transports that addresses:

- Identification and training of transport personnel
- Mobile equipment for safety and monitoring during move
- Pre-transport communication and strategies for coordination of move
- Careful documentation

Serious physiologic deterioration may occur during transport of seriously ill children, dependent on severity of illness and duration of transport. Use of hospital policies and procedures and adherence to evidence-based guidelines for safe transport will lead to an organized, efficient process conducive to patient safety.

Falls

Hospitalized or ill children are at high risk for falls. The following factors contribute to the risk:

- Pain medication
- Post-surgery status
- Loss of memory
- Seizure history
- IV tubing
- Changes in vision
- Difficulty hearing
- History of falls

These children may find it difficult to maintain their balance, with subsequent difficulty walking or even just standing. When a child is at risk for falls, special considerations include

- Hanging signs that alert caregivers of the risk,
- Educating children and parents or caregivers to use call lights to ask for help when getting out of bed,
- Placing children on special beds with bed alarms, and
- Educating families about the importance of asking nurses for assistance.

Fall prevention is a team effort that includes the child, family, and the healthcare team! (Jamerson, Graf, Messmer, et al., 2014).

De-escalation

While most children and adolescents proceed through their developmental stages without significant incidents, illness and stress may lead to disruptions that threaten the child's and family's stability, requiring the support of professionals who respond in a professional manner. The most effective care is collaborative care using a team approach that involves the child, family, and an interdisciplinary healthcare team to resolve issues.

The goal of de-escalation is safety, not only for children, but for others in the immediate environment. Multiple factors can contribute to the concern for safety:

- Patient aggression, which may be verbal or physical. While verbal aggression seems to be the safer of the types of aggression, it can lead to physical aggression, which may be aimed at property, self, or others. Suicide and homicide are also possible responses to physical aggression.
- Possible triggers for aggression include youth's family dynamics, mental health factors, developmental delays, attention deficit disorders, oppositional defiant disorders, living arrangements, traumatic experiences, fear, frustration, grief, shame, hurt, sadness, and isolation from peers.
- Responses to the aggression should be nonjudgmental, empathic, and calm; recognize emotional reactions such as anger and embarrassment, and avoid defensive stances.

Possible steps to take:

- Ignore verbal aggression initially
- Stay calm
- Use distraction
- Stay calm
- Start a conversation about something of interest
- Stay calm
- Use humor appropriately
- Stay calm
- Set boundaries and be directive
- Stay calm
- Remove items that could harm self or others
- Stay calm

Restraints

Although there are times when it is necessary to restrain a child for his or her own safety, it is a very stressful strategy for children. Children and adolescents may need to be restrained for disruptive behavior or risk of harm, but the use of restraints requires safe application and use of reassessment guidelines. Restraints should be used only when other methods are not successful. Restraints may be physical or chemical. Use of physical or mechanical devises to minimize movement is called physical restraint, while use of psychotropic drugs, sedatives, or paralytic agents constitutes chemical restraint.

Physical restraints may be cloth, leather, metal, car seats, or seat belts. The Joint Commission describes the use of restraint as a special treatment that requires justification for its use (Niespondiziani & Hepola, 2011). A practitioner's verbal or written order must be obtained for use of restraints, and periodic observations according to the organization's policies should be completed. Typically, policies for the use of physical restraint include

- An explanation to the child, parents, or both of the rationale for use of restraints,
- A verbal or written order describing type of restraint and time period for its use, and
- Assessments according to hospital policies to examine skin integrity and neurovascular status (Brenner, Parahoo, & Taggart, 2007).

III. FAMILY-CENTERED CARE

A. ADVOCATING FOR THE FAMILY

Child advocacy typically includes the efforts of individuals, healthcare professionals, and advocacy groups who promote optimal development and care of children. They may modify a plan of care with a goal of protecting a child's rights, which may have been abridged or abused.

One form of child advocacy gives voice to an individual or group when interests are not being heard. This may involve ensuring that children have access to positive influences or services such as schools, childcare, or constructive parenting. Another type of child advocacy occurs at the policy level and works through lobbying, research, and lawsuits to change governmental policies or even transnational policies.

Individualized plans of care

Plans of care should be developed using evidence-based guidelines with bundled care, clinical pathways, and order sets. Continuity of care across the continuum of care will include the child, family, and the interdisciplinary team, working together to ensure goals are realistic, understandable, measureable, behavioral, and achievable. Work with community resources will assist the child and family toward independence. Technology may be useful as developmentally and medically age-appropriate.

- Use of evidence-based interventions
  - Prevent infection (e.g., chlorhexidine baths, contraindications)
  - Therapeutic holding
  - Oral sucrose
- Risk of potential treatment interactions
  - Food, herbs, and medications
  - Fluid resuscitation and renal failure
- Risk of infection
  - Use of evidence to minimize risk of infections (e.g., chlorhexidine baths)
  - Nosocomial infections (acquired in the hospital or another healthcare agency)
  - Cost of these infections is both money and lives
  - Infection control guidelines established by the CDC
  - Potential routes of infection
    - Contact with a contaminated surface
    - Airborne transmission of an organism through tiny droplets of the infectious agent suspended in the air
    - Contact with blood and other body fluids, including droplets
    - Ingestion of food and water
    - Via animal or insect vectors

B. METHODS AND MODES OF EDUCATION

Teach-back: a method of education used by healthcare providers to confirm that they have explained use of medications, procedures, health promotion, or other healthcare information in a way that the child or family can understand. If the child or family member can, in his or her own words, describe the discussed information to the healthcare provider, the teach-back method has successfully been applied (Parnell, 2015).

SMART Objectives

A well-written objective is

- Specific: includes who, what, when, and how
- Measurable: uses action verbs that can be assessed
- Attainable: includes a goal that can be reached
- Realistic: is within the realm of possibility for the child for whom the objective is written
- Time-bound: has a constrained timeframe

Age and developmentally appropriate techniques

Effective teaching in a healthcare environment involves choosing a strategy to fit a specific situation and considering the developmental level of the child. This list of strategies may be useful, but remaining flexible and vigilant is essential.

- Acknowledge the child and provide positive attention, which may be done through words or mere presence with the child.
- Encourage effort rather than only praising positive results.
- Be specific in providing feedback so improvements can be made.
- Be a great role model in attitudes as well as behaviors.
- Demonstrate the correct way to do a procedure.
- Add one step at a time, so a child can experience success, but is challenged for the next step.
- Ask questions that stimulate thought.
- Provide subtle hints or cues when needed.
- Give direct information and facts.
- Provide specific directions to accomplish a goal.

Adapting for factors that may influence learning

- Sensory impairment: When one sense is compromised, children rely more heavily on other senses.
- Cognitive deficits: Medications or illness may necessitate specifically timed teaching interventions.
- Environment: Remember that a quiet, nondistracting environment is conducive to learning.
- Cultural differences: Consider a child's culture when discussing healthcare issues.

C. TECHNOLOGY

Based on factors such as sensory and cognitive deficits, technology may be useful in providing graphic depictions when words are difficult to understand.

IV. PROFESSIONAL ROLE

A. HEALTHY WORK ENVIRONMENT

Lateral violence and bullying

Lateral violence in nursing refers to acts that occur between or among colleagues; bullying describes acts inflicted by one with a higher level of authority. Some acts are covert while others are overt acts of either verbal or nonverbal aggression (Dellasega, 2009). The ANA (ANA, 2012) reported the following statistics:

- 48% of nurses, pharmacists, and other healthcare professionals reported strong verbal abuse
- 43% of nurses, pharmacists, and other healthcare professionals reported threatening body language
- 53% of student nurses reported being "put down" by a staff nurse

Possible solutions reported in the literature (Yoder-Wise, 2014) include

- Zero tolerance toward violent or abusive behavior,
- Protection from retribution if reported,
- Use of employee assistance program,
- Interruption of the violence, and
- Brainstorm solutions and encourage dialog.

Team-building

Teamwork is a critical element in a healthcare setting. Effective teamwork promotes quality care through a shared vision, positive attitudes, skilled work, and mutual respect. Key characteristics of quality teams are positive attitudes, effective leadership, successful collaboration, and therapeutic communication. Not only do children and families benefit from effective teamwork, but employee satisfaction generally increases and turnover decreases. The following strategies may be helpful in promoting team building:

1. Clearly communicate the mission of the organization.
2. Recognize important contributions to quality care of children and their families.
3. Assist new employees to integrate into the team.
4. Be a compassionate and effective role model.
5. Ask for feedback and listen to staff.

Diversity

The literature shows a strong connection between a culturally diverse nursing workforce and high-quality, culturally competent patient care. The U.S. Census Bureau indicates racial and ethnic minority groups accounted for 37% of the U.S. population in 2012 with predictions that minority populations will exceed 50% of the population by 2043 (U.S. Census Bureau, 2012). Professional nurses need to demonstrate cultural awareness, sensitivity, and competence to provide high-quality care across settings.

B. LEADERSHIP DEVELOPMENT

Roles of the leader (Yoder-Wise, 2014):

- Mentor: a role model and advocate for a mentee's personal and professional development. An effective mentor is available, responsive, professional, and supportive.
- Preceptor: an individual who demonstrates competence and serves as a teacher, leader, facilitator, and role model for students rotating into clinical areas.
- Clinical content expert: an individual with a specific area of clinical expertise. One example is a clinical nurse specialist who is an expert at diagnosing and treating illness in a specific area. Clinical nurse specialists may focus on one of three main specialty areas: patients and their families, nurse management, or administration.
- Change agent: an individual who facilitates change within professional organizations and activities to advance nursing practice. In the current healthcare environment, change is constant. A nurse manager needs strong leadership skills to navigate change without losing sight of the quality of nursing care. A change agent is often referred to as a coach, with skills including inspiration, facilitation, guidance, and support.
- Shared governance: Tim Porter-O'Grady (2009) describes shared governance as a professional practice model founded on partnership, equity, accountability, and ownership that form a culturally sensitive and empowering framework. He posits that the concept of shared governance enables sustainable and accountability-based decisions to support interdisciplinary collaboration and quality patient care .
- Clinical ladders: Planned, coordinated academic programs were developed in the 1960s to help students move up the academic hierarchy in steps. This concept was then applied to nursing so staff nurses learn new skills and gain new knowledge to advance their careers.

Quality improvement

Continuous quality improvement includes the concepts of quality assurance, problem resolution, and improved care. These initiatives are driving changes in the American healthcare system at a rapid pace. The goals mirror the National Quality Strategy's three aims to improve the patient care experience, improve the population's health, and reduce healthcare costs (Weston & Roberts, 2013).

Risk management

The overall goal of risk management in nursing is to reduce or prevent any type of risk to a healthcare facility. These risks might include preventable patient or staff injuries, preventable accidents, and financial loss. Main categories of risk management include

- Risk avoidance,
- Risk identification,
- Risk analysis, and
- Risk abatement.

C. DELIVERY MODELS

- Mobile clinics: healthcare facilities on wheels. A van or truck provides exam rooms, diagnostic services, and treatment facilities to people in areas lacking access to healthcare.
- Home visits: nurses may visit children and families in their homes to assess needs or to provide services when families are not able to travel to the healthcare facility. These nurses work closely with the family to create a plan of care that supports an independent lifestyle, promotes developmentally appropriate growth, and fosters teamwork.
- Telehealth: nurses who speak with children and families over the phone to provide nursing care. Current technology allows nurses in a variety of settings to see, monitor, and interact with families in remote locations.
- Parish nurse: focuses on spiritual care as part of promoting holistic health and minimizing illness in a faith community; initiated by Granger Westberg in the 1980s. Roles of the parish nurse include
  - Health advisor,
  - Educator on health issues,
  - Home visitor of church members,
  - Provider of referrals to community resources,
  - Developer of support groups,
  - Trainer and coordinator of volunteers, and
  - Provider of health screenings (King, 2011).
- Food banks: nonprofit organizations that provide food, free of charge, to those in need. Many food banks operate as food storage and distribution stations and provide resources to nonprofit community and governmental agencies.
- Homeless shelters: temporary housing to help protect vulnerable populations while reducing the environmental impact on a community. Often a separate shelter exists for families and for youth.
- Special Supplemental Nutrition Program for Women, Infants, and Children (WIC): federally funded program that allows states to provide supplemental foods, healthcare referrals, and nutrition education for low-income pregnant, postpartum, and breastfeeding women, and for infants and children up to age five who are at nutritional risk (O'Malley, Luckett, Dunaway et al, 2015).

- Children's health insurance program (CHIP): health coverage for nearly eight million children in families with incomes too high to qualify for Medicaid but who can't afford to purchase private coverage. Signed into law in 1997, CHIP provides federal matching funds to states to provide this coverage (AAP, 2014).
- Child protective services: state agencies that respond to reports of child abuse or neglect. Some states use other names such as "Department of Children and Family Services (DCFS)" or "Social Services."
- Healthy People 2020 initiatives: The Department of Health and Human Services launched Healthy People 2020 (Koh, Blakey, & Roper, 2014) in December, 2010, to address public health needs. The four overarching goals of the document are
  - Attain high-quality, longer lives free of preventable disease, disability, injury, and premature death;
  - Achieve health equity, eliminate disparities, and improve the health of all groups;
  - Create social and physical environments that promote good health for all; and
  - Promote quality of life, healthy development, and healthy behaviors across all life stages.

REFERENCES

American Academy of Pediatrics. Children's Health Insurance Program (CHIP): Accomplishments, challenges, and policy recommendations. (2014). *Pediatrics, 133*(3), E784–793.

American Nurses Association (2012). *Bullying in the workplace: Reversing a culture.* Silver Spring, MD: American Nurses Association.

Brenner, M., Parahoo, K., & Taggart, L. (2007). Restraint in children's nursing: Addressing the distress. *Journal of Children's and Young People's Nursing, 1*(4), 159–162. doi: doi:10.12968/jcyn.2007.1.4.24406

Bruns, E. (n.d.). Managing verbal and physical aggressiveness. *Nationwide Children's.* Retrieved from www.nationwidechildrens.org/medical-professional-publications/managing-verbal-and-physical-aggressiveness?contentid=62898

Ceballos, C., Bau, R., Dunkin, D., Sond, Y., Lil, X., & Venkov, K. (2014). Complementary and alternative medicine use at a single pediatric inflammatory bowel disease center. *Gastroenterology Nurse,* 37(4), 265–271.

Cohen, M. H., Kemper, K. J., Stevens, L., Hashimoto, D., & Gilmour, J. (2005). Pediatric use of complementary therapies: Ethical and policy choices. *Pediatrics, 116*(4), e568–e575. doi: 10.1542/peds.2005-0496

Davis, M. P., & Darden, P. M. (2003). Use of complementary and alternative medicine by children in the United States. *Archives of Pediatrics and Adolescent Medicine, 157*(4), 393–396. doi: 10.1001/archpedi.157.4.393

De Vita, C. J., & Mosher-Williams, R. (2001). *Who Speaks for America's Children?: The Role of Child Advocates in Public Policy.* Washington, DC: Urban Institute Press.

Dellasega, C. A. (2009). Bullying among nurses. *American Journal of Nursing, 109*(1), 52–58. doi: 10.1097/1001.NAJ.0000344039.0000311651.0000344008

Donley, R., & Flaherty, M. J. (2008). Promoting professional development: Three phases of articulation in nursing education and practice. *OJIN: The Online Journal of Issues in Nursing, 13*(3), Manuscript 2. doi: 10.3912/OJIN.Vol13No03Man02

Emerich, M., Braeunig, M., Clement, H. W., Ludtke, R., & Huber, R. (2014). Mode of action of cupping—local metabolism and pain thresholds in neck pain patients and healthy subjects. *Complementary Therapies in Medicine, 22*(1), 148–158.

Freeman, J. M., Kossoff, E. H., & Hartman, A. L. (2007). The ketogenic diet: One decade later. *Pediatrics, 119*(3), 535–543. doi: 10.1542/peds.2006-2447

Gilmour, J., Harrison, C., Cohen, M. H., & Vohra, S. (2011). Pediatric use of complementary and alternative medicine: Legal, ethical, and clinical issues in decision-making. *Pediatrics, 128*(Supplement 4), S149–S154. doi: 10.1542/peds.2010-2720B

Gold, J. I., Nicolaou, C. D., Belmont, K. A., Katz, A. R., Benaron, D. M., & Yu, W. (2009). Pediatric acupuncture: A review of clinical research. *Evidence-Based Complementary and Alternative Medicine,* 6(4), 429–439. doi: 10.1093/ecam/nem181

Golianu, B., Yeh, A., & Brooks, M. (2014). Acupuncture for pediatric pain. *Children, 192*, 134–148. doi: 10.3390/children1020134

Griffin, M. (2004). Teaching cognitive rehearsal as a shield for lateral violence: An intervention for newly licensed nurses. *Journal of Continuing Education in Nursing, 35*(6), 257–263.

Grossoehme, D. H., Cotton, S., & McPhail, G. (2013). Use and sanctification of complementary and alternative medicine by parents of children with cystic fibrosis. *Journal of Health Care Chaplaincy, 19*(1), 22–32. doi: 10.1080/08854726.2013.761007.

Hannan, J., (2007). Minority mothers' healthcare beliefs, commonly used alternative healthcare practices, and potential complications for infants and children. *Journal of the American Association of Nurse Practitioners.* doi: 10.1002/2327-6924.12153.

Harris, T. S. (2010). Bruises in children: Normal or child abuse? *Journal of Pediatric Health Care, 24*(4), 216–221. doi: 10.1016/j.pedhc.2009.03.007

Helman, C. (2007). *Culture, health, & illness: An introduction for healthcare professionals*, 5th edition. London: Hodder Arnold.

Italia, S., Wolfenstetter, S., Teuner, C. (2014). Patterns of complementary and alternative medicine (CAM) use in children: A systematic review. *European Journal of Pediatrics, 173*(11), 1413–1428.

Jamerson, P., Graf, E., Messmer, P., Fields, H., Barton, S., Berger, A., Daraiseh, N., Fix, M., Huth, M., Latta, L., et al. (2014). Inpatient falls in freestanding children's hospitals. *Pediatric Nursing, 40*(3): 127–135.

King, M. (2011). Parish nursing: Holistic nursing care in the faith communities. *Holistic Nursing Practice, 25*(6), 309–315.

Koh, H., Blakey, C., & Roper, A. (2014). Healthy People 2020: A report card on the health of the nation. *Journal of the American Medical Association, 311*(24), 2475–2476.

Ladas, E. J., Lin, M., Antillion, F., Rivas, S., Chantada, G., Cacciavillano, W., Ortiz, R., Stein, K., Castillo, L., Rocha, V., Fu, L., Rodriquez, H., & Kelly, K. M. (2014). Improving our understanding of the use of traditional complementary/alternative medicine in children with cancer. *Cancer.* doi: 10.1002/cncr.29212

Levy, S., & Hyman, S. (2015). Complementary and alternative medicine treatments for children with autism spectrum disorders. *Child and Adolescent Psychiatric Clinics of North America, 24*(1), 117–143.

Loman, D. G. (2003). The use of complementary and alternative health care practices among children. *Journal of Pediatric Health Care, 17*(2), 58–63. doi: 10.1067/mph.2003.29

Longo, J. (2007). Horizontal violence among nursing students. *Archives of Psychiatric Nursing, 21*(3), 177–178. doi: 10.1016/j.apnu.2007.02.005

Manikandan, N., & Chandrasehara, K. (2014). Influence of simplified Kundalini Yoga with medication on selected physiologic variables among diabetic patients. *International Journal of Recent Research and Applied Studies, 1*, 4(9), 42–44.

National Association for the Education of Young Children. (2009). 10 effective DAP teaching strategies. *NAEYC.* Retrieved from www.naeyc.org/dap/10-effective-dap-teaching-strategies

Ndetan, H., Evans, M., Williams, R., Woolsey, C., & Swartz, J. (2014). Use of movement therapies and relaxation techniques and management of health conditions among children. *Alternative Therapies in Health and Medicine, 20*(4), 44–50.

Niespondiziani, C., & Hepola, B. (2011). *The CMS-Joint Commission Crosswalk.* HCPro, Inc.

O'Malley, K., Luckett, B., Dunaway, L., Bodor, J., & Rose, D. (2013). Use of a new availability index to evaluate the effect of policy changes to the Special Supplemental Nutrition Program for Women, Infants, and Children (WIC) on the food environment in New Orleans. *Public Health Nutrition, 18*(1), 25–32.

Pauley, B., Houston, L., Dunlei C., & Johnston, D. (2014). Clinical relevance of the Humpty Dumpty Falls Scale in a pediatric specialty hospital. *Pediatric Nursing, 40*(3), 137–142.

Parnell, T. (2014). *Health literacy in nursing: Providing person-centered care.* New York, NY: Springer Publishing Co.

Perry, R., Hunt, K., & Ernst, E. (2011). Nutritional supplements and other complementary medicines for infantile colic. *Pediatrics, 127,* 720–733.

Phillips, A. (2009). Realistic team building in a nurse managed clinic setting. *Internet Journal of Advanced Nursing Practice, 10*(1), 1–14.

Porter-O'Grady, T. (2009). *Interdisciplinary shared governance: Integrating practice, transforming health care.* Burlington, MA: Jones & Bartlett Learning.

Stefancyk, A., Hancock, B., & Meadows, M. T. (2013). The nurse manager: Change agent, change coach? *Nursing Administration Quarterly, 37*(1), 13–17. doi: 10.1097/NAQ.0b013e31827514f4

U.S. Census Bureau. (2012). *Statistical abstract of the United States.* U.S. Government Printing Office.

Valji, R., Adams, D., Dagenais, S., Clifford, T., Baydala, L., King, W. J., & Vohra, S. (2013). Complementary and alternative medicine: A survey of its use in pediatric oncology. *Evidence-Based Complementary and Alternative Medicine.* doi: 10.1155/2013/527163.

Vinson, R., Yeh, G., Davis, R. B., & Logan, D. (2014). Correlates of complementary and alternative medicine use in a pediatric tertiary pain center. *Academic Pediatrics, 14*(5), 491–496.

Weston, M., & Roberts, D. W. (2013). The influence of quality improvement efforts on patient outcomes and nursing work: A perspective from chief nursing officers at three large health systems. *OJIN: The Online Journal of Issues in Nursing, 18*(3), Manuscript 2. doi: 10.3912/OJIN.Vol18No03Man02

Woolf, A. D. (2003). Herbal remedies and children: Do they work? Are they harmful? *Pediatrics, 112*(1 Pt 2), 240–246.

Yoder-Wise, P. (2014). *Leading and managing in nursing.* St. Louis, MO: Mosby.

Wynia, M., Papadakis, M., Sullivan, W., & Hafferty, F. (2014). More than a list of values and desired behaviors: A foundational understanding of medical professionalism. *Academic Medicine, 89*(5), 712–714.

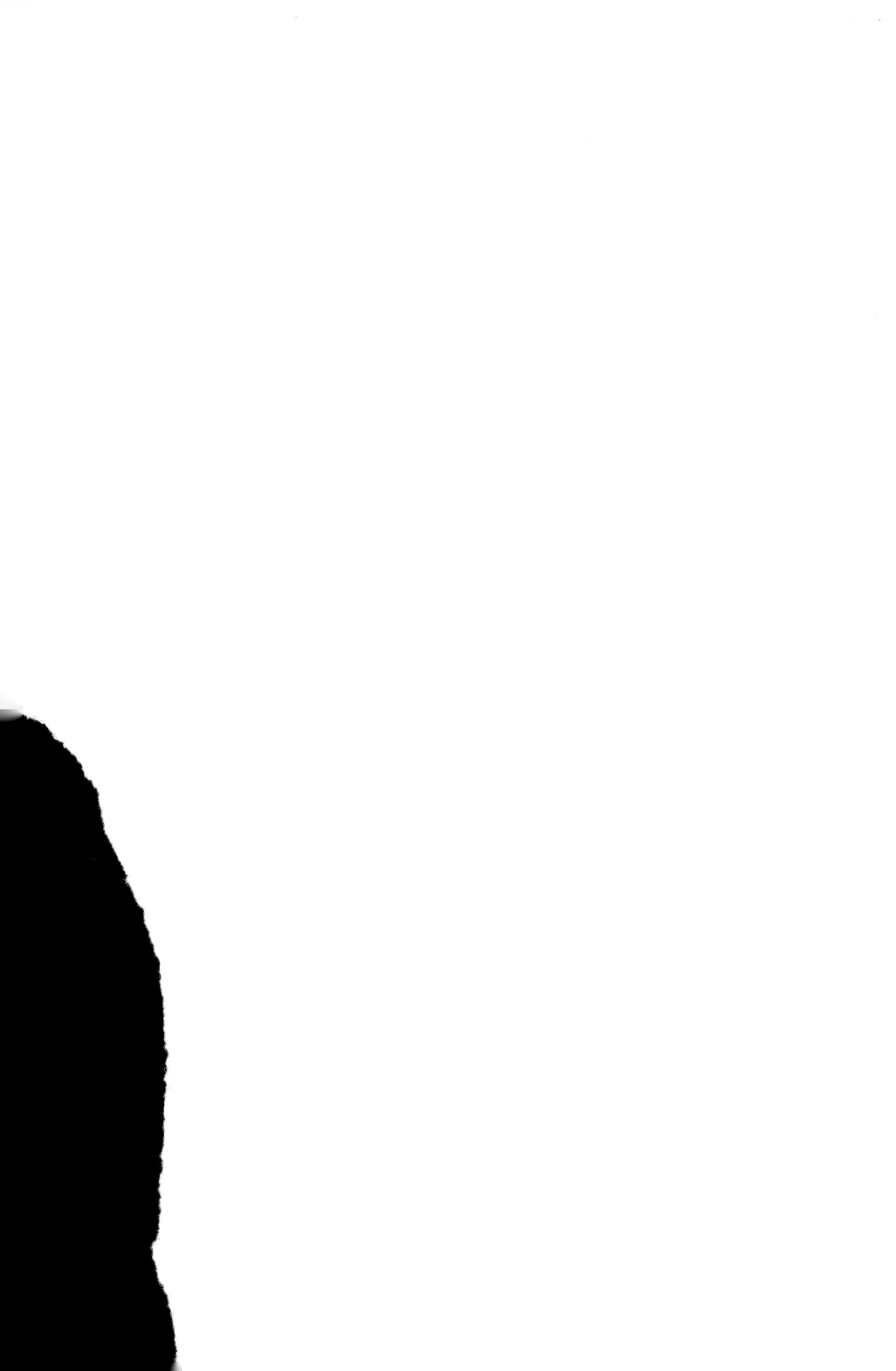

Made in the USA
Middletown, DE
27 September 2021